The Story of Taxol:
Nature and Politics in the Pursuit of
an Anti-cancer Drug

Taxol is arguably the most celebrated, talked about, and controversial natural product in recent years: Celebrated because of its efficacy as an anti-cancer drug and because its discovery has provided powerful support for policies concerned with biodiversity. Talked about because in the late 1980s and early 1990s, the American public was bombarded with news reports about the molecule and its host, the slow-growing Pacific yew. Controversial because the drug and the tree became embroiled in several sensitive political issues with broad public policy implications.

Taxol has revolutionized the treatment options for patients with advanced forms of breast and ovarian cancers and some types of leukemia; it shows promise for treating AIDS-related Kaposi's sarcoma. It is the best-selling anti-cancer drug ever, with world sales of $1.2 billion in 1998 and expected to grow. Goodman and Walsh's careful study of how taxol was discovered, researched, and brought to market documents the complexities and conflicting interests in the ongoing process to find effective treatments. From a broader perspective, *The Story of Taxol* uses the discovery and development of taxol as a paradigm to address current issues in the history and sociology of science and medicine.

Jordan Goodman is Senior Lecturer in History at the Manchester School of Management, University of Manchester Institute of Science and Technology. Goodman's previous books include *Tobacco in History* (1994) and *Consuming Habits: Drugs and History in Anthropology* (1995).

Vivien Walsh is Reader in Technology Management at the University of Manchester Institute of Science and Technology. She has been researching the pharmaceutical and chemical industries for years and is currently working on globalization of innovative activity in the chemical, pharmaceutical, and agro-food industries. Walsh has been a consultant to the European Commission and to the Organisation for Economic Cooperation and Development.

The Story of Taxol

Nature and Politics in the Pursuit of an Anti-cancer Drug

JORDAN GOODMAN

VIVIEN WALSH

University of Manchester Institute of Science and Technology

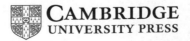
CAMBRIDGE
UNIVERSITY PRESS

PUBLISHED BY THE PRESS SYNDICATE OF THE UNIVERSITY OF CAMBRIDGE
The Pitt Building, Trumpington Street, Cambridge, United Kingdom

CAMBRIDGE UNIVERSITY PRESS
The Edinburgh Building, Cambridge CB2 2RU, UK
40 West 20th Street, New York NY 10011-4211, USA
10 Stamford Road, Oakleigh, Victoria 3166, Australia
Ruiz de Alarcón 13, 28014 Madrid, Spain
Dock House, The Waterfront, Cape Town 8001, South Africa

http://www.cambridge.org

First published 2001

Printed in the United States of America

Typeface   Palatino 10/12 pt   *System*   3B2 6.03   [KWP]

A catalog record for this book is available from the British Library

Library of Congress Cataloging-in-Publication Data

Goodman, Jordan.
The story of taxol : nature and politics in the pursuit of an anti-cancer drug / Jordan
Goodman, Vivien Walsh.
p. cm.
Includes bibliographical references.
ISBN 0-521-56123-X
1. Paclitaxel – Research – Political aspects – United States. 2.
Paclitaxel – Research – Economic aspects – United States. 3.
Cancer – Treatment – Research – Political aspects – United States. 4. Pacific
yew – Harvesting – Northwest, Pacific. I. Walsh, Vivien. II. Title.
RC271.P27 G66 2000
616.99′406–dc21   00-034200

ISBN 0 521 56123 X hardback

For Danny and Ben

For Daniel and in memory of Jacky Weiss

CONTENTS

ACKNOWLEDGEMENTS

We are indebted to a great number of individuals and institutions without whose generous assistance the research leading to the writing of this book could never have been undertaken.

The evidence that we have accumulated comes from three main sources: unpublished primary material – letters, memos, reports, and the like; published secondary and technical material; and oral testimony. A few individuals, of inestimable generosity, furnished us with precious primary material and shared their thoughts and memories with us, giving of their time and emotional energy. To them the biggest thanks of all. They are: Fred Boettner, Chuck Bolsinger, Pat Connolly, Gordon Cragg, John Destito, Jim Duke, Hal Hartzell, Jim Mead, Bob Perdue, Stan Scher, Richard Spjut, Monroe Wall and Wendell Wood.

Other individuals, no less generous in giving of their precious time, also shared their thoughts and memories with us. We thank them for all their help. They are: at the University of Toronto, Toronto, Canada – Frank DiCosmo; at the Albert Einstein College of Medicine, New York – Susan Horwitz; at Columbia University – Koji Nakanishi; at SHARE, New York – Alice Yaker; at Gilda's Club – Joanna Bull; at the New York Botanical Garden – Douglas Daly; at the Agricultural Research Service, United States Department of Agriculture, Ithaca, New York – Donna Gibson; at Phyton Catalytic, Ithaca – Venkataraman Bringi and John Bela; at the Worcester Foundation for Experimental Biology, Worcester, Massachusetts – Richard Vallee; at Boehringer-Ingelheim – Vittorio Farina; at Bryn Mawr College – Charles Swindell; at SmithKline Beecham – Randall Johnson; at Bristol-Myers Squibb – Joe Salenitri and Dianne De Furia; at Rhône-Poulenc Rorer, Collegeville, PA – Luz Hammerschaimb, Meg Martin and Jean-Pierre Bizzary; at the National Cancer Institute – Jill Johnson, David Newman, Saul Schepartz, Dale Shoemaker, Ken Snader and Matt Suffness(†); in North Bethesda, Maryland – Georgia Persinos; in Greenbelt, Maryland – Arthur Barclay; at the Environmental Defense Fund, Washington, DC – Michael Bean;

in Washington, DC – James Love and Bruce Manheim; at Virginia Polytechnic Institute – David Kingston; at the Research Triangle Institute – Jane Righter and Mansukh Wani; at Emory University – Bill McGuire; at Florida State University – Bob Holton; at the University of Mississippi – Ed Croom; at the University of Kansas – Valentino Stella; at Middle Tennessee State University – Kurt Blum; at Michigan State University – Steve Heidemann; at NaPro Therapeutics – Sterling Ainsworth and Jim McChesney; at Hauser Chemical Research – David Bailey and Randy Daughenbaugh; at Arizona State University – Bob Pettit; at the University of Arizona – Jack Cole; in Southern California – Janice Thompson; at the Scripps Research Institute – K.C. Nicolaou; at the University of California Santa Barbara – Mary Ann Jordan and Leslie Wilson; at Stanford University – Paul Wender; at the University of Southern California – Frank Muggia; in Foster City, California – Walter Goldstein; in Sutter Creek, California – Shimon Schwarzschild; in Days Creek, Oregon – Ed Reed; in Medford, Oregon – Floyd Ehrheart and Bob Warner; at the Oregon Natural Resources Council, Eugene, Oregon – Doug Heiken; at *The Register-Guard*, Eugene, Oregon – Lance Robertson; in Portland, Oregon – Jerry Rust; at Oregon State University – Daniel Luoma; in Beaverton, Oregon – Fred Page; at the Bureau of Land Management, Portland, Oregon – John Allegria; at the Forest Service, Portland, Oregon – Sally Campbell, Lisa Naylor, Diane Smith and John Teply; at *The Seattle Times* – Eric Nalder; at Weyerhaeuser – Nick Wheeler; at the University of British Columbia – Neil Towers; at the University of Victoria – Nancy Turner; at the Pacific Forestry Centre, Canadian Forest Service, Victoria, British Columbia – Alan Mitchell; at Phytogen Life Sciences, Delta, British Columbia – Bryan Wilson; at Yew Tree Pharmaceuticals, Ware, Hertfordshire, England – Tom Donovan; at the CNRS Institut de Chimie des Substances Naturelles, Gif-sur-Yvette, France – Pierre Potier; at the Laboratoire d'Etudes Dynamiques et Structurales de la Sélectivité, Université Joseph Fourier, Grenoble, France – Andrew Greene; at Rhône-Poulenc Rorer, Antony, France – Jean-Louis Fabre; at Rhône-Poulenc Rorer, Vitry-sur-Seine, France – François Lavelle; and at INDENA, Milan – Ezio Bombardelli.

We would also like to thank the staff of the Library and Information Section, National Cancer Institute, for allowing us access to the NCI Archives and the staff the Inter-Library Loans Section, Joule Library, University of Manchester Institute of Science and Technology, for help in getting scarce material.

Susan Hutton transcribed the taped interviews and Sofie Verzylbergen translated some Dutch material for us. Thank you for your help.

Early versions of parts of the book were given as lectures and as seminar papers at the University of California, Berkeley, the University of Cambridge, Columbia University, Cornell University, the University of Edinburgh, the University of Lancaster, the Massachusetts Institute of Technology, the University of Manchester, the University of Manchester Institute of Science and Technology, Mount Holyoke College and the University of Sussex; and as conference papers at the London School of Hygiene and Tropical Medicine, Keele University and the Wellcome Trust. We are grateful to our colleagues in these and other institutions, and especially to David Edge, Rebecca Eisenberg, Jean-Paul Gaudillière, Sarah Green, Jim Hanson, Donna Haraway, Nick Lawrence, Ilana Löwy, Richard Nelson, Paolo Palladino, Max Parrott, Judith Reppy and Marilyn Strathern for their very helpful contributions.

The manuscript was read, in all or in parts, by Andrew Greene, Nick Lawrence, Bob Perdue, Georgia Persinos, Dallas Sealy, Stan Scher and Michael Unger. Earlier plans and drafts were read by Michel Callon and Nelly Oudshoorn. We thank them for their time and extremely helpful suggestions.

The research was made possible by the generous financial assistance of the Nuffield Foundation and the Wellcome Trust.

ABBREVIATIONS

Primary Material

BOL	Papers in the possession of Chuck Bolsinger
CON	Papers in the possession of Patrick Connolly
DST	Papers in the possession of John Destito
EDF	Papers in the Environmental Defense Fund
FRD*	Papers in the Natural Products Branch, National Cancer Institute
GCB	Papers in the Grants and Contracts Operations Branch, National Cancer Institute
NPB*	Papers in the Natural Products Branch, National Cancer Institute
NPB(S)*	Papers in the Natural Products Branch, National Cancer Institute
PER	Papers in the possession of Robert Perdue
SCH	Papers in the possession of Stanley Scher
SPJ	Papers in the possession of Richard Spjut
UDA	Papers in the Agricultural Research Service, United States Department of Agriculture
WLL	Papers in the possession of Monroe Wall
WOD	Papers in the possession of Wendell Wood

* Primary materials in the Natural Products Branch do not have designations. These are ones devised and used by the authors to organize the material.

xiii

Introduction

One of the few organic compounds, which, like benzene and aspirin, is recognizable by name to the average citizen.[1]

... taxol is the first naturally occurring plant-derived drug product to gain FDA approval in more than a quarter of a century.[2]

This book is the history of taxol, the anti-cancer drug, and of the tree, *Taxus brevifolia*, the Pacific yew, from which it derives. Our story begins in the 1960s when Western science 'discovered' the existence of taxol in the yew bark and ends, for our purposes, in the 1990s when corporate capitalism took over the drug and abandoned the tree. Taxol is arguably the most celebrated, talked about and controversial natural product in recent years: celebrated because of its efficacy as an anti-cancer drug and because its discovery has provided powerful support for policies concerned with biodiversity; talked about because in the late 1980s and early 1990s, the American public was bombarded with news reports and special programmes about the molecule and its host; and controversial because during the early 1990s the drug and the tree became embroiled in a number of very sensitive political issues with wide implications for the conduct of public policy.

Taxol is currently available in clinics throughout the world for the treatment of ovarian and breast cancer. It is approved for use against non-small cell lung cancer and Kaposi's sarcoma in the United States; approval in other countries is pending. Clinical trials for other types of cancer continue world-wide; however, from early results, it is expected it will be approved for other uses. It is the best-selling anti-cancer drug ever. World sales reached $1.2 billion in 1998 and are expected to continue growing for the foreseeable future.[3] Taxol is made and sold by Bristol-Myers Squibb, the world's largest supplier of anti-cancer drugs, and the fourth largest pharmaceutical company in the world.[4] Taxol is Bristol-Myers Squibb's second biggest pharmaceutical earner, accounting for about ten per cent of the company's total pharmaceutical sales.[5] The drug is widely available but at a price basically set by Bristol-Myers Squibb, although the first thirty years of the research and development of taxol was carried out in the public sector, and managed and funded by the United States Government.

As the source of taxol, the Pacific yew, *Taxus brevifolia*, has also had its share of fame. For a while in the early 1990s it became a symbol of the value and precariousness of the old-growth forest in the Pacific Northwest. Although the media portrayed a battle between the defenders of the habitat of the spotted owl, and the oncologists and their patients who needed the tree bark for making taxol, in the Pacific Northwest it was hoped that the harvesting of *Taxus brevifolia* for taxol might provide a new source of revenue for a depressed area, and possibly an example of how to use and preserve a forest habitat. These hopes were dashed when Bristol-Myers Squibb adopted a semi-synthetic method of production that did not use *Taxus brevifolia* or any other American tree.

Much has been written about taxol, but mostly in newspapers, magazines or journals.[6] Less ephemeral accounts, sometimes by participants in the story, have told only part of the tale. Looking back, the story of taxol can be told either as a triumph of science and individual effort or dismissed in a few words as it was by Bruce Ross, who held a highly responsible position at Bristol-Myers Squibb in 1992. In 1998, he was quoted as saying: 'Taxol was developed in the early 1960s and languished for almost 30 years because nobody could make it.'[7]

Ross's dismissive attitude to the work of the National Cancer Institute is representative of Bristol-Myers Squibb's version of the history of taxol. In a published report the company writes: 'It was not until 1971 that both chemical and biological testing enabled the isolation of paclitaxel, initially described as "compound 17", as the molecule responsible for remarkable antitumor effects against murine tumors and leukemias. In this effort, Dr. Wall was helped by his collaborator Dr. Mansukh C. Wani.'[8] In fact Monroe Wall named the bioactive compound from the bark of *Taxus brevifolia* 'taxol' in 1967.[9] Wall and Wani published their account of the structure of taxol in 1971, but had been submitting their accounts of the compound to the National Cancer Institute under the name 'taxol' since 1967. The first published use of the name 'taxol' was in 1969.[10] It was only in 1990 that Bristol-Myers Squibb applied to trademark the name 'taxol', and the name was not registered until 1992. It was then that taxol became Taxol® and the generic name of 'paclitaxel' was approved. Since that time Bristol-Myers Squibb have insisted that the molecule be referred to as paclitaxel and that the drug is called Taxol®, even, as the excerpt from their report shows, when it means rewriting history.

When this kind of misrepresentation is perpetrated it is essential that a properly documented account of what actually happened is published. Fortunately not only are many of the protagonists of the taxol story alive, but many kept documents, letters and memos, as well as publications, and have been generous in sharing them with us. We have been able to use material from the National Cancer Institute and the United States Department of Agriculture, as well as congressional hearings, newspaper reports, unpublished papers, papers in journals, and articles in magazines. The breadth and depth of these sources, the way in which they reinforce and interact with one another, offers the best hope of presenting as complete and coherent a version of the taxol story as possible.

How to organize such a large amount of material, oral and verbal, published and unpublished, and to make it as comprehensible and fascinating as it deserves to be, is a problem. Taxol is an entity with multiple identities, a natural product, an anti-cancer drug, a complex organic molecule, a biomedical research tool, an agent of political leverage, an object of hope and a bone of contention. Perhaps a biography of taxol would be the answer. Igor Kopytoff writes:[11] '...an eventful biography of a thing becomes the story of the various singularizations of it, of classifications and reclassifications in an uncertain world of categories whose importance shifts with every minor change in context. As with persons the drama here lies in the uncertainties of valuation and of identity.'

This is suggestive, and the method has been very successfully used by art historians in recounting the histories of art objects, but the model of personal biography does not quite accommodate taxol's peculiar state of coexistence with its source *Taxus brevifolia*, or its ability to appear in different roles in different milieus at the same time.[12] A more useful approach would be to combine biography with the approach of actor–network theory, in which the distinction between objects and humans is not given, but made and remade, and which offers the research and narrative strategy of following the object wherever it leads, thus allowing a relationally based biography to be constructed.[13] Instead of settling on one trajectory in time, or dissecting the object and its situation into different categories or compartments, one can, as Bruno Latour suggests, simply follow the 'fragile thread' of the object's associations through the various networks of which it is part.[14] 'The only task of the analyst is to follow the transformations that the actors convened in the stories are undergoing.'[15]

A major advantage of actor–network theory is its capacity to encompass transformation and change. As Michel Callon says 'the actor network should not ... be confused with a network linking in some predictable fashion elements that are perfectly well defined and stable, for the entities it is composed of, whether natural or social, could at any moment redefine their identity and mutual relationships in some new way and bring new elements into the network. An actor network is simultaneously an actor whose activity is networking heterogeneous elements and a network that is able to redefine and transform what it is made of.'[16] An actor, in this theory, can, of course, be a thing; humans are not privileged. Although, as Callon says 'by themselves, things don't act. Indeed, . . . there are no things "by themselves." . . . instead, there are relations, relations which (sometimes) make things.'[17]

All the interests of the other actors, people and things, techniques, instruments, etc. are inscribed on the object. The object becomes an archive, a text of all the actors and events that have gone before, but it is in no way static.[18] The elements are constantly regrouping and forming new objects and new networks. This recognition of the inherent instability and contingency of the actors and their networks is a central tenet of the theory.[19] Other notions specific to the theory are those of 'enrolment', 'translation', and 'obligatory points of passage'. 'Enrolment' is the process whereby one actor attempts to enlist other actors for some purpose involving imposition rather than mere invitation. The enroller is active in constructing the network, assuming the role of spokesperson, and assigning roles to the other actors; this activity is termed 'translation'. Crucial to the idea of 'translation' is the creation of 'obligatory points of passage', i.e. 'unavoidable conduits through which they (the actors) must pass in order to articulate both their identity and their raison d'être'.[20]

We have found these ideas of great value both in researching and writing about such a complex and diverse body of material. Actor–network theory is implicit throughout the text, and occasionally explicit. Welcome to the taxol/*Taxus brevifolia* network of which we are all now part.

Notes

1 Nicolaou, Dai and Guy, 'Chemistry and biology', p. 15.
2 Kinghorn and Balandrin, 'Preface', p. xi.
3 'Bristol-Myers Squibb reports record fourth quarter and annual sales (1998)', http://www.prnewswire.com/cgi-bin, 20 January 1999.
4 Barker, 'Merck', p. 39. This ranking is based on prescription sales.
5 Calculated from 'Bristol-Myers Squibb reports record fourth quarter and annual sales (1998)' http://www.prnewswire.com/cgi-bin, 20 January 1999.
6 The newspaper coverage of taxol in the early 1990s was enormous. In 1991 and 1992, for example, *The Oregonian*, Oregon's major newspaper and published in Portland, ran a 'taxol' story more than once a week on average.

Between 1990 and 1995, according to the medical database MEDLINE, about 250 biomedical articles appeared annually on the subject of taxol. Many of these accounts provided a short background to taxol's history, focusing primarily on the biological, clinical and chemical work since the 1980s. The first accounts to concentrate on the history of taxol before the 1980s were by Persinos, 'Taxol' and 'The Pacific yew and cancer'. The first review of taxol by participants in its development at the National Cancer Institute and the Research Triangle Institute began to appear from 1993. See: Suffness and Wall, 'Discovery and development'; Wall and Wani, 'Paclitaxel'; Suffness, 'Taxol'; Suffness, 'Overview'; and Cragg, 'Paclitaxel'. Joyce, *Earthly Goods*, pp. 235–248 and Fellers, 'The medicine market' are two recent general treatments that discuss taxol. See also Parks, 'Taxol' for a wide-ranging discussion of taxol based on published materials.

7 Quoted in Fellers, 'The medicine market', p. 24. Ross, according to this article, was Bristol-Myers Squibb's chief negotiator in a meeting with the National Cancer Institute in July 1992 concerned with setting a price for taxol.

8 Bristol-Myers Squibb, 'The development of Taxol® (paclitaxel)', March 1997.

9 A full account of Wall's work with taxol in the 1960s can be found in Chapter 2.

10 Perdue and Hartwell, 'The search for plant sources'.

11 Kopytoff, 'The cultural biography', p. 90.

12 In 1995, the Association of Art Historians had 'Objects, histories and inter-pretations' as the theme of their annual conference, in London. A whole session was devoted to the life histories of artefacts. Debbora Battaglia argued this point in her paper, 'Do objects have individual histories: a cri-tical examination from postcolonial New Guinea'. We have shown, in other places, that the biography of an object is written by the network dynamics of which the object is a participant. See: Goodman, 'Plants, cells and bodies'; Walsh, 'Industrial R&D', pp. 323–334; and Goodman and Walsh, 'Attaching to things'. Contingency, or non-essentialism, is central to Kopytoff's ideas about the biography of objects. This seems to have been overlooked in a recent attempt to apply Kopytoff's ideas to the case of pharmaceuticals. Instead of contingency the reader is offered a programmatic biography, following life cycles within prescribed stages and teleological in character – see Van der Geest, White and Hardon, 'The anthropology of pharmaceuticals'.

13 Following 'actors' was proposed by Bruno Latour as a research methodol-ogy in Latour, *Science in Action*. The literature on actor–network theory is vast, growing and changing. Aside from the writings of Michel Callon, Bruno Latour and John Law, those most frequently associated with this analytical tool, there are a number of good studies using it, and a number of good overviews. On case studies, two of the best are also early examples of this kind of analysis: Callon, 'The state' and Callon, 'Some elements'. Other notable case studies are: Singleton and Michael, 'Actor–networks and ambivalence' and Prout, 'Actor–network theory'. Both cover the literature well. As for overviews, one of the best is also one of the most recent. Though written primarily for an audience of geographers, the coverage of actor–network theory is excellent. See Murdoch, 'Inhuman/nonhuman/human'. Another useful overview and critique can be found in a special issue devoted to the topic 'Humans and others: the concept of "agency" and its attribution,' *American Behavioral Scientist* **37** (1994), 731–856. In 1997, the Centre for Social Theory and Technology at Keele University, UK, hosted a

workshop entitled 'Actor Network Theory and After'. The internet site for the workshop which contains several of the plenary papers and links to bibliographical information is at http://www.keele.ac.uk/depts/stt/stt/ant. Some of the papers have been published in Law and Hassard, *Actor Network Theory*. See also Law, 'Notes on the theory'.

14 Latour, *We Have Never*, pp. 2–3. Latour's thoughts on following actors also appears in anthropology as 'multi-sited ethnography' – see Marcus, 'Ethnography'.

15 Latour, *The Pasteurization*, p. 10.

16 Callon, 'Society in the making', p. 93.

17 Callon and Law, 'Agency', p. 485. See also Michael, 'Narrative space'. On identity, see Michael, *Constructing Identities*, pp. 79–104.

18 For similar ideas, see Latour, 'Do scientific objects' who writes: '... the meaning of the word *substance* changes profoundly and becomes the gradual attribution of stable properties attached by an institution to a name lastingly linked to a practice, the whole circulating in a standardized network,' – p. 85. See also Strathern, 'What is intellectual property after?' and Law, *Organizing Modernity*. Marilyn Strathern, referring to John Law's concept of relational materiality, has given the following interpretation of objects. 'If people were not divided into different kinds of experts then we would not have an expert description of the substance divided up like that. Moreover because experts get themselves into permanent positions of competence, as the authority on this or that aspect, they presuppose that there is no substance which could not be divided up thus. Any organic substance can have a biochemical analysis done on it. Whether anyone wishes to will depend on other interests, but properties attributed to the thing will summon forth their own experts, and thus justify the divisions between people. Things come to seem heterogeneous this way ... the thing itself will identify what people have to be mobilised.' – pp. 172–173.

19 An appeal to take account of and incorporate contingency in historical studies of science (and technology) is not new. See, for example, Shapin, 'History of science'; MacKenzie, 'Marx and the machine'; Noble, 'Social choice'; and David, 'Clio'. For environmental history, see also: Taylor, 'Making salmon'; Dann and Mitman, 'Essay review'; and McEvoy, *The Fisherman's Problem*. Donna Haraway has also made a plea for contingency over essentialism in cultural studies of science – see Haraway, 'Universal donors'. On contingency from a philosophical perspective see Ben-Menahem, 'Historical contingency' and Rorty, *Contingency, Irony, and Solidarity*. For contingency in the writing of natural history, see Gould, *Wonderful Life*, pp. 284–285.

20 Singleton and Michael, 'Actor–networks and ambivalence', pp. 229–230.

Part I

Agents

1

Cancer Chemotherapy:
Plant Knowledge and Practice

In 1960, the National Cancer Institute (hereafter NCI) and the United States Department of Agriculture (hereafter USDA) began an inter-agency programme to procure and screen plant products as potential anti-cancer agents. It was an ambitious programme that would consume vast amounts of labour and laboratory time. The programme lasted just over twenty years and, although a huge number of plants were screened, no plant product reached the clinic during the period of the programme's existence. Though samples of the Pacific yew, *Taxus brevifolia*, were procured in 1962, taxol, the tree's promising compound, had not yet reached clinical trials by the time that the programme was wound up.

To follow and understand taxol's path through the American cancer research and biomedical community, it is necessary to explore, in some detail, two principal contexts: the history and development of cancer chemotherapy and its target; and the structure and strategy of the NCI–USDA plant screening programme.

Cancer Chemotherapy and the Malignant Cell

The years from roughly 1945 to 1970 were formative in the history of cancer chemotherapy in two principal senses.[1] First, chemotherapy came to achieve status as a therapeutic regimen for the cure or at least the palliation of cancer, towering over surgery and radiotherapy, during this period.[2] Secondly, chemotherapy became a research regimen in biomedicine that mirrored, incorporated and modified models of large-scale cooperative ventures in other scientific endeavours.

The medical literature abounds with reviews of the historical development of cancer chemotherapy. The general consensus of the literature is that 'modern' cancer chemotherapy emerged from research in gas warfare by the Americans and British during World War II.[3] The landmark papers on nitrogen mustards contributed to a heightened interest and belief in chemical agents rather than radiotherapy and surgery as the techniques of choice in cancer treatment:[4] attacking the 'biochemical soil' in which cancers arose, as a leading advocate of chemotherapy put it.[5] Wartime programmes devoted to the large-scale production of penicillin and antimalarial drugs built on the success of the sulpha drugs of the late 1930s in convincing many people that disease could be eradicated by chemical means.[6]

The bulk of experimental and clinical research on chemotherapeutic agents from roughly 1945 to 1960 focused on two kinds of chemicals and two mechanisms of action: alkylating agents that combine chemically with cellular constituents, and antimetabolites that compete with the substrate of an enzyme system for engagement in metabolism.[7] Steroid hormones and antibiotics were also examined for chemotherapeutic potential. Cortisone, for example, was studied for its ability to regress tumours long before its more famous effects on arthritis were observed.[8] Among antibiotics, the only one to be used clinically was actinomycin D.[9]

Cancer chemotherapy was not then the core activity it would become. Research glided between experimental (laboratory) activities, predominantly biological work on animal tumours, and clinical trials on humans.[10] Until the 1940s, experimental cancer chemotherapy was carried out by many different investigators in many different disciplinary specialties – biology, physiology, pharmacology and botany, and in many different sites – pathology laboratories, hospitals, universities, and private biological research institutes.[11] One of the most important of the latter type was the Rockefeller Institute which, for many decades, had been actively engaged in experimental cancer research. James Murphy, who was with the Institute from 1911 to his death in 1950, summed up the achievements of cancer research during his period of activity.[12] According to Murphy, the chief insights included: (i) that tumours could be transplanted, a fact that demonstrated that malignancy was centred in the cells; (ii) that genetic factors influenced cancer but that they varied within the population; (iii) that there were certain agents called carcinogens that induced tumours; and (iv) that in the change from normality to malignancy, the cell was altered and that proliferation became automatic and therefore no longer dependent on the causative agent.[13]

With the ending of World War II, the diffracted nature of experimental and clinical cancer chemotherapy gave way to a more standardized practice. As architects of early post-war American chemotherapy, Cornelius Packard 'Dusty' Rhoads and the Sloan–Kettering Institute were instrumental in this change. Rhoads began his professional career in haematology at the Rockefeller Institute in 1928,[14] and in 1933 was put in charge of the clinical haematology service where he remained until 1940 when he was made director of the Memorial Hospital for Cancer and Allied Diseases.[15] Within a very short time of the date of this appointment, Rhoads became the Chief of the Medical Division of the Chemical Warfare Service of the United States Army. Rhoads assembled under him an impressive array of medical scientists. Many of them joined him after the war at the Sloan–Kettering Institute and those that did not found their way into other cancer research centres in the United States.[16]

It was during his time as Chief of the Division that experiments were conducted with nitrogen mustards, investigating their pharmacology, toxicology and mechanism of action: according to one commentator, nitrogen mustards became 'a model for the study of antitumor drugs'.[17] Once the war ended and the ban on public statements about this research was lifted, it was Rhoads who made the knowledge public to the American Medical Association.[18] At the close of the war, the work on nitrogen mustards came under the direction of the Committee on Growth of the National Research Council who, in turn assigned the work to three institutions, one of which was the Memorial Hospital.[19]

The Sloan–Kettering Institute was founded in 1945 and rapidly became the largest private cancer research institute in the United States. In tracing the first few years of its history, the historian Robert Bud reminds us that the institute was founded on industrial principles of organization and practice.[20] Not only were its founders and many of the trustees industrialists – Alfred P. Sloan and Charles F. Kettering of General Motors, Frank Howard of Standard Oil – but it also expressly adopted a programme of research modelled on the industrial laboratories of such companies as Bell, DuPont, General Motors, etc.[21] The press release announcing the founding of the institute contended that its task was to 'concentrate on the organization of industrial techniques for cancer research'.[22]

Precisely what was meant by the 'organization of industrial techniques' would only become apparent as the system of research evolved over the years. What was emphatically clear, however, was that the centrepiece of the entire organization was the cell. Rhoads had a deep conviction of the truth of the central tenet of chemotherapy, namely that there were chemical agents that could selectively destroy or control the cancer cell, in contrast to the prevailing focus on surgery and radiotherapy. This was founded on his own experience with nitrogen mustards and laid the foundation of what he called 'an empiric attack on cancer'.[23] The laboratories at the institute began to construct an organization and programme to fulfil the promise. The structure of the organization followed on from the strategy of testing as many substances as possible against a number of experimental tumour models.[24]

The screening of potential anti-cancer compounds began in 1947 and, by 1955, it was estimated that 20,000 chemical agents (synthetic and natural) had been tested: this represented three-quarters of the total American chemotherapy screening capacity.[25] Rhoads drew up contracts with many suppliers who submitted confidential materials for screening in return for a full evaluation of their anti-cancer potential. The top American chemical and pharmaceutical companies were well represented: Du Pont, American Cyanamid, Eastman Kodak, Dow Chemical and Union Carbide on the chemical side: Parke, Davis, Merck Sharp and Dohme, Lederle, Lilly, Abbot Laboratories, Pfizer, Upjohn and Searle, to name but the best known, on the pharmaceutical side. These were obvious choices but the screening strategy cast an even wider net. Universities and hospitals were invited to submit materials: the Department of Agriculture sent samples of natural products; and invitations were made to similar institutions abroad, in England, Ireland, France, Germany, Switzerland, India and Australia.[26]

This was one very important aspect of the industrialization of cancer chemotherapy. Another aspect of the same process concerned the screening techniques and here the strategy was based on contemporary ideas of industrial efficiency; namely, standardization, throughput and a managerial structure capable of achieving the stated objectives.[27] To standardize testing runs, for example, the Sloan–Kettering used only one screen, the sarcoma 180 mouse tumour (S-180).

The Sloan–Kettering system industrialized the organization of experimental cancer chemotherapy into a linear research configuration. It bore a striking and not coincidental similarity to an assembly line. Compounds were screened at one end of the process, and those showing promise were tried out in clinics in the adjoining Memorial Hospital.

The newly established NCI also had its own research programme dating back to the 1930s and screened material in a manner similar to that of the Sloan–Kettering. Compounds were either purchased on the open market or donated by investigators.[28] By the early 1950s the laboratory, with Murray Shear in charge, had screened more than 3,000 chemicals and some plant material.[29] But success in the laboratory did not spill over into the clinic. Despite a desperate search for partners, Shear was only able to enrol the Lankenau Hospital in Philadelphia into the programme.[30] By the time Shear's outfit was wound up in 1953, only two potential anti-cancer agents had got as far as clinical testing.[31]

Although he never achieved it in practice, Shear understood well that successful experimental cancer chemotherapy depended on the articulation of laboratory and clinic. As he put it:

> Those chemical agents that produce results of sufficient interest
> in the cancer patient are then to be brought back to the laboratory
> for further study and modification in the light of the clinical
> effects observed. ... In other words, the work of the research
> laboratory in chemotherapy is not ended when it sends a sterile
> vial over to the clinician, with a label giving the formula and
> the concentration of the agent. For, once a material is accepted
> for research in patients with advanced cancer, the second stage
> of the work of the research laboratory now begins, in intimate
> collaboration with the clinical investigator.[32]

By the time Shear wrote the above words – 1951 – cancer chemotherapy had already become the leading edge of cancer research, in two
senses. First, research on cancer chemotherapy had become respectable.
As Shear reminded his readers, cancer chemotherapy had been in the
past a highly discredited and unpopular field of scientific endeavour,
with little chance of funding: Peyton Rous of the Rockefeller Institute
expressed similar sentiments.[33] Secondly, within cancer research, the
search for chemical treatments had come to dominate other concerns.
In an analysis of 1,000 research projects supported by the NCI, the
results pointed clearly to treatment as the main activity; second in
importance was research on cancer growth, and prevention hardly
got a look-in.[34]

There were several reasons for the change in emphasis to chemotherapy rather than other methods of treatment. The presence of the
Sloan–Kettering certainly helped to raise the standing of experimental
cancer chemotherapy. Moreover, public agitation to do something
about cancer was becoming much more vocal and effective; in particular, there was the growing lobbying power of the American Cancer
Society, especially that of Mary Lasker, President of the Albert and
Mary Lasker Foundation, and a long and very active member of the
board of the American Cancer Society.[35] Additionally, and as a consequence of the heightened public awareness, an increasing amount of
money was put into cancer research. The budget of the NCI grew
exponentially from less than $0.5 million at its founding in 1937, to $1.75
million in 1946 and then $14 million in 1951 – it was $110 million in 1961;
the total amount of research grants of the National Institutes of Health
(NIH) earmarked for cancer rose from $85,000 in 1945 to $4.92 million in
1953; the total value of funds awarded by both government and private
sources for cancer research increased more than ten times between 1946
and 1951; and NCI grant money increased from $77,000 in 1946 to $9.26
million in 1955.[36] By 1948 cancer had become America's best funded
disease entity and much more money was on its way.

In quite a different and more profound way, cancer chemotherapy also drew increasing social prestige by embracing or enrolling other scientific interests, especially in biology and particularly cell and molecular biology, in pursuit of its objective.[37] One aspect of this process of enrolment was to transform the language of cancer research in order for it to be better understood especially by cell biologists who, armed with new and powerful instruments such as the electron microscope, were rapidly becoming a powerful disciplinary force.[38]

Roscoe R. Spencer who worked in the Cancer Control Branch of the NIH summed it up this way:

> Cancer is a process in which certain cells of an organized cell group have become parasitic on and finally fatal to the mother organism. These cells are truly traitors from within, in contrast to those responsible for communicable diseases, which are all invasive gangster cells (bacteria, protozoa, viruses) from without ... Although I hesitate to introduce new terms, one may think of cancer as an 'autoparasite'.[39]

The metaphor of the traitor is revealing (and worthy of further research), but the cellular definition was also something more than metaphor.[40] As Spencer put it, cancer was 'basically a problem in growth, and a study of growth leads naturally into practically every field of biology'.[41] He was also in no doubt that government and private funding notwithstanding, what explained the acceleration in cancer research since 1945 was that:

> the cancer process, involving as it does problems in cell division, in metabolism, in regeneration and in the differentiation and organization of tissues, is of deep interest to all workers in experimental biology and medicine. No other disease problem has created such widespread interest among nonmedical investigators. Thus, cancer research is activating numerous other fields of biology, and herein lies, I think, its basic importance and its true meaning.[42]

Embedded in this statement is not only a description of cancer but a clear direction for a cancer research programme which would enlist a variety of scientific disciplines and actors. Spencer's views should be taken as representative of an attempt to make cancer into an integrative force in biomedicine.[43]

Many of those involved in experimental chemotherapy research viewed their activities as grounded in basic biomedical sciences and, therefore, central to cancer research. In this manner, they promoted themselves as superior to radiotherapists and surgeons who treated cancer in a crude and empirical way. David Karnofsky, a leading authority on cancer chemotherapy at the Sloan–Kettering Institute, for example, stated boldly, as he himself recognized, that the object of research in cancer chemotherapy was to find a universal cure for the disease.[44] Less self-consciously, he also remarked that 'cancer chemotherapy as a subject is the synthesis and represents the goal of all cancer research'.[45] He repeated the claim, in an altered form, in an essay he wrote with his colleague Joseph Burchenal. While acknowledging that chemotherapy had until then only had limited success, they applauded the interest shown in it and offered an explanation: 'This interest is entirely justified, however, because chemotherapy, in principle, offers the best hope of controlling cancer, the various aspects of chemotherapeutic research represent a cross section of modern science, and the clinical material available for study offers an endless variety of fascinating problems'.[46]

Karnofsky and Burchenal were clearly reflecting and reinforcing the power of their own institution, the Sloan–Kettering. They were also suggesting that a cancer chemotherapy programme both had significant social value and represented a major challenge to a range of disciplines, to be brought together in a new alliance. The likely shape of such a programme emerged from a series of meetings that were held on Gibson Island, Maryland in 1945 and 1946. Dean Burk, the conference chairman, summed up the meeting's aspirations: he had no doubt that the problem of cancer had a chemical solution, that biochemistry would provide the necessary insights and that this would bring an end to the use of 'the knife and the ray'.[47]

Cancer Chemotherapy and the NCI

In July 1953, the United States Congress directed the NCI 'to explore the feasibility of an engineered, directed extramural research programme in the chemotherapy of acute leukemia'.[48] Behind this decision was a powerful lobby composed on the medical side by the leading advocates of the chemotherapeutic solution to leukaemia, Cornelius Rhoads of the Sloan–Kettering Institute in New York, Sidney Farber of the Children's Cancer Research Foundation in Boston and on the political side by Mary Lasker of the American Cancer Society.[49] The directive turned out to be controversial and met with resistance. Many scientists, it appeared, did not want a repetition of wartime programmes for penicillin and malaria chemotherapy – in the words of one commentator: 'their (i.e. the wartime programs) urgency and secrecy had left a bitter taste'.[50] The National Advisory Cancer Council, the advisory body for the NCI, was opposed to an engineered programme.[51] These voices were silenced, however, by those advocating a strong national programme: principally, Mary Lasker, Sidney Farber and

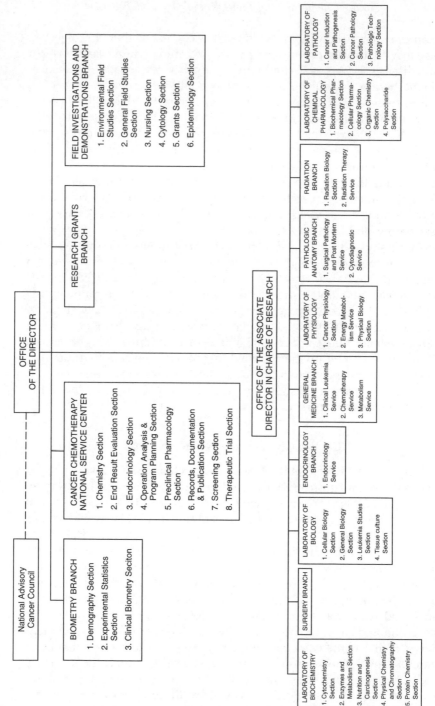

Figure 1.1 The National Cancer Institute (circa 1957). (Source: Heller, 'The National Cancer Institute', p. 187.)

Cornelius Rhoads. Congress yielded to their lobbying power despite the public disapproval of the programme by the National Advisory Cancer Council and put up $1 million for leukaemia research in 1953.

Initially, the NCI was able to interpret Congress's will in its own way and settled for a system of voluntary cooperation. But the state seemed to have other ideas and pushed for a much more rigid programme. One of the results was the creation within the NCI of the Cancer Chemotherapy National Service Center (CCNSC) in April 1955 directed by Kenneth Endicott (see Figures 1.1 and 1.2).

The CCNSC was the nation's answer to the private initiative of the Sloan–Kettering Institute's chemotherapy programme. Its early strategy was to act as a public screening facility for compounds submitted voluntarily by institutions and companies. Materials submitted in the first few years of operation were synthetics and fermentation products whose chemical structures were known: in 1960, the programme extended to natural, that is plant and animal products, in which the structures were unknown.[52] In this same year, barely five years into the programme, the CCNSC was screening more than 30,000 compounds annually – ten times the volume of the Sloan–Kettering. Moreover, in the meantime, the CCNSC had become transformed from a service into a 'targeted drug development program'.[53]

What this meant, in effect, is that cancer chemotherapy had begun to take on a certain logic and momentum, separate from other approaches to cancer treatment. In the words of Robert Coghill, the deputy for industrial research: 'The CCNSC, after several years of tooling up, has a massive machine in operation – from animal breeding to clinical trials. The machine has built up a tremendous momentum, as a result of which its direction cannot be changed overnight'.[54] Its screening programme of 30,000 compounds had vast repercussions throughout the biomedical community and in several ancillary activities. Thirty thousand compounds translated into almost 300,000 tests; these tests used three mouse tumours: Carcinoma 755, Leukemia L1210 and Sarcoma 180. Whereas the latter could be transplanted in non-genetically defined mice, the first two required in-bred lines: the Roscoe B. Jackson Laboratories were enlisted as suppliers of in-bred mice and, thanks to a grant from the NCI, were able to guarantee a supply of 100,000 mice annually from 1956.[55] More than that, the CCNSC established banks of frozen animal and human tumours, and the world's largest computerized data base for experimental drugs. The scale and methods of clinical trials were also profoundly affected by the existence of the CCNSC.[56] In the words of one the leading scientists in the NCI:

> Not only have these resources permitted the conduct of the NCI program, but they have also provided both material and data to

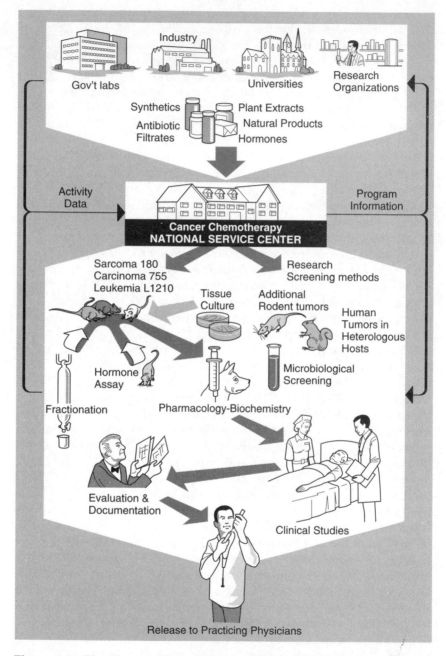

Figure 1.2 The Cancer Chemotherapy National Service Center. (Source: Endicott, 'The chemotherapy program', p. 279.)

oncologists throughout the world. This highly organized program at the NCI has become a focal point for the entire chemotherapy effort in the United States and is in active collaboration and well-coordinated with preclinical and clinical chemotherapy programs on a world-wide basis.[57]

With the participation of more than 3,400 suppliers (including all of the world's leading pharmaceutical companies, many of the world's major chemical companies, government agencies, universities and private research institutes) and the disbursement of an enormous and exponentially growing amount of funds in the form of grants and contracts, it is not surprising that cancer chemotherapy and its institutional embodiment became the bandwagon for researchers throughout biomedicine.[58]

Plants and the NCI

By 1955, only six anti-cancer drugs, all of them synthetic compounds (antimetabolites and alkylating agents), had been approved for clinical use in the United States.[59] Not surprisingly, therefore, the first compounds to be screened by the newly created CCNSC were synthetic ones, furnished primarily by industrial contacts. Owing to past successful experience with micro-organisms as antibiotics, in the same year, a small number of fermentation products were also screened. The number was increased substantially in the following year and for the next few years remained at a very high level. Altogether, in the first five years of the programme, almost 115,000 synthetic and fermentation compounds were screened.[60] Plants were not screened during these first few years of the programme because, as an annual report on the activities of the CCNSC maintained, other raw materials were more readily available.[61]

The absence of plants from the CCNSC screening programme needs some comment. Biologists distinguish between primary metabolites – compounds essential to the life and functioning of the organism and formed in a process known as primary metabolism – and secondary metabolites – compounds without essential functions and formed in a process called secondary metabolism.[62] These terms were introduced at the end of the nineteenth century and have been in general use ever since, although they often cause as much confusion as clarity – some compounds can be classed as either.

Though there is no general agreement on what specific role secondary metabolites play in the living organism, it is widely accepted that they perform both ecological and internal roles.[63] They improve the organism's survival fitness, by serving as competitive and defensive weapons against other organisms; they are agents of plant–microbe relations and insect–microbe symbiosis; and they act as sexual hormones and metal-transporting agents.[64] Most organisms produce secondary metabolites, but they are most common in plants and microorganisms.[65]

As far as humans are concerned, secondary metabolites, especially those from plants, have been a rich source of useful compounds. Natural dyes, oils, resins, tannins, flavours and fragrances, for example, are secondary metabolites.[66] Because secondary metabolites are relatively scarce, they have been highly valued throughout human history. The greater the extent of biodiversity, the larger the range of secondary metabolites. Societies inhabiting biodiverse environments have typically used a greater variety of secondary metabolite compounds than those who do not. It is for this reason that rainforests are particularly rich in secondary metabolites.[67]

Some secondary metabolites are bioactive to humans. Whether in their crude or in the extracted and purified form, they have been and continue to be used as medicinal preparations throughout the world. For most of human history, the plant world has reigned supreme as a source of therapeutics. It is only in the twentieth century, in the West, that its role came to be severely challenged by the advent of synthetic preparations and fermentation products, particularly antibiotics.

At the time when the CCNSC was established, only a very small fraction of the world's plants had been investigated systematically for their bioactivity. For more than a century, it was known that many plant alkaloids – nitrogenous-based secondary metabolites – were bioactive, yet in 1952, only two per cent of the world's plant species had been screened for their alkaloid content.[68] Even less was known about the cytotoxic and antitumour possibilities of plant products.[69]

To get plants assessed as part of the CCNSC screening programme was a challenge taken up by Jonathan Hartwell, an organic chemist who, in 1958, had become Assistant Chief for Program Analysis Activities of the CCNSC.[70] After graduate studies at Harvard, Hartwell worked for a short time in industry before becoming, in 1938, a research fellow at the newly created NCI. In 1942 he was promoted to the post of chemist and in 1947 to the head of the organic chemistry section of the Laboratory of Chemical Pharmacology. He moved to the CCNSC in 1958.[71]

Jonathan Hartwell could not have been a better choice for convincing the NCI to include plants in their screening project. His experience and knowledge in natural product chemistry and his interest in plants as chemotherapeutic agents were arguably unsurpassed by anyone else at the NCI. In his first few years at the NCI, Hartwell had worked closely with Murray Shear who had become absorbed in studying polysaccharide fractions of the toxin of the bacterium *Bacillus prodigiosus*. Known more popularly as Coley's toxin, after William B. Coley, a New York surgeon who had observed the regression of malignant tumours of cancer patients after they developed a severe streptococcal infection, it had become well-known earlier in the twentieth century as a treatment for cancer.[72] Thanks to work in the 1930s, there was growing evidence that bacterial toxins might have antitumour effects.[73] Shear isolated lipopolysaccharide and demonstrated that it was the biologically active substance in Coley's toxin and that it induced necrosis of mouse tumours.[74]

Hartwell was thus introduced, albeit indirectly, to natural products as possible anti-cancer agents, but much stood in the way of realizing this. The plant world, as we have seen, had hardly been investigated systematically for bioactivity. Moreover, until the outbreak of World War II, the bulk of screened compounds were inorganic and synthetic organic chemicals, primarily toxic dyestuffs.[75]

One of the only plant products to be considered as a potential anti-cancer agent that would influence Hartwell in the future was colchicine.[76] First isolated by Joseph Pelletier and Joseph Caventou in Paris in 1820, colchicine's cytological activity became widely acknowledged during the 1930s as a result of research in Brussels and London. Unlike bacterial toxins which induce cell death through haemorrhaging, colchicine kills cells by preventing mitosis (cell division). Colchicine was the first natural product recognized as a mitotic poison, although it soon proved to be far too toxic for clinical use.

Hartwell, in common with others who were attracted by its antimitotic properties, turned to colchicine during the late 1940s in an attempt to improve it as a potential anti-cancer agent.[77] Earlier he and Shear had begun to work on podophyllin, a crude natural product made from parts of *Podophyllum peltatum*, a small herb growing in the United States and known as the May apple.[78] Their interest in podophyllin was aroused by several articles published early in the 1940s that reported dramatic results obtained by using the preparation against venereal warts which, following treatment, disappeared entirely, leaving no trace of their existence.[79] Attracted by the idea of a preparation that regressed growths, Hartwell and Shear demonstrated in the late 1940s that podophyllin and its principal component podophyllotoxin severely damaged sarcomas in laboratory mice.[80] They had thus established that another natural product had antitumour effects. Very soon comparative studies of the cytology of podophyllin and colchicine began to appear.[81] Hartwell continued into the early 1950s to pursue podophyllin from a chemical perspective, isolating more substances and elucidating their structures.[82]

Because of his expert knowledge of the only two plant-derived products known to possess antitumour properties, Hartwell was in a unique position in the cancer research community of the 1940s and early 1950s. His training in organic chemistry was fundamental to his approach. But there was also something else in his range of knowledge and interests that was to be particularly relevant though, given his training and appointments, it was both unusual and unpredictable.

Arising from his work on podophyllin in the late 1940s, Hartwell became interested in the folk knowledge concerning the use of plants for medicinal purposes. The review of the biology and chemistry of podophyllin that appeared in 1954 and summed up a huge body of basic research, was introduced, interestingly, by several pages outlining its use in folk medicine.[83] Hartwell's interest in folk medicine, particularly as it applied to cancer treatment, was enlarged even more by scores of unsolicited letters received by the NCI. Arriving on Hartwell's desk from 1953 onwards, the letters recounted tales of wonderful plant treatments for cancer, giving information on the plant, its habitat, how it was to be used, and so forth.[84] He took them very seriously both in the sense of noting the pathological condition and the claimed effects of the remedy, and the description of the plant. Indeed, his interest led him to botanists at the Plant Introduction Section of the USDA in an attempt to establish scientific nomenclature for local names and vague descriptions. His communications with the USDA botanists grew in frequency over the 1950s as he attempted to make sense of what he called his 'cancer plants'. The links he built with the USDA were to prove extremely important later.

With the help of these letters, other unpublished sources and a wealth of published material, Hartwell began to compile a comprehensive survey of cancer treatments world-wide arranged, interestingly, by botanical classification.[85] Beginning in 1967 and continuing over the next four years he published eleven instalments of a magisterial survey of plants used against cancer as they were described in plant folklore and the historical literature.[86] Despite his enormous interest in plant folklore and folk medicine as leads to particular plants used in the treatment for cancer, however, it remained a scholarly rather than a practical pursuit.[87] We will return to this point later.

Questions about plant folklore was only one of Hartwell's reasons for contacting the USDA. In the early 1950s, the Laboratory of Chemical Pharmacology of the NCI undertook a systematic study of the damaging capacity of plant materials known to have some kind of biological activity. The plants were grouped into cathartics, diuretics and pesticides and the modestly encouraging results appeared in 1952 and 1953.[88] One of the plants investigated in the course of this programme was the savin, a small juniper bush, *Juniperus sabina*. It showed activity against the sarcoma 37 mouse tumour screen, and on that basis the search was extended to a variety of conifers growing in the United States. Needles and berries were tested. The results were mediocre, with one notable exception: the active material in the positive tests on three juniper species turned out to be podophyllotoxin.[89] In the next few years the search for active conifers extended beyond the United States and specimens were collected for testing at the NCI from Australia, New Zealand, New Guinea and South America. Of thirty-six genera of conifers tested, only five showed activity: in several species podophyllotoxin was shown to be the active material.[90]

The NCI–USDA Plant Screening Programme

To get enough specimens and to get the botanical information correct, Hartwell turned to the USDA for help. His relationship with botanists there appears to have been cordial and friendly. Certainly Hartwell got what he wanted from them.[91] But as the frequency and workload of requests began to grow in the last few years of the 1950s, officials at the USDA became less willing to undertake Hartwell's work. Towards the end of 1959, Carl Erlanson, Chief of the New Crops Research Branch, advised Hartwell that he could no longer fulfil the latest request, made on 26 October 1959, for plant procurement. If Hartwell wanted to have future relationships, these would need to be organized in an official interagency programme with which the USDA had years of experience.[92]

One of the most important functions of the USDA was in collecting, identifying, storing and cultivating plant materials as part of their task of introducing beneficial plants into American agriculture. From the beginning of this programme in 1898, the USDA had built up a wealth of information and expertise in plant exploration.[93] For most of its history, plant introduction concentrated on edible and industrial crops, seeking to increase the germplasm stock available to American farmers.

After World War II, the USDA embarked on a special assignment, in an interagency programme with the NIH. The goal of the programme, initiated by a decree from President Truman in 1950, was to search for plants native to the United States or easily imported or cultivated as a starting material for making the drug cortisone.[94] Eight botanists from the Section of Plant Introduction were assigned to the programme responsible for procuring the plant material. Screening and chemical isolation were the responsibility of the USDA's Eastern Utilization Research Branch (formerly the Eastern Regional Research Laboratory) located in Philadelphia where Monroe Wall was the chemist in charge of analysing the plant extracts.[95]

After the plant extracts were analysed for their potential as the starting material for making cortisone, those that were rejected were typically thrown away but many were saved. According to Monroe Wall, Hartwell learned of the analysis of plant extracts in Philadelphia and paid him a site visit in 1957.[96] Some 1,000 samples of plant extracts that had been saved were prepared so that they could be screened by the NCI in an *in vivo* assay. About a year later, the results showed that seventeen samples were active, especially the leaves of a tree native to China, *Camptotheca acuminata*, which was growing in the Plant Introduction Station of the USDA in Chico, California.

Upon receiving the results of the tests, Hartwell wrote on 26 October 1959 to Quentin Jones at the USDA: 'We wish to confirm this activity on fresh specimens large enough to permit of chemical fractionation if still found active. Ideally, a new specimen should be obtained from the same locality as the old, and at the same time of year'.[97] It was this memo and the workload implicit in the request that prompted the branch Chief, Carl Erlanson, to bring a halt to the ad hoc arrangements between the NCI and the USDA that had been made since Hartwell's first communications earlier in the decade.

By late 1957, Hartwell had become widely involved in a number of investigations into the chemotherapeutic value of plant extracts. These included Wall's extracts as well as several hundred more supplied by the University of Arizona and others.[98] Additionally, Hartwell had interested several other groups, notably at the University of Maine and at Florida State University, to investigate specific families of plants for antitumour activity: these were families which were prominent in the folk literature that he was already collecting.[99]

There is little doubt that such a flurry of activity would have set Hartwell thinking about a more systematic programme for investigating plant materials. A timely review of the CCNSC activities in 1959 recommended that 'plants be explored more extensively as a source of agents with antitumour activity'.[100] What direct role Hartwell played in this initiative is unknown but his influence and experience must have helped its recommendation. By late June of that year, negotiations and clarification of operations were already underway between the NCI and the USDA.[101] The process was slow and problematic, at least from the USDA's point of view.

In March of the following year, 1960, Hartwell invited Quentin Jones, a botanist from the New Crops Research Branch of the USDA and with experience of plant screening programmes, to join a team inspecting the facilities of the University of Wisconsin and the University of

Arizona.[102] Both universities had put forth proposals to the NCI to procure plant materials and to fractionate and isolate active extracts. Hartwell made it clear that he wished the team to constitute 'an ad hoc committee to advise the Cancer Chemotherapy National Service Center on setting up its plant program . . . This committee will report directly to the staff of the CCNSC thru me'.[103] Jones reported to Erlanson that in requesting his participation, the NCI was making no assumptions about the willingness or otherwise of the New Crops Research Branch, of which Erlanson was Chief, to become involved in the cancer screening project.[104] Though showing little personal desire to make the trips, Jones did feel that his participation would be of value to the Branch in reaching a decision whether or not to join the NCI in the programme. Jones was somewhat ambivalent about the programme: he did not want to do it if it competed for staff time with ongoing cooperative programmes; at the same time, he saw it as an opportunity 'for gaining some immediate additional support for our overall botanical program, including screening programs'.[105] Jones was referring primarily to several programmes at the USDA, begun in 1956 and 1957, to search for new industrial crops, principally vegetable oils, pulp crops and protein sources.[106] These programmes enhanced the agency's long experience in exploring for and procuring plant materials, but it also tied up substantial staff time. Erlanson, however, appears to have been more enthusiastic about an interagency programme.[107]

Hartwell was ready to move with a firm proposal, including financial arrangements, once the site visits were over. In April 1960 he wrote to the Administrator of the Agricultural Research Service, asking for the New Crops Research Branch to procure plants for anti-cancer screening by the NCI, in a cooperative programme.[108] By the end of June, the proposal had been approved and signed by both agencies and in July of the same year the programme was up and running.[109] Hartwell was to organize operations from the NCI and the botanist Robert Perdue, also a Harvard PhD, assigned to the post by Erlanson, was to do the same at the USDA. One of the first meetings between the two groups, held at the end of July, stressed the absolute need to identify plants precisely noting genus, species, description of plant part, date of collection and location details. It was noted that the extracts sent by Wall's laboratory to the CCNSC for testing several years earlier had been inadequately identified.[110]

Despite the optimism evident in Hartwell's various communications, and perhaps more generally in the cancer research community, about the potential of plants as anti-cancer agents, there was nothing inevitable about the plant screening programme. In his official proposal to the USDA, Hartwell was indirectly alluding to the fact that there was no institution, other than the USDA, with the capacity and expertise to handle the flow of materials. The University of Arizona, one of the only universities in the country with the capacity to procure plants and prepare extracts of plant materials, and under contract to the NCI at the time, could handle only fifteen per cent of the total number of plant extracts envisioned in the programme annually.

The choice of the USDA in a cooperative venture was based not only on its expertise and experience. It also rested on the manner in which submissions of materials were made to the CCNSC. As mentioned before, pharmaceutical and chemical companies voluntarily submitted material to be screened by the CCNSC for their possible anti-cancer properties. The procedure was handled, in principle, in the strictest confidence to avoid any leakage of proprietary information. In practice, however, pharmaceutical and chemical companies were less than confident of the NCI's protocols. The absence of formal arrangements for protecting proprietary rights and a clear patent policy in the early years of the CCNSC's existence, in particular, delayed the full partici-pation of industry for several years. In 1958, the Department of Health, Education and Welfare revised its policies regarding patents on prod-ucts or processes developed by industry, and in that year, it enlisted the support of more than 100 companies who sent synthetic chemicals and fermentation products for anti-cancer screening.[111]

As plants were, by definition, not proprietary, the idea of voluntary submission could not work, except on a small-scale. A comprehensive programme (for that was what was needed) could only come about through a contractual agreement to submit an agreed number of plant samples in an agreed amount of time. A commercial supplier, such as a nursery or a firm specializing in botanicals, was a possibility. If a plant or plant extract showed promise, the commercial supplier would probably be able to supply a large amount of requisite material. Standing against this, however, was a major disadvantage. Relying on commercial growers and firms specializing in botanicals severely restricted the search to cultivated plants and those extracts already shown to have some kind of biological activity. The diversity of plant material would not be tapped. As Hartwell's informants demonstrated and his researches into plant folklore confirmed, there were plants growing in the wild with promise as anti-cancer agents. The USDA with its long history of plant exploration and its far-flung botanical (and political) connections throughout the world was, therefore, an obvious partner.

Even though Hartwell was enthusiastic about the programme and even though on a formal level, the NCI had given its blessing to a plant screening programme, the potential of such a venture was far from clear. During the 1950s, as we have seen, many plant extracts had been submitted for screening at the NCI. Few showed any marked activity. At the University of Texas, another group had been screening plant extracts since 1952 – in the late 1950s and early 1960s, this group tested more than 1,500 extracts prepared in the search for steroidal sapogenins also tested at CCNSC. The great majority of the tests were negative, except in the case of one member of the family Compositae, a family of plants which Hartwell had encouraged a group at Florida State University to investigate in collaboration with the CCNSC.[112] In addition, all of the approved anti-cancer drugs before 1960, it will be recalled, were synthetic products. Antibiotics as possible anti-cancer agents were generally a better bet than plants, first because the pharmaceutical industry was already heavily involved in producing them for other therapeutic uses, and second because strong activity had already been demonstrated in the case of the antibiotic actinomycin D both experimentally and clinically.

The Vinca Alkaloids

Against this rather pessimistic background for launching a plant programme outlook, a real breakthrough did occur in the hopeful search for plants as anti-cancer agents, although it was not a result of the NCI–USDA plant screening programme. Two groups, one at the University of Western Ontario, and the other in the laboratories of Eli Lilly in Indianapolis, independently responded to separate reports from Jamaica and the Philippines, respectively, of the alleged beneficial effects of the leaves of the Madagascar periwinkle (*Catharanthus rosea* but incorrectly referred to as *Vinca rosea*, at the time) in treating diabetes in the absence of insulin.[113] The Western Ontario group started working on the problem in 1952 but, despite spending substantial time on research, they could find no effect on blood sugar by administering a water extract of the leaves on laboratory animals. Instead, and by chance it appears, they observed that after giving rats an intraperitoneal injection of a concentrated version of the extract, the white blood counts were enormously reduced and the bone marrow destroyed.[114]

By 1955, the group had abandoned the diabetes problem and began to think about leukaemia instead: they also began to try to isolate the active ingredient in the periwinkle responsible for the dramatic effects on the white blood count.[115] In 1957, Charles Beer of the Western Ontario group succeeded in isolating the active fraction and the group named it vincaleukoblastine: the results of the research were presented to the New York Academy of Sciences in 1958 and published in the same year.[116] The group at Eli Lilly had similar negative results with extracts for the treatment of diabetes, and in 1957 submitted the sample for cancer screening. In 1958 and 1959, they too worked on isolating the active agent and revealed a substance they named leurosine.[117] The Eli Lilly group subsequently isolated a more active alkaloid which, in 1961, they named leurocristine, more commonly known as vincristine.[118] This, together with vincaleukoblastine, renamed vinblastine, entered into clinical evaluation and became available by 1964 for clinical use: vincristine for acute childhood leukaemia and vinblastine for lymphomas, especially Hodgkin's disease.[119]

Before the 1962 Kefauver–Harris amendments tightened the regulatory process, active compounds could move from the laboratory with remarkable speed.[120] This was true for both vinblastine and vincristine, both of which gained FDA approval within three years of their discovery.[121] Vinblastine was the first plant product to reach this stage.[122] That the discovery of the vinca alkaloids as clinically useful anti-cancer agents was a real breakthrough and raised the hopes of those searching for plant sources is beyond doubt. To claim, however, as some writers do, that the discovery of the vinca alkaloids was the impetus for the discovery of other plant agents would be to simplify an otherwise complicated situation as the previous discussion has argued.[123]

The process of the discovery of the vinca alkaloids also had a moral to it but one not particularly comforting to those who believed in folk medicine as a tool to guide the explorer to specific active plants. The sting was delivered by the Western Ontario group when they presented their results in New York in 1958. 'The results of our research', they wrote, 'which are presented here for the first time, should not be considered in terms of a new chemotherapeutic agent, but rather in terms of a chance observation that has led to the isolation of a substance with potential chemotherapeutic possibilities'.[124] They were claiming, in other words, that had they restricted their search to plants with suspected anti-cancer properties, they would have missed the Madagascar periwinkle.

Procuring Plants

The issue of how to select plants for screening would be raised several times during the course of the NCI–USDA cooperative programme. The USDA, however, had a very clear idea of how to procure plant samples, garnered over decades of experience and, in the case of medicinal research, particularly in recent years. Hartwell envisioned an annual procurement of about 1,000 plant species. The preferred collection strategy when the type of compound to be extracted was unknown was of the general kind – all identifiable material is collected and prepared for further evaluation.[125] That is, the approach was one of 'chemical prospecting' rather than pre-selection based on the annals of folk medicine or expectations of activity among certain genera of plants. The USDA plant explorers had developed networks of contacts and co-operators throughout the world. There would be no problem satisfying the NCI's requests. Two points, however, were stressed. The first was that the USDA expected to work in close association with the chemists on the programme; and second, that from the point of view of the USDA, this was primarily an exercise in botany. That is, as far as the plant explorers were concerned, they were adding to or amending botanical knowledge. Time-consuming post-procurement activities (as they were called) had to be recognized by the NCI as essential operations, although not strictly part of the plant screening programme.[126]

Apart from Perdue, no botanists were assigned to the plant screening programme on a full-time basis in its early years. Rather, they collected plants while assigned to other programmes, in those parts of the world in which they had expertise. One of the first to be engaged in the programme was Arthur Barclay whose main area was south-western and western United States, although eventually his trips included visits to Mexico, Chile, Colombia and South Africa. He exemplified the part-time nature of the procurement of plants for the NCI. For most of the 1960s, his chief exploration work (and publications) concerned sources of oil seeds, particularly the plant *Lesquerella*, a major preoccupation of New Crops Research Branch.[127] Lloyd Spetzman joined in the search for plants in other parts of the country in 1967 as did Ed Terrell. Perdue concentrated on Africa. Following the passage of the National Cancer Act of 1971, several more botanists were brought in and Barclay was made full time.[128]

Random selection of plants for screening remained the collection method for the entire period of the programme. Perdue and Hartwell did, however, discuss the comparative merits of random searching versus selective searching.[129] Selective searching – targeting a specific family or genus, for example – would, it was acknowledged, lead to a higher number of hits, but by the same token, it would not uncover substances possessing entirely new structures and mechanisms of activity.[130] And that was the key to a successful programme. As the NCI–USDA plant screening programme was envisioned to be long-term (at least ten to fifteen years, initially), Perdue and Hartwell insisted that broad, random screening was the best way to uncover compounds of hitherto unknown types of activity.[131] As Perdue and his co-authors from the NCI put it: 'The key to the discovery of an array of useful antitumor agents in plants is to detect activity in as many species, genera and families as possible'.[132]

During the life of the programme, as data accumulated on plants and their activity, proposals to alter the collection strategy were proffered. One such proposal related to the observation that a high degree of activity was present in a few families; in other words, a few families of plants appeared to produce secondary metabolites more likely to be bioactive than other families. An experimental programme to investigate this began in 1972 and plants of six families were targeted.[133] During its three years of operation, the programme substantiated the earlier observation of the concentration of compounds in particular families. New compounds were discovered, but most were related to ones already known.[134] The main point, however, was the one that Perdue and Hartwell had already recognized at the beginning of the cooperative programme; namely, that any kind of limitation by a systematic pre-screen would cut out really novel leads. Retrospective studies of the relationship between bioactivity and taxonomy and bioactivity and folklore concluded that both had advantages over random collection but, in a long-term programme, could not substitute for the broad sweep.[135]

Perdue outlined detailed procedures for procurement in a programme guide distributed to all collectors, first prepared in 1967 and revised on several occasions during the period of the programme.[136] The programme guide covered all aspects of collecting including the important job of recording collection information. It also drew attention to another and vital issue, that of secrecy. Perdue explicitly urged his staff to understand that 'the fact that a plant is a confirmed active is confidential. This is primarily to protect the interest of the chemist'. There was, of course, no way to police confidentiality but the association between federal agencies gave some minimal guarantee that 'the information does not get into the wrong hands'.

Extracting and Screening

Procuring the plant was only the first step in the NCI's programme to discover clinically useful anti-cancer drugs.[137] All of the other steps were handled by NCI contractors whose operations were approved by the NCI. The Wisconsin Alumni Research Foundation (WARF) prepared the crude plant extracts.[138] Their contract with the NCI began in 1961 and continued until the end of the programme. Until 1974, extraction was based on a procedure developed by the chemist Morris Kupchan then at the University of Wisconsin and subsequently at the University of Virginia; after 1974, WARF used a modified and more complicated system.[139] The crude plant extracts were then sent to a number of laboratories where they were tested in various bioassay systems: among the laboratories contracted by the NCI for this purpose were Arthur D. Little, Hazleton Laboratories, Microbiological Associates, Southern Research Institute and the University of Miami.[140]

Once a plant extract had been prepared, a sample was screened to see if it had potential as an anti-cancer agent. When the plant screening programme first began, material was tested in one *in vitro* screen, KB cell culture, and three *in vivo* screens (tumours transplanted in laboratory mice); S-180, a sarcoma; CA-755, an adenocarcinoma; and L1210, a lymphoid leukaemia.[141] The purpose of the screen was to eliminate the vast majority of inactive materials and identify the few that had potential as anti-cancer agents. Screens are only predictors of anti-cancer activity: no single screen is infallible.

The screening methodology changed frequently.[142] By 1962, plant extracts were routinely tested against KB cell culture, L1210 and two randomly selected transplantable tumour systems. In 1966, after it had been discovered that both S-180 and CA-755 were sensitive to extensive plant constituents, particularly tannins and phytosterols, and were, therefore, producing many false positives, they were replaced by Walker 256, a rat tumour system. Walker 256 only lasted until 1969 as a screen for plant extracts because it, too, was sensitive to tannins and other inactive plant constituents. P388, a new *in vivo* leukaemia screen, was introduced to take its place. L1210 was phased out in the early 1970s, leaving KB cell culture and P388 as the screens for plant extracts – the one testing for cytotoxicity and the other for antitumour activity.[143]

Those crude extracts satisfying the criteria for activity and confirmed as active on a second sample were then candidates for fractionation, leading to the isolation of the active compounds.[144] Before this could proceed, however, it was necessary to re-collect the plant in substantially larger quantities (fifty pounds was the preferred amount but, in rare cases, it could reach 500 pounds).[145]

Fractionation and isolation were handled by a small number of chemical laboratories. In the first years of the programme, these were the University of Wisconsin, succeeded by the University of Virginia when Morris Kupchan moved to the latter, and the University of Arizona under the direction of Jack Cole. The third laboratory was the Research Triangle Institute which, in 1960, one year after it opened its doors, hired Monroe Wall, from the USDA laboratories in Philadelphia, as head of its Natural Products Laboratory.[146] Towards the end of the programme, these chemists were joined by colleagues at Arizona State University (Bob Pettit) and the University of Illinois (Norman Farnsworth).[147] Once the pure active compound was isolated and its structure was determined, it returned to the NCI for a further series of screening and preclinical and clinical evaluations.

The Demise of the NCI–USDA Plant Screening Programme

Between 1960 and 1975, Hartwell and Perdue remained in charge of the plant screening programme at the NCI and at the USDA, respectively.[148] But then big changes occurred. Hartwell retired in 1975. John Douros, who had been working under Hartwell since 1972, succeeded him as Head of the Natural Products Section of the Division of Cancer Treatment. In 1976 the section changed its name to the Natural Products Branch and Douros became its Chief.[149] He was assisted by Matthew Suffness, in his capacity as Head of the Plant and Animal Products Section. At the USDA, there were organizational and personnel changes as well. In 1972, following a reorganization of the Agricultural Research Service, a new facility, the Medicinal Plant Resources Laboratory, was created with Perdue as head. This carried on the plant screening programme previously housed in the New Crops Research Branch.

At the end of March 1978, the USDA received a letter from the NCI on the subject of the plant screening programme. It stated that the inter-agency agreement would not be renewed unless certain problems within the USDA's sphere of operations were solved.[150] In this letter, the NCI accused USDA personnel of a number of failings: a lack of flexibility in relation to NCI needs, unauthorized communication with NCI contractors, excessive delays to NCI requests for plant collection and re-collection, and an excessive reliance on subcontractors.

According to Saul Schepartz, then the Deputy Director of the Division of Cancer Treatment, the NCI had been having difficulties with the plant collections for several years.[151] The finger pointed directly at the USDA's Principal Investigator, Robert Perdue. But that was only one side of the story. Perdue, for his part, was also concerned that the programme was not bearing results. He pointed especially to a failure in the screening programme to detect active plants. As early as 1972, Perdue expressed great concern about the decline in the number of materials showing KB activity. Increasing the productivity of the programme, he argued, depended on solving this problem. Referring to a graph showing the number of KB actives since the start of the programme, Perdue pointed to the sharp fall from a high point around 1964. 'It seems reasonable', he argued, 'that the yield of KB-actives should be much higher. If this matter can be resolved in the near future; procurement of confirmed-actives can be increased . . .'.[152] No action was taken, although it was repeated to the Chief of the Drug Development Branch in 1974 and to Matthew Suffness at the Natural Products Branch in 1976.[153]

In his letter to the Chief of the Drug Development Branch, Perdue also suggested that the use of P388 as a general screen should be

reduced thereby saving money and increasing the screening productivity. Throughout the 1960s and 1970s, the NCI showed a clear
preference for *in vivo* screens, despite the fact that they were time-
consuming and expensive.[154] Perdue maintained that most of the plant
compounds then under consideration for clinical evaluation were
active in KB, an argument he repeated to Matthew Suffness two years
later.[155] Perdue's recommendations, however, fell on deaf ears during
the time he was with the programme. The NCI stuck to P388, despite its
cost and slow turnaround.[156] Some of Perdue's concerns were vindicated when in 1979, the General Accounting Office produced evidence
of the cost-effectiveness of an *in vitro* screen: it also stressed that the
P388 was probably not sensitive enough to detect active plant agents
because of their low concentrations.[157] The concentration on P388 in the
1970s is now viewed as having been a serious shortcoming in the
programme: 'continued use of the primary P388 mouse leukaemia
screen appeared to be detecting only previously identified active
compounds or chemical structure-types having little or no activity
against solid tumors'.[158]

The USDA's response to the NCI's complaints was to move Robert
Perdue out of the plant screening programme.[159] Barely one month
after the NCI's letter, Perdue was reassigned to the post of Chief of the
Plant Taxonomy Laboratory.[160] After eighteen years service, Robert
Perdue ended his relationship with the plant screening programme.
James Duke, the Laboratory's previous Chief, took Perdue's position at
the Medicinal Plant Resources Laboratory and changed its name to the
Economic Botany Laboratory.

For the time being, the NCI got its way and was in the driving seat. In
his New Year's message to his staff in the following year, Duke focused
his staff on their duties: 'We are expected to move into the future with
the cancer program, conforming as closely as possible to the wishes of
the cancer institute. This means fewer collections with more select-
ivity . . . It is a new ball game for the cancer program, and that is what
was wanted by the NCI. I have discussed these ideas with Dr. Suffness.
He wants us to collect new genera and species, not to evaluate the
history of the program. I concur.'[161]

The new team and the new association did not improve matters. It
also hardly had a chance to find its feet. On 2 October 1981, the Board of
Scientific Counselors of the Division of Cancer Treatment, by a vote of
six to four, decided to abolish the NCI–USDA plant programme in its
entirety.[162] The decision was opposed by many scientists involved in
cancer research and medical botany. Both the American Society of
Pharmacognosy and the Society for Economic Botany responded to the
announcement with shock and anger. Harry Fong, President of the

Society for Economic Botany, remarked in an open letter to the Society's members that, according to his information, the vote was taken without all the facts being presented to the meeting. He went so far as to state that 'the plan to guillotine the plant program...was carefully and cleverly orchestrated in advance of the meeting.'[163] The decision to axe the programme was wrong, he maintained. The NCI was the only institution in the United States which could be expected to support natural products research.[164] Pharmaceutical companies, he remarked, had a dismal record in the cancer field, let alone natural products. Even Eli Lilly and Co., with its winning combination of vinblastine and vincristine, had left the field, as far as research and development was concerned. Though they urged their members to raise political voices, nothing came of it and in the following year all of the operations were wound up.[165]

In more than twenty years, the programme screened over 114,000 plant extracts, representing about 35,000 samples.[166] How many species these figures represent is unclear because, for larger plants, more than one part was collected. A reasonable estimate might be 15,000 species.[167] Estimates of the number of species of higher plants in existence vary between 230,000 and 500,000, although the figure of 250,000 seems acceptable.[168] On these estimates, the programme tested six per cent of the world's plant species.

Just over four per cent of the extracts were confirmed actives.[169] Each year many pure compounds were isolated and tested against the tumour screen and, each year, some of these would go forward to further stages of study. Each review of the programme contained a list of active compounds which cascaded into the following review. Many compounds went through toxicity studies, fewer entered into Phase I clinical trials and even fewer into Phase II clinical trials. By the time the programme wound up it could not boast a single plant-based approved anti-cancer drug. Of those plant-derived compounds that were discovered in the programme and were in advanced clinical development – ellipticine, taxol, homoharringtonine, tripdiolide and bouvardin – only taxol would continue advancing until it achieved FDA approval in 1992.[170] The great hopefuls of the late 1960s and 1970s such as emetine, thalicarpine, bruceantin and maytansine all dropped out.[171]

Despite its failure in bringing a plant extract to a marketable drug during its time, the plant screening programme innovated and expanded knowledge in many different areas.[172] The data on medicinal plants simply from a botanical point of view grew prodigiously through the period. The methods of procurement, of the organization of information, of re-collections, all of these were improved upon as the scale of the operations grew. For the chemists involved in fractionation and isolation, the opportunities to improve their techniques were also substantial given the nature of the throughput. They also developed a substantial knowledge base around the structure and activity of natural products. Pressures on the screening system, inherited from a period when the amount and diversity of material was small, have already been remarked upon. Finally, the programme offered a great deal of experience in constructing interagency cooperative ventures in bio-medicine.

These were all beneficial effects. But, because of the failure to bring an extract to the clinic, the programme did not even pose two crucial questions, never mind find the answer to them. These were: first, what were the problems associated with the commercial production of an NCI-developed plant compound? and second, what were the problems associated with supplying enough of the raw materials to make such a compound?

These questions would only begin to appear in the late 1980s as taxol was making its way towards its transformation into an anti-cancer agent. That decade turned out to be crucial in the form the answers would take. No one was prepared for what was to happen: everyone was taken by surprise. But first, back to 1960.

Notes

1 See, for example, Bud, 'Strategy in American cancer research', p. 440.
2 Although the term 'chemotherapy' refers generally to the use of chemical agents in the treatment of diseases, in this text we are using it in the narrower sense of treating cancer with chemical agents.
3 The research was conducted from 1942 but the results could not be published until after the war: see Zubrod, 'Historic milestones', p. 491. The various studies on mustard gas during World War I did not uncover its cytotoxic properties – Macgregor, 'The search for a chemical cure', p. 380. The major publications from American researchers on nitrogen mustards reporting on their wartime and post-war activities are: Goodman et al., 'Nitrogen mustard therapy'; Rhoads, 'Nitrogen mustards'; Karnofsky, 'The nitrogen mustards'; and Gilman and Philips, 'The biological actions'. For an account of the explosion in 1943 of 100 tons of mustard gas in the port of Bari and its impact on research into malignant growths see Rhoads, 'The sword', pp. 299–302 and Infield, *Disaster*.
4 James Patterson refers to the heightened interest in cancer chemotherapy as part of a broader fascination with 'chemical marvels' – see Patterson, *The Dread Disease*, pp. 195–196.
5 Quoted in Hess, *Can Bacteria*, p. 70.
6 See Helfand et al., 'Wartime industrial development' and Neushul, 'Science, government'. The wartime antecedents of cancer chemotherapy are often emphasized in general accounts of developments. See, for example, Zubrod et al., 'The chemotherapy program'.

7 For a review of screened agents until the late 1940s, see Dyer, *Index*.

8 Zubrod, 'Historic milestones', p. 492.

9 Waksman and Woodruff, 'Bacteriostatic and bactericidal substance'. Neither penicillin nor sulphanilamide showed cancer chemotherapeutic activity – see Lewis, 'The failure of purified penicillin' and Lewis, 'Inertness of sulfanilamide'.

10 In the case of nitrogen mustard therapy, the experimental research was reported in one journal and the clinical work in another, in the same year: see respectively Gilman and Philips, 'The biological actions' and Goodman et al., 'Nitrogen mustard therapy'.

11 At the end of their report of the clinical results on nitrogen mustard, Goodman and Gilman wrote: 'Chemicals discovered to be therapeutically active in neoplastic disease deserve close study by clinicians, experimental pathologists, enzymologists and others interested in cancer and in cellular biology.' Goodman et al., 'Nitrogen mustard therapy', p. 132.

12 For a short biography of Murphy see Little, 'James Bumgardner Murphy'. For an excellent discussion of Murphy's work on lymphocytes and their role in immune reactions – and much more besides – see Löwy, 'Biomedical research'.

13 Murphy, 'An analysis', p. 111.

14 Corner, *A History*, p. 271. Other information about Rhoads can be found in Patterson, *The Dread Disease* and Hess, *Can Bacteria*.

15 Corner, *A History*, p. 477.

16 See Zubrod, 'Historic milestones', p. 491 and Rusch, 'The beginnings of cancer research'.

17 Zubrod, 'Historic milestones', p. 491.

18 Rhoads, 'Nitrogen mustards'.

19 Rhoads, 'The sword', p. 308.

20 Bud, 'Strategy in American cancer research'.

21 Bud, 'Strategy in American cancer research', p. 433. For industrial laboratory research and organization see: Dennis, 'Accounting for research'; Smith, 'The scientific'; and Hounshell, 'Interpreting the history of industrial research'. On the Sloan foundation and its other interests, see Kevles, 'Foundations'.

22 Bud, 'Strategy in American cancer research', p. 433.

23 Rhoads, 'Rational', p. 77.

24 Stock, 'Aspects of approaches', p. 659.

25 Zubrod et al., 'The chemotherapy program', p. 351 and Stock et al., 'Sarcoma 180 screening', p. 193.

26 See an example of the list of suppliers in Stock et al., 'Sarcoma 180 screening', pp. 195–202 and Stock et al., 'Sarcoma 180 inhibition', pp. 182–187.

27 See the discussion on these elements of American industrial capitalism in Chandler, *Scale and Scope*, pp. 90–193.

28 Shear, 'Some aspects', p. 240.

29 Zubrod et al., 'The chemotherapy program', p. 350.

30 Shear, 'Some aspects', p. 238. See also Bud, 'Strategy in American cancer research', pp. 445–446.

31 Zubrod et al., 'The chemotherapy program', p. 350.

32 Shear, 'Role', p. 570.

33 Shear, 'Role', p. 571 and Rous, 'Concerning', p. 335. Rous was firm on what should be done to raise the interest in cancer chemotherapy: 'attempts to find ways to cure cancer', he wrote, 'are generally shunned (save by quacks),

and this will continue to be the case until the public decides to subsidize such efforts broadly, rewarding for acumen and enterprise as such until they bring success' – p. 335. The *Annual Report of the Chemotherapy Section, NCI, 1947–8* (in National Library of Medicine, Murray Shear Papers, Box 16) reads: 'Contrary to all *a priori* objections raised by the timid to this line of investigation (chemotherapy), gratifying findings were made.' An article on Shear in the *Saturday Evening Post*, 31 December 1959 (in NCI Archives, AR-2541) remarked that he was told, when entering the field of cancer research, that he would not find a chemical to hit a tumour because 'cancer is blood of our blood, bone of our bone, and flesh of our flesh.'

34 Steiner, 'Emphasis', p. 1213. For a recent assessment of the direction of cancer research since 1945 see Proctor, *Cancer Wars* and Gaudillière, 'Essay'.

35 This aspect of the history of cancer chemotherapy has been very well covered in the literature. See Patterson, *The Dread Disease*, pp. 114–200; Strickland, *Politics*; and Rettig, *Cancer Crusade*, pp. 1–41. For the early years of the American Cancer Society, see Triolo and Shimkin, 'The American Cancer Society'. For a more critical analysis, see Moss, *The Cancer Industry*, pp. 399–406.

36 Patterson, *The Dread Disease*, pp. 171–172; Endicott and Allen, 'The growth of medical research', p. 341; Deignan and Miller, 'The support of research', pp. 330–332 and Baker, 'Cancer research', p. 652.

37 Evelyn Fox Keller argues that physics contributed to the success of molecular biology by giving it 'social authority and social authorization'. See Keller, 'Physics', p. 390.

38 See Bechtel, 'Integrating sciences'; Bechtel, 'Deciding on the data'; Rasmussen, 'Facts'; and Rasmussen, 'Mitochondrial structure'.

39 Spencer, 'The meaning, p. 1362.

40 See Erwin, 'The militarization'. Erwin sees the National Cancer Act of 1971 as the starting position for what she calls medical militarization. This may be somewhat too simplistic and requires further research. Metaphors in cancer is a huge subject but one that has only received some scholarly attention. Military metaphors have certainly prevailed since World War II. Words such as 'weapons', 'task force', 'enemy', 'the front' and many more are used commonly in the medical and popular press. On military metaphors in biomedicine, see: Montgomery, 'Codes'; Ross, 'The militarization'; and Erwin, 'Militarization'. The classic study of metaphors in cancer as a disease is Sontag, *Illness*, but see also Stacey, *Teratologies*, especially Chapter 2. On metaphors in biology, see Maasen, 'Who is afraid?'. On metaphors in general, see Lackoff and Johnson, *Metaphors* and Leary, 'Naming and knowing'.

41 Spencer, 'The meaning', p. 1363.

42 Spencer, 'The meaning', p. 1363.

43 See Bechtel, 'Integrating sciences' for a similar argument concerning cell biology.

44 Karnofsky, 'The bases', p. 260.

45 Karnofsky, 'The bases', p. 268.

46 Karnofsky and Burchenal, 'Present status', p. 778.

47 Burk, 'Foreword'.

48 Endicott, 'The chemotherapy program', p. 275.

49 Rettig, 'Cancer crusade', pp. 56–59. See also Löwy, 'Nothing more', pp. 212–219. As it turned out, the NCI's chemotherapy programme's greatest success came in the treatment of acute lymphoblastic leukaemia in children in the

period after 1962. The chemotherapeutic success in this area rested on previous work done in the NCI's endocrinology department on the use of methotrexate, a folic acid antagonist, in the treatment of choriocarcinoma, a rare cancer affecting the cells that secrete gonadotrophin, a sex hormone. See Löwy, 'Nothing more', pp. 216–217.

50 Zubrod, 'Origins and development', p. 11.
51 Zubrod, 'Origins and development', p. 11 and Zubrod et al., 'The chemotherapy program', p. 354.
52 Zubrod et al., 'The chemotherapy program', p. 373; McCracken, 'Introduction', p. 974.
53 Schepartz, 'History of the National Cancer Institute', p. 975.
54 Coghill, 'Preclinical program', p. 40.
55 Zubrod et al., 'The chemotherapy program', pp. 363–364. On the problem of supplying genetically defined mice see Gaudillière and Löwy, 'Disciplining cancer' and Rader, 'Making mice'.
56 This is a point made and elaborated upon in Löwy, 'Nothing more', pp. 215–221.
57 Goldin et al., 'Historical development', p. 171.
58 Wood, 'Selection of agents', p. 15. The total amount of funds increased as follows: 1955 $8.4 million; 1960 $31.7 million; 1965 $103 million; and 1975 $270 million. Throughout this whole period, therapy and tumour development applications accounted for about two-thirds of monies granted: diagnosis and epidemiology together rarely over five per cent – see Baker, 'Cancer research', p. 653. We are using the term 'bandwagon' in a similar way to which it is used in Fujimura, 'The molecular biological bandwagon'.
59 DeVita et al., 'The drug development and clinical trials programs', p. 206. The success of synthetic compounds as chemotherapeutic agents underpinned the general belief in the value of these compounds and the research and practice culture that produced them in the chemical and pharmaceutical industry. For a discussion of the rise and success of synthetic compounds as pharmaceuticals, see: Liebenau, 'Industrial'; Liebenau, 'Paul Ehrlich'; Lesch, 'Chemistry and biomedicine'; Goodman and Walsh, 'Little and big heuristics'; Walsh, 'Demand'; Goodman, 'The pharmaceutical industry'; and Swann, 'The biomedical industries'. For a discussion of pharmaceuticals as the embodiment of cultural practices, see Goodman, 'Can it ever be pure science?'
60 Zubrod et al., 'The chemotherapy program', p. 373.
61 NCI, AR-6304-002480, 'NCI Report on CCNSC', 17 April 1963, p. 3.
62 There is no general consensus as to the definition of this metabolic process. The one given here is taken from Demain, 'Microbial secondary metabolism', p. 21.
63 Demain, 'Functions of secondary metabolites' and Waterman, 'Roles for secondary metabolites'.
64 See Bentley, 'Secondary metabolites', p. 199; Vining, 'Roles of secondary metabolites'; Williams et al., 'Why are secondary metabolites biosynthesized?' and Jacobson, 'Plants, insects, and man'.
65 Bentley, 'Secondary metabolites', p. 198.
66 Bentley, 'Secondary metabolites'; Balandrin et al., 'Natural plant chemicals'.
67 See, for example, Plotkin and Famolare, *Sustainable Harvest* and Schultes and Raffauf, *The Healing Forest*.

68 Willaman and Schubert, 'Alkaloid hunting', p. 141. Very little seems to have changed over the subsequent decades. A recent estimate is that only five to fifteen per cent of the approximately 250,000 species of higher plants have been systematically investigated for biological activity – see Balandrin, Kinghorn and Farnsworth, 'Plant-derived natural products', p. 8.

69 For the sake of consistency we have used the following technical words in the text in the following senses: CYTOTOXICITY – Toxicity to tumour cells in culture – *in vitro*: ANTITUMOUR – Activity in experimental systems – *in vivo*: ANTICANCER – Activity in human clinical trials. See Suffness and Douros, 'Current status', p. 4.

70 NCI, AR-6402-004322, 'Curriculum vitae: Jonathan L. Hartwell', February 1964.

71 NCI, AR-6402-004322, 'Curriculum vitae: Jonathan L. Hartwell', February 1964.

72 Löwy, 'Innovation and legitimation', pp. 338–339.

73 Löwy, 'Innovation and legitimation', p. 341.

74 Löwy, 'Innovation and legitimation', p. 341. Coley's toxin has been the subject of substantial controversy as an anti-cancer treatment. For recent assessments see Hess, *Can Bacteria*, pp. 10–19 and Moss, *Cancer Industry*, pp. 119–129.

75 Dyer, *Index* and Goodman, 'Plants, cells and bodies'.

76 The following section is based on Goodman, 'Plants, cells and bodies'.

77 Pettit, 'The scientific contributions', p. 360.

78 Pettit, 'The scientific contributions', p. 359.

79 See, for example, Culp, Magid and Kaplan, 'Podophyllin treatment'.

80 Pettit, 'The scientific contributions', pp. 359–360.

81 Kelly and Hartwell, 'The biological effects', pp. 973–977.

82 Pettit, 'The scientific contributions', pp. 359–360.

83 Kelly and Hartwell, 'The biological effects', pp. 967–969.

84 Some of these letters can be found in PER1. The American public's interest in the chemotherapy of cancer was partly driven by the substantial funds that the NCI was placing in this research area and partly by the outspoken, influential and well-connected scientists who brought it to their attention – see Patterson, *The Dread Disease*, p. 196.

85 For a description of his sources and methodology, see Hartwell, 'Plants', pp. 379–385.

86 The articles were published in the journal *Lloydia* in volumes 30–34. They were collected and republished in a single volume – Hartwell, *Plants*.

87 In the introduction to his first article dealing with the folk knowledge of cancer treatments, Hartwell states that 'the possibility arose that these records might be useful in providing leads for the laboratory investigation of other plants and the development of useful drugs in the therapy of human cancer' – Hartwell, 'Plants', p. 379. There were other researchers, notably Richard Schultes, pressing for a closer appreciation of the ethnobotanical record in the search for medicinal plants: see, for example, Schultes, 'Tapping our heritage' and 'The role of the ethnobotanist'.

88 Belkin and Fitzgerald, 'Cathartics'; Belkin, Fitzgerald and Felix, 'Diuretics'; and Belkin and Fitzgerald, 'Pesticides'.

89 Fitzgerald, Belkin, Felix and Carroll, 'Conifers'.

90 Fitzgerald, Hartwell and Leiter, 'Distribution of tumor-damaging lignans',

91 Hartwell to Schubert, 10 December 1953 and Schubert to Hartwell, 9 May 1957, both in PER1.

92 Jones to Hartwell, 16 November 1959, PER1.

93 A short history of the plant introduction programme of the USDA is given in Klose, *America's Crop Heritage*. See also Hodge and Erlanson, 'Plant introduction' and Pauly, 'The beauty and menace'.

94 Hodge and Erlanson, 'Plant introduction', p. 194 and Correll et al., 'The search'. Cortisone was the new wonder drug of the period. Its dramatic effects on patients suffering with rheumatoid arthritis were first made public in 1949. Originally isolated from the adrenal cortex, by the early 1950s it was being made by synthesizing bile acids of cattle but in scarce amounts. Thanks to the work of Russell Marker, who had been working in this area since the late 1930s, it was known that some plants contained steroids called sapogenins, and that these could be used as a starting material for synthesizing cortisone. For cortisone, its history and politics, see: Marks, 'Cortisone'; Cantor, 'Cortisone and the politics of drama' and 'Cortisone and the politics of empire'. See also Lehmann, Bolivar and Quintero, 'Russell E Marker'.

95 See Wall et al., 'Steroidal sapogenins'.

96 Interview with Wall, 15 September 1997. In published accounts of this episode, the number of extracts is put at 600. See Ross, 'Recent advances', p. 374 and Pettit, 'The scientific contributions', p. 361. Both accounts incorrectly refer to the Eastern Utilization Research and Development branch of the USDA as being responsible for the plant collection. It was, in fact, the Plant Introduction Section that did the collection.

97 Hartwell to Jones, 26 October 1959, PER1.

98 Ross, 'Recent advances', p. 374.

99 Pettit, 'The scientific contributions', p. 361 and interview with Pettit, 22 October 1997.

100 Sessoms, 'Review', p. 27.

101 Jones and Schubert to Erlanson, 30 June 1959, PER2.

102 Hartwell to Jones, 24 March 1960, PER1.

103 Hartwell to Jones, 24 March 1960, PER1.

104 Jones to Erlanson, 30 March 1960, PER2.

105 Jones to Erlanson, 30 March 1960, PER2.

106 There are various accounts of these programmes. See, for example: Wolff and Jones, 'Cooperative new crops'; Jones and Wolff, 'The search'; Barclay, Gentry and Jones, 'The search'; and Princen, 'New oilseed crops'.

107 Perdue, e-mail, 5 June 1999.

108 Hartwell to Shaw, 25 April 1960, PER2

109 Brander (Operations Officer, CCNSC, NCI) to Spencer (Acting Administrator, Agricultural Research Service, USDA), 21 June 1960, PER2.

110 Fitzgerald to Leiter, 28 July 1969, PER2.

111 Zubrod et al., 'The chemotherapy program', pp. 361, 366–367. 'Progress report on national programme of research in cancer chemotherapy', 10 March 1958, AR-2546, NCI.

112 The Texas group published the results of its work variously in *Texas Reports on Biology and Medicine* between 1952 and 1962, the senior authors being Alfred Taylor and George McKenna. For Compositae, see Pettit, 'The scientific contributions', p. 361. See also Farnsworth et al., 'Biological and phytochemical evaluation'.

113 Noble, Beer and Cutts, 'Role of chance', p. 882 and Johnson et al.,

'Experimental basis', p. 830. The error in referring to the plant as *Vinca rosea* was pointed out in Farnsworth, 'The pharmacognosy of the periwinkles'. It is called the Madagascar periwinkle because it likely originated there but by the time of this work it was growing throughout the world; in Europe and the United States it was an ornamental plant.

114 Noble, 'The discovery of the vinca alkaloids', p. 1345.
115 Noble, Beer and Cutts, 'Role of chance', p. 883 and Noble, 'The discovery of the vinca alkaloids', pp. 1345–1346.
116 Noble, Beer and Cutts, 'Role of chance'.
117 Johnson, Wright and Svoboda, 'Experimental basis', p. 830 and Neuss et al., 'The vinca alkaloids', p. 135.
118 Neuss, Gorman and Johnson, 'Natural products', pp. 644–649 and Svoboda, 'Alkaloids of vinca rosea'.
119 Neuss et al., 'The vinca alkaloids', p. 172. A recent review of vinca alkaloids can be found in Neuss and Neuss, 'Therapeutic use'.
120 For an excellent overview of drug development and regulation before and after 1962, see Lasagna, 'Congress'.
121 Driscoll, 'The preclinical new drug research program', p. 75. For a review of the clinical progress of vinblastine and vincristine to the mid-1970s, see Carter and Livingston, 'Plant products'.
122 DeVita et al., 'The drug development and clinical trials programs', p. 206.
123 See, for example, Tyler, 'Medicinal plant research', p. 98; Schepartz, 'History of the National Cancer Institute', p. 976; and Noble, 'The discovery of the vinca alkaloids', p. 1349. In an interview, Schepartz reiterated that the discovery of the vinca alkaloids was important but not the only reason in getting the plant programme going – interview with Schepartz, 14 March 1995.
124 Noble, Beer and Cutts, 'Role of chance', p. 882.
125 Hyland to Hartwell, 2 July 1959, PER2.
126 Hyland to Hartwell, 2 July 1959, PER2.
127 Arthur S. Barclay's curriculum vitae, GCB1. See also A.S. Barclay, special assignments, 1960–1976, SPJ3 and 'USDA explorers to 1985', SPJ3.
128 The botanists were Richard Spjut, Peter Ensor, Sandra Saufferer and Gudrun Christenson – see Perdue and Christenson, 'Plant exploration', pp. 70–78.
129 Perdue and Hartwell, 'The search for plant sources', pp. 36–37. According to Perdue, Hartwell wanted the USDA botanists to make a special effort to collect plants recorded in the literature on folk medicine, but Perdue argued that they would be collected, in any case, in a broad sweep.
130 For arguments in favour of selective screening, see Willaman and Schubert, 'Alkaloid hunting' and Raffauf, 'Plants' and 'Mass screening'.
131 Perdue and Hartwell, 'The search for plant sources', p. 37. In the negotiations leading to the 1960 agreement to go ahead with the cooperative programme, Hartwell informally mentioned this time span to Jones – see, Jones to Erlanson, 30 March 1960, PER2. In later years, some critics of the chemotherapy screening programme in general referred to the effort as 'nothing-is-too-stupid-to test' – quoted in Patterson, *The Dread Disease*, p. 197.
132 Perdue, Abbott and Hartwell, 'Screening plants', p. 1.
133 This was called the FOSI (Families of Special Interest) programme – see Suffness and Douros, 'Drugs of plant origin', p. 78.

134 Suffness and Douros, 'Drugs of plant origin', p. 78 and Spjut, letter, 20 March 1997. One of the payoffs of the programme was the identification of the plant *Maytenus buchananii* as a superior source for the compound maytansine.

135 See Barclay and Perdue, 'Distribution of anti-cancer activity' and Spjut and Perdue, 'Plant folklore'. Support for Perdue and Hartwell's philosophy came in Spjut, 'Limitations of a random screen', p. 280 and Suffness and Douros, 'Drugs of plant origin', p. 79.

136 Perdue, 'Program guide', SPJ3.

137 A description of how plants were procured can be found in Perdue, 'Procurement'. This article and others on the mechanics of plant exploration – see for example, Creech, 'Tactics of exploration' and Perdue and Christenson, 'Plant exploration' – do not convey the actual practices, difficulties as well as achievements. Much of the history of plant exploration has been romanticized. For an example of this in the field of medical botany, see Kreig, *Green Medicine*.

138 A crude plant extract is the soluble residue removed from a solid mixture of ground plant material by means of a solvent.

139 Statz and Coon, 'Preparation of plant extracts', Suffness and Douros, 'Drugs of plant origin', pp. 82–83.

140 The protocols for test screening were published on several occasions, in 1959, 1962 and 1972. These protocols provide a thorough review of the testing procedures and choice of test system. For the 1972 edition, see Geran et al., 'Protocols for screening'. A short synopsis of the screening system can be found in Abbott, 'Bioassay'.

141 Abbott, 'Bioassay', p. 1007. For the history of the development of the screening methodology during the 1950s, leading up to the protocol of 1959, see Zubrod et al., 'The chemotherapy program', pp. 362–365.

142 The following is taken from: Abbott, 'Bioassay'; Hartwell, 'Types of anti-cancer agents'; and Suffness and Douros, 'Drugs of plant origin', p. 84.

143 Abbott, 'Bioassay', p. 1009; Geran et al., 'Protocols for screening', p. 1; and Perdue and Hartwell, 'The search for plant sources', pp. 41–43. See also Venditti and Abbott, 'Studies on oncolytic agents' and Goldin, Carter and Mantel, 'Evaluation of antineoplastic activity', pp. 13–14. The KB cell culture was derived from the biopsy of a nasopharynx carcinoma from a 54-year-old man in 1954 – Eagle, 'Propagation'.

144 Fractionation uses the different physical properties of substances to separate them from a mixture.

145 Perdue and Hartwell, 'The search for plant sources', p. 44.

146 Wall, it will be recalled, was the head of the plant steroid section of the Eastern Regional Research Laboratory of the USDA in Philadelphia, engaged in the cortisone programme. This was terminated in 1959. Wall recounts that he became extremely curious to discover the compound in the leaves of *Camptotheca acuminata*, that had shown antitumour activity in 1959. He could not work on this problem at the USDA but was encouraged to do this at the Research Triangle Institute. See interview with Wall, 15 September 1997, Wall and Wani, 'Camptothecin', p. 2 and Larrabee, *Many missions*, pp. 43–48.

147 Schepartz, 'History of the National Cancer Institute', p. 977. A description of fractionation and isolation as done in one of the contract laboratories can be found in Wall, Wani and Taylor, 'Isolation and chemical characterization'.

148 Between 1965 and 1972, the CCNSC, together with the Intramural Laboratory of Chemical Pharmacology and the Medicine Branch, formed the National Chemotherapy Program of the NCI.

149 In 1972, the CCNSC's work was subsumed within the newly created Division of Cancer Treatment, as part of the reorganization of the NCI following the passage of the National Cancer Act of 1971. The Division of Cancer Treatment, one of four divisions of the NCI, became responsible for co-ordinating cancer research within the NCI. The Developmental Therapeutics Program, one of its major subdivisions, administered the search for new anti-cancer agents, and one of its sections/branches, the Natural Products Branch, arranged for acquiring plant and animal products.

150 Palmieri to Finney, 30 March 1978, SPJ3.

151 Schepartz to Paul G. Rogers (House of Representatives, US Congress), 10 May 1978, NCI Archives, D-7805-2896. Rogers, a Democrat from Florida, played a crucial role in the story of the National Cancer Act of 1971. On this, see Rettig, *Cancer Crusade*.

152 Perdue, 'Proposal for procurement', PER6. In order to make this argument, Perdue had to eliminate conifers and other plant families from the screening data. Conifers were unusually active against KB. In the early 1970s, these and plants from other families were collected not at random as had been the practice in the past. Once they were excluded from the analysis, the data showed an unmistakable fall in the number of KB actives from a high point around 1964 – see Perdue, 'KB cell culture'.

153 Perdue to Wood, 7 January 1974, Perdue to Suffness, 18 November 1976, PER5. There was another problem with KB which went unnoticed. Reports of cross-contamination of cell cultures, including KB, had been growing in number since the late 1960s. One of the first to raise the alarm was Stanley Gartler – see Gartler, 'Apparent HeLa cell contamination'. An article in *Science* published in 1981 presented evidence gathered since the 1960s that the KB cell culture had been contaminated with HeLa cells – see Nelson-Rees, Daniels and Flandermeyer, 'Cross-contamination'.

154 It is important to understand that screening was big business. In this period, screening and the industry of producing laboratory animals were inseparable. In the 1970s, the great leap forward was the development of the nude mouse giving rise to the ability to transplant human tumours into laboratory mice. For an excellent discussion of the role of the laboratory mouse in constructing research practices in the NCI see Löwy and Gaudillière, 'Disciplining cancer'. For a good review of *in vitro* screening, see Hakala and Rustum, 'The potential value'. Debates concerning screening systems were certainly polarized during the 1970s. See Weisenthal, '*In vitro* assays'.

155 Perdue to Wood, 7 January 1974, Perdue to Suffness, 18 November 1976, PER5. In 1982, Perdue published an analysis of screening with KB cell culture. In it he remarked that, 'KB activity of crude products would have led to the discovery of . . . the antitumour agents now under development toward or in clinical evaluation'. Had KB alone been used, then the large resources devoted to the *in vivo* screens could have been diverted to procurement, extraction and more KB screening – see Perdue, 'KB cell culture', p. 425.

156 According to the General Accounting Office, the cost of a P388 screen was $80.28 while that of KB was $19.40. P388 results took thirty days while KB

results were available in one or two days. The difference in the amount of test material each screen consumed was also highly significant: P388 used one to two grams while KB used five to ten milligrams – from Comptroller General of the United States to the Chairman, Subcommittee on Health and Scientific Research, United States Senate, 28 February 1980, p. 8, in NCI Archives, LT-8004-000501.

157 Comptroller General of the United States to the Chairman, Subcommittee on Health and Scientific Research, United States Senate, 28 February 1980, pp. 7–9, in NCI Archives, LT-8004-000501.

158 See Cragg, Newman and Weiss, 'Coral reefs', p. 159 and Grindey, 'Current status'. On the basis of evidence of the bias and high costs of P388, the Board of Scientific Counselors of the Division of Cancer Treatment gave approval, on 29 October 1979, to develop new *in vitro* screens. In 1985 the NCI reorganized its screening methodology so that it now consisted solely of *in vitro* human cancer cell lines. See Boyd, 'Status of implementation'. Boyd's discussion points clearly to the bias to select lymphoma/leukaemia active agents inherent in P388.

159 'We have had several discussions with senior USDA officials during the past several months, in the course of which we informed the USDA that the agreement would have to be terminated unless the problems . . . were remedied. The USDA agreed that the action was necessary and proposed to change the Principal Investigator (Robert E. Perdue, Jr), a decision with which we concurred.' Schepartz (Deputy Director, Division of Cancer Treatment, NCI) to Paul Rogers (House of Representatives, US Congress), 10 May 1978, NCI Archives, D-7805-2896.

160 Hanson to Moseman, 18 April 1978, SPJ3.

161 Duke to Economic Botany Laboratory Staff, 31 December 1979, SPJ3.

162 Saul Schepartz, the Deputy Director of the Division of Cancer Treatment, when asked to explain the decision to cut the programme answered by saying that 'more pure materials are provided to us through literature surveillance and contacts with independent academic and industrial investigators in this country and abroad than we have been able to obtain through our contract-supported projects.' Schepartz, open letter, 1981/1982, in NCI Archives, DC-8206-005799.

163 Fong to colleagues, 10 October 1981, PER2.

164 Fong to colleagues, 10 October 1981, PER2.

165 Varro Tyler, quoting remarks made by Monroe Wall and Norman Farnsworth, suggested that the programme failed because of the lack of effective co-operation of researchers in a variety of fields – chemistry, botany, biology and medicine. A close look at the programme for most of its history shows this view to be exaggerated, at best. See Tyler, 'Plant drugs', p. 280.

166 Suffness and Douros, 'Current status', p. 1.

167 In many reviews, the figure of 35,000 is reported as being the number of species. This is wrong. Gordon Cragg, e-mail, 25 March 1998, puts the figure at between 10,000 and 13,000 species.

168 Farnsworth and Soejarto, 'Potential consequence', p. 185.

169 Suffness and Douros, 'Current status', p. 1

170 Douros and Suffness, 'The National Cancer Institute's', pp. 38–39 and Cragg et al., 'Role of plants'. Camptothecin, the active compound of *Camptotheca acuminata* (active in the first batch of plants from the cortisone

programme), advanced to clinical trials in the 1970s but was dropped because of toxicity – semi-synthetic derivatives are clinically active and, one of them, topotecan is now approved and available. Etoposide and teniposide, semi-synthetic derivatives of podophyllotoxin (Hartwell's discovery), are also in regular clinical use. So are the vinca alkaloids. These examples of plant-derived anti-cancer drugs did not strictly result from the NCI-USDA programme. There is little doubt, however, that *Camptotheca acuminata* would have been picked up in the course of the programme as samples of the bush were growing in a USDA station in California.

171 Cragg et al., 'Role of plants', p. 85.
172 The progress of the plant programme can be reconstructed through the following: Hartwell and Abbott, 'Antineoplastic principles'; Hartwell, 'Types of anti-cancer agents'; and Douros and Suffness, 'The National Cancer Institute's'. The 16th Annual Meeting of the Society for Economic Botany focused on the plant programme and its achievements. The papers were published in a special issue of *Cancer Chemotherapy Reports*, vol. 60, no. 8, August 1976.

Part II

Practices

2

Act I: 1962–1975

The Pacific yew, *Taxus brevifolia*, is a very slow-growing conifer found principally in the understory of old-growth forests in the Pacific Northwest, from northern California to Alaska. In 1962, as part of their sweep through California, Oregon and Washington, collecting plant material at random for the NCI–USDA interagency plant screening programme, a USDA botanist, together with three graduate student helpers, sampled parts of *Taxus brevifolia*. They bagged, tagged and shipped the collection back to the East Coast for further analysis. Four years later, chemists at the Research Triangle Institute in North Carolina isolated a cytotoxic compound from the bark. The following year, 1967, they named the compound taxol. It had antitumour activity against L1210.

This chapter follows *Taxus brevifolia*, taxol and those responsible for writing their stories from 1962 until 1975. Over this period, *Taxus brevifolia* was made to reveal its molecular secret to the cancer research community and taxol was shown to be a promising agent. Science was doing its work. But there was more to it than that. Both small and large decisions were being made by key individuals at key points that tempered the science with unpredictability, gave it political substance and closed certain paths of development while opening others. Tensions pervaded the networks of researchers, government officials, and bark collectors into which the molecule, the tree, the forest and the laboratory were sucked. Collective memories of suggestions, claims and knowledges were eroded and forgotten as those tensions led to changes in personnel, organizations and programmes.

Monroe Wall headed the fractionation and isolation laboratory at Research Triangle Institute in North Carolina. He, it will be recalled, had been contracted by the NCI as a fractionator in 1960 after a long spell of employment with the USDA, working for nine years on the cortisone programme as head of the chemistry section. Wall recounts that he left the USDA because he wanted to work on *Camptotheca acu-minata*, which, as we have seen, was one of the many plants collected and screened in the cortisone programme, and which showed pre-liminary activity against a number of tumour systems.[1]

In the first few years of the plant screening programme, Wall, in common with the other two fractionators, routinely received plant material as they were collected. As the scale of operations increased, however, Hartwell changed the routine. He diverted all the plant col-lections to the Wisconsin Alumni Research Foundation (WARF) where a crude extract was prepared and screened. If the crude extract was found to be active in the KB *in vitro* screen then further extracts were prepared from the same plant extract and subjected to further *in vivo* tests.[2] Plants passing these tests were referred to as confirmed actives. In April 1964, Hartwell notified the chemists that from this date forward, they were to be assigned only confirmed actives from the WARF output.

Confirmed activity would, according to the system in operation, automatically result in action to re-collect the plant; that is, a USDA botanist would attempt to duplicate the original collection, by returning to the original site of collection at the same time of the year and col-lecting as much material as possible.[3] Hartwell informed Perdue that, because of the change in the role of WARF, all re-collections as of April 1964 would go directly to the chemists.

Arthur Barclay joined the New Crops Research Branch of the Agri-cultural Research Service of the USDA as a botanist at the age of twenty-seven, armed with a PhD from Harvard University. He was introduced to the practices of the Branch by Howard Scott Gentry who had arrived at the USDA in 1950 and, because of his knowledge of Mexican and south-western plants, especially the agave, was put straight on to the cortisone programme.[4]

Exploring for the NCI plant screening programme was, as we have seen, conducted alongside other USDA plant exploration programmes. Barclay's first assignment was in February 1960, in the company of Gentry, to collect samples of *Lesquerella*, a promising plant for oilseeds, in south-western United States. His first collection for the NCI had been done with Gentry in the Republic of South Africa while they were selecting plants, particularly of the family Compositae, for seed screening.[5] On returning to the United States early in 1961, Barclay continued to collect oilseeds for the seed screening programme and plants for the NCI plant screening programme, in both the south-east and the south-west of the country as well as in Mexico.

In the following year, 1962, Barclay travelled to the western United States, still collecting for both programmes. He began his searches in northern California on 19 June, eventually extending into Oregon and north-west Nevada. He travelled into Washington State around the middle of August and was in the Gifford Pinchot National Forest by 20 August. The following day Barclay, assisted by three students on a field trip, travelled to a spot in the forest, seven miles north of the small town of Packwood. At an elevation of 1,500 feet, the party found in dense forest a twenty-five-foot-high Pacific yew tree, *Taxus brevifolia*, designated as B-1645.[6] They made two collections: twigs, leaves and fruit, which they bagged as accession number PR-4959, and stembark, bagged as PR-4960.[7] This was almost the last of their collections before winter. The trip lasted just under four months. Barclay's herbarium labels for the trip show that he collected a variety of plants, mostly herbaceous and some shrubs and trees. No collections were particularly heavy, ranging around two pounds in weight. He probably collected samples from about 200 different plant species.

There seems to have been no particular reason why Barclay sampled *Taxus brevifolia*. Very little was known about the tree apart from some basic taxonomic information. It belonged to the genus Taxus, the yew, one of five genera of the family Taxaceae. The yew is native to the Americas, Europe and Asia. In Europe the native variety is *Taxus baccata*, in North America it is *Taxus canadensis* (Canadian yew), *Taxus floridana* (Florida yew), *Taxus globosa* (Mexican yew), and *Taxus brevifolia* (Pacific yew). The map in Figure 2.1 shows the distribution of the different yew species in North America. It was generally known that the tree was of medium height, the bark of a reddish to purple colour and very thin, with flat, slightly curved needles, no more than an inch long. It was an understory tree, living in the shade of the giant conifers, on the banks of streams, deep gorges and damp ravines. Though its range was large, it was not particularly frequent in any one place. Its wood, hard, heavy and slow to rot, found limited use.[8]

By the time of Barclay's collection, there were only two published articles in recent times on *Taxus brevifolia*. Neither gave any indication that the tree was interesting from the point of view of cancer. Indeed, one of them dismissed *Taxus brevifolia* as a likely candidate. The first corrected previous research that suggested *Taxus brevifolia* lacked alkaloids. Verro Tyler, then at the College of Pharmacy, University of Washington, reported that he had isolated an alkaloid from the needles and twigs of *Taxus brevifolia*, collected in the state of Washington.[9] Though it was only present in tiny amounts, Tyler was able to show that it was identical to an alkaloid present in all other species of the genus. This did not bear either way on *Taxus brevifolia* as a source of anti-cancer agents. But the second article focused on just this point and its conclusions were disheartening. Ironically, the research leading to this conclusion had been done in Jonathan Hartwell's laboratory.[10] As a

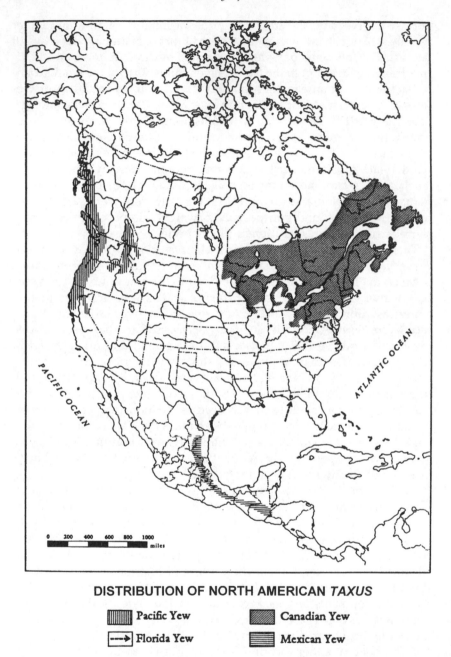

DISTRIBUTION OF NORTH AMERICAN *TAXUS*

Pacific Yew   Canadian Yew

Florida Yew   Mexican Yew

Figure 2.1 Distribution of North American *Taxus*. (Source: Hartzell, *The Yew Tree*, p. 59; reproduced by permission of Harold R. Hartzell, Jr.)

result of their successful work, which showed several species of juniper to be active against experimental tumours, Hartwell's group had decided to extend their search to other conifers. They examined a number of species of Taxaceae, including *Taxus brevifolia*. They injected an aqueous suspension of dried, powdered needles from the species into mice bearing Sarcoma 37. *Taxus brevifolia* needles, they concluded, had no activity whatsoever.[11]

Most scientific interest in the yew focused on *Taxus baccata*, the European yew.[12] The widespread mythological associations of the yew with death and the substantial number of stories and cases of yew poisoning undoubtedly contributed to this strong interest.[13] An alkaloid, named taxine, responsible for the tree's poisonous nature, was isolated in 1856.[14] Between then and the 1960s, countless other alkaloids were isolated from *Taxus baccata* and a number of other yew species by Basil Lythgoe, Koji Nakanishi and others.[15] In the eighty-plus articles on yew, indexed by *Chemical Abstracts* between 1947 and 1966, fewer than five dealt with *Taxus brevifolia*. *Taxus cuspidata*, the Japanese yew, and *Taxus media*, a cultivated variety, were much better served by the botanical and chemical literature.

The procedure for testing plant materials for activity was based on a system of contracting the stages of the process to specialist outfits.[16] Preparing the crude plant extract, the first step in the process, was contracted to WARF as of August 1961.[17] Both of Barclay's samples were sent to WARF for extraction.[18] Of the two samples of *Taxus* material, PR-4960, the stembark of the tree, was found to be cytotoxic as defined by its activity against KB on 22 May 1964.[19] The *in vivo* tests, carried out between April and November of the same year, were less revealing.[20] L1210 activity was present at one dose schedule but not at another; the Dunning leukaemia model and the P1798 lymphosarcoma system showed no antitumour activity.

Though the *in vivo* tests on L1210 that were done in April and May produced contradictory results, PR-4960 was retested against KB in June 1964 and, on 14 July, its activity was confirmed.[21] This evidence of reproducible activity justified further chemical analysis. As Perdue and Hartwell argued, the screening experiments were 'not designed to detect highly spectacular anti-cancer activity, but to detect activity of a lower order that [was] significant and reproducible.'[22] Certainly *Taxus brevifolia* conformed to these expectations, as far as cytotoxicity was concerned. In accordance with CCNSC protocol, the crude plant extract was designated as NSC670549. One week later, Hartwell told Perdue that he should take steps to re-collect large quantities of bark from the tree.[23]

Barclay was asked to return to the spot where he had originally collected PR-4960. On 8 September 1964, Barclay, together with

Juan Argüelles, who had been Gentry's assistant on Mexican trips, collected thirty pounds of stembark from *Taxus brevifolia*, recorded as accession number PR-8059 of NSC670549.[24] In accordance with the new rules concerning re-collections, the stembark went immediately to the Research Triangle Institute, in the safe-keeping of Monroe Wall and his colleagues. This was Barclay's last contact with *Taxus brevifolia*. He continued to collect plants for the cancer programme into the 1970s in the United States, Mexico and Colombia. The thirty pounds of bark left the forest unnoticed. For the time being, its future lay in the hands of chemists.

The absence of information on *Taxus brevifolia* was certainly not an obstacle, at this point at least. The objective, from the NCI's perspective, was to reveal the compound responsible for the activity of the crude plant extract. That it was *Taxus brevifolia*, a relatively unknown understory tree growing in the Pacific Northwest, was immaterial. Its identity was neither here nor there. On the instructions of Hartwell, Perdue assigned the re-collected sample, designated as PR-8059 to Wall's laboratory. At the same time, early in September 1964, Wall was also asked to fractionate and isolate six other confirmed actives.[25]

Wall's laboratory was mostly preoccupied with *Camptotheca acuminata* that had been confirmed active in 1962.[26] There was an urgency surrounding *Camptotheca acuminata* over the following year because of a lack of supplies of the plant material.[27] In addition, the laboratory appears to have been swamped with work, preparing extracts for a considerable number of samples.[28] The arrival of a bag-load of confirmed active plant material was, therefore, a mixed blessing. At a meeting of programme participants on 21 November 1963, convened at the CCNSC, Jonathan Hartwell emphasized that there was no shortage of confirmed actives in the programme. The head of the CCNSC, Joe Leiter, reminded the meeting, however, that enough time had elapsed in the programme for results to show. Current expenditure on the programme was running at $1,600,000 annually but no more expansion would occur, he warned, 'until something comes out the other end in the form of agents for clinical trial'.[29]

Chemists looked for good activity in the early stages of fractionation as it was known that activity rarely improved in the latter stages.[30] The fractionation process was guided by the compound's bioactivity with assays – *in vitro* against KB and *in vivo* against P1534 (a leukaemia system) and W256 (a carcinosarcoma system) – in order to determine which fractions contained the active agent. The assays were, however, not performed by the chemist but by NCI contract biological laboratories scattered throughout the country.[31] The results of *in vitro* assays were available within one or two days and those of *in vivo* assays in about one month. Active fractions were separated into even further fractions with more complex procedures and instruments until the process zeroed in on the compound or compounds in the plant source responsible for the activity. For a plant with one or two compounds of interest, a rule of thumb was the separation of the crude extract into about fifty fractions.[32]

Wall's laboratory began fractionating a crude extract prepared from PR-8509 late in 1964 or early 1965. By late December 1965, they reported that they were able to increase the potency of the crude extract 1000 times in the first chloroform fraction F021. In January of the following year, Wall informed Hartwell of the excellent results he had received from Hazleton Laboratories, one of the main biological screeners.[33] In a report dated 20 May 1966, Wall could not withhold his enthusiasm that they were on to something good. F021 was active in a number of *in vivo* systems, including P1534, the test system that had been used to detect the activity of the vinca alkaloid at Eli Lilly and Company. 'This is the broadest spectra of activity we have ever noted in our samples and the first time we have observed activity in P4 [P-1534]', he wrote.[34] Wall had already shared his enthusiasm with Hartwell in a communication in the previous month.[35] He also expressed confidence in using the KB *in vitro* screen as a predictor of activity. As he put it: 'we can conclude that activity "in vivo" is following activity in 9KB "in vitro" screens'.[36]

Notwithstanding the optimism, progress over the next few months was not as rapid or as easy as the laboratory would have liked. In particular, Wall and his co-workers encountered several setbacks using the bioassay system to guide the isolation. In their May 1966 report, Wall revealed that the process was more trial and error than textbook.[37] Trial and error took its toll on plant material. Wall had run out of material by December 1965.[38] Hartwell responded by passing the request on to Perdue: because of winter, the collection could not happen before March.[39] In May, he received a consignment of *Taxus brevifolia* plant material, consisting of 45 pounds of stembark, 135 pounds of twigs and leaves and 55 pounds of stemwood.[40] At the end of July 1966, Wall reconfirmed that the active fraction was in the stembark and that 'we are steadily closing in on the substance'.[41] But he also reported that, once again, he was running out of plant material: he told Hartwell he wanted Perdue to re-collect several hundred pounds of *Taxus brevifolia*. Hartwell responded by authorizing Perdue to make another, larger collection, scheduled for the following year, 1967.[42]

The year 1966 turned out to be good for the Research Triangle Institute. Wall and his co-workers were making good progress. In September, they managed to isolate from one of the fractions a crystalline substance that they designated K172 (in accordance with NCI nomenclature in which pure compounds were identified with a 'K' prefix).[43] The molecular formula of $C_{23}H_{26}O_7$ was tentatively proposed. Good news on the isolation but the chemists were uncovering an uncomfortable fact. They were consuming large amounts of plant material. Wall realized that the yield of K172 was very low, 'as bad or worse than camptothecin'. By March of 1967, Wall was again requesting more material. 'We need a lot more...if we are going to get enough product even for preliminary chemistry and the necessary preliminary antitumor studies to allow for a judgement of the utility of the substance.'[44] Wall continued to work on the isolation procedure and repeatedly isolated a substance identical to K172. The isolation work confirmed that the pure substance was present in only minute amounts. Twelve kilograms of dried bark produced 0.5 grams of the pure substance – a yield of 0.004 per cent.[45]

It was common practice for the laboratory to name the pure compound isolated from the plant material assigned to them: in June 1967, Wall decided on the name taxol.[46] In explaining why he chose the name, Wall recounts that, although he and his co-workers did not know its complete structure, they were certain the molecule contained hydroxyl groups that signified it was an alcohol.[47] As it was common to name a molecule after the genus of the plant in which it was found, the molecule became known as taxol – *tax*- for *Taxus* and -*ol* for alcohol.[48] 'It had a nice ring to it', remarks Wall.[49] Many years later, others would feel the same way.[50]

The road from receipt of the confirmed active re-collection to the isolation of the active substance was long. For *Taxus brevifolia* it was about two years. The main reason for the delay was a cumbersome bureaucratic machine that subcontracted biological laboratories across the country to perform the assays. Each fraction had to be screened before the fractionate could proceed. When all the paperwork was taken into account, chemists had to wait a month for *in vitro* results and up to three months for *in vivo* results.[51]

Wall and his co-worker Mansukh Wani made their work with *Taxus brevifolia* public at the annual meeting of the American Chemical Society in April 1967, although the main focus of their talk was *Camptotheca*. Little was said about the structure of taxol. Biological activity was the main issue but structural elucidation was the main problem. By September, they were already revising their thoughts about the molecular formula of taxol: they were now certain that it also contained nitrogen.[52] Wall and Wani spent the next few years, first, deciding on a molecular formula and, secondly, attempting to develop a structural formula – a structure for the molecule that fitted the number of atoms in the molecular formula but in addition described an arrangement of the atoms in space. One of the main methods for determining the structure of crystalline substances available at the time was X-ray crystallography, a specialist activity they could not do themselves. They enlisted the help of other researchers, including Andrew McPhail, a former colleague, to whom they sent taxol crystals for X-ray analysis at his laboratory at the University of Sussex in England.[53] At the end of January 1969, Wall disclosed all of the data he had on taxol to the NCI, including his procedure for extraction and isolation.[54] In return, the NCI officially adopted taxol as its molecule by assigning it the number NSC125973.[55] NSC670549, the crude extract of *Taxus brevifolia*, had now been supplanted and laid to rest.

By early 1970, Wall and Wani concluded that taxol had a molecular formula of $C_{47}H_{51}NO_{14}$. They proposed one of two structures for taxol, and in April, they informed Robert Engle, head of the Chemical and Drug Procurement Section of the CCNSC, that they had decided on one of these (see Figure 2.2).[56] The proposed skeleton for taxol was of a similar basic shape to that of several compounds obtained from various *Taxus* species. This was a feature noted a few years earlier by Basil Lythgoe and colleagues at the University of Leeds in England and named the 'taxane ring system'.[57] In May 1971, Wall and co-workers published the results of their work on taxol as a communication to the editor of the *Journal of the American Chemical Society*.[58] As the title of the article made clear, the chief importance of their work was that this molecule exhibited antileukaemic and antitumour activity. Many compounds were isolated by other researchers in England, Japan and the United States from other *Taxus* species – especially *Taxus baccata* – at the same time as Wall and Wani were working with *Taxus brevifolia*, but taxol was the only one to exhibit this unique biological activity.[59]

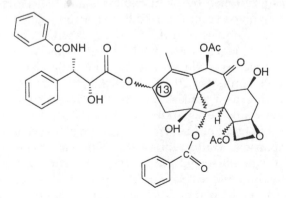

Figure 2.2 The structural formula of taxol.

In the manner of a relay race, *Taxus brevifolia* passed its bark to Arthur Barclay in 1962 who in turn passed it to Monroe Wall in 1964. With the 1971 publication of the structure of taxol, Monroe Wall passed the molecule to the NCI to be put through further analysis. The change in title to the object was signified by changes in names. B-1645, a USDA number designating Barclay's collection of *Taxus brevifolia*, a named species; PR-4959 and PR-4960, accession numbers to distinguish different samples from the same collection; B-670549, the CCNSC number designating the active sample of the collection; and finally, NSC125973, the NCI number for the molecule also known as taxol.

In most accounts of the discovery and development of taxol, *Taxus brevifolia* fades rapidly into the background as science is shown triumphantly to reveal the tree's innermost molecular secret.[60] In most accounts of the discovery and development of taxol, the voice of *Taxus brevifolia* is only heard in the late 1980s and early 1990s when, in the latter stages of taxol's progress towards clinical use, the tree found itself in the middle of several heated controversies. This narrative ploy results in a misunderstanding and foreshortening of that voice over time. It seeks to emphasize, in other words, the inevitable march of scientific knowledge, rather than its contingencies, focusing attention on the molecule and sidelining other actors, silencing their voices. By allowing *Taxus brevifolia* to take its rightful place as an actor in this drama, we can recover its voice and the contingent nature of taxol's development. *Taxus brevifolia* appeared as an actor in the historical performance of the drama of taxol the instant that Barclay and his helpers stripped a few pounds of bark from the tree in August 1962. Its voice continued to be heard, in the forest and in the laboratory, throughout the period.

Barclay's sampling of *Taxus brevifolia* parts, collected in 1962, was a botanical act as performed by plant explorers and collectors for centuries. The act involved several carefully rehearsed steps: identifying the species, taking samples of different parts, labelling, bagging and recording the collection. The 1964 re-collection was also a botanical act, a confirmation of the first collection. At that point, Barclay's work was done and he could continue with other tasks. *Taxus brevifolia* appeared in Wall's laboratory as a subject for isolation work, from which its constituent parts would be separated.

In March 1966 Robert Perdue arranged for a new collection of *Taxus brevifolia* in response to Wall's request for more plant material. As we have seen, Wall had exhausted the thirty-pound supply collected by Barclay. The amount requested was 375 pounds of *Taxus brevifolia* material. This was no longer an exercise in botany, but one of logistics. The amount of material was more than ten times the amount last collected. What did it mean to collect 375 pounds of this material from that tree? Would it be difficult? Who, other than a botanist, would be able to locate the tree/trees? Remember that hardly any detailed information existed on *Taxus brevifolia*. Perdue could have assigned one of his staff to do the new collection but, given the heavy workload that the programme was experiencing – several thousand plant samples were being collected annually – it made more sense to use botanists where they had a comparative advantage.[61] Barclay had made his two collections on public land, so Perdue turned for assistance to the Forest Service, who owned the land, and to the District Ranger, who was responsible for timber sales in that part of the forest where Barclay explored. The 1966 collection was the first of a series of collections in which the practice entailed a new dialogue with the forest.

The Forest Service and the Bureau of Land Management are the stewards of nationally owned forests in the United States. The two agencies belong to different branches of government: the Forest Service is part of the Department of Agriculture (USDA), and the Bureau of Land Management is part of the Department of the Interior. Of the two, the Forest Service is the larger and the more important. In 1891, Congress had legislated that the President could, by executive order, establish reserves of forests, retained permanently and protected as public property rather than being sold privately.[62] Thus was born the National Forest system. In 1905, Gifford Pinchot was appointed the first Chief Forester of the Forest Service, the custodian of the national forest system. The first national forests were carved out of federal lands in the west. By 1907, 150 million acres of land had been designated national forests in the west.

Until World War II, the Forest Service provided a custodial role, protecting the natural resources entrusted to them. Though some timber was harvested from this land, the amount was small. Most commercial forest was held then (as now) in private hands. Federal timber sales were generally opposed by the timber industry on the grounds that it would flood the market and depress prices. All of this changed abruptly with the coming of the war and the post-war economic boom. Instead of the possibility of glutted markets, the reverse was possible, a timber famine. Timber interests looked to the federal government to help, by opening its vast timber reserves to the industry. And so it did. Timber sales in the whole national forest service surged ahead at unprecedented rates. Between 1945 and 1965, for example, the sale of timber from Forest Service lands on the westside of Oregon and Washington alone shot up from 900 million board feet to just under 5 billion board feet – a board foot is a unit of wood a foot square and an inch thick.[63]

Large timber companies were the main buyers of the National Forest trees. In accordance with the contemporary practices of the timber companies and associated with the increase in the demand for its trees, the Forest Service began to embrace the idea of even-age management.[64] This entailed a view of the forest as an industrial resource in which the forest area would be organized in units of uniform age. To achieve uniformity, the forest needed to be cleared of existing stands of trees of varying ages and replanted with desirable species. The industry's preferred cutting method to achieve the conditions for and the reproduction of even-age management was clear-cutting – a harvest in which the entire stand of trees is removed at one time. By the 1960s, more than half of the national forest harvests had been removed in this manner.[65] The proportion climbed over the following decades before reaching a peak of over seventy per cent in 1987.[66]

As privately owned forests had been subject to some form of even-age management practices since the turn of the twentieth century, by the time of World War II, variegated forests were only to be found on reserves held as public property, administered by the Forest Service and the Bureau of Land Management. These forests were complicated ecosystems – referred to as old-growth.[67] They contained many varieties and ages of trees; some, such as the Douglas fir, the Sitka pine and the western cedar of enormous commercial value, and others, of no known value. Dying trees, dead standing trees and decaying fallen trees were enveloped by the living biomass. Even-age forests, by contrast, contained only commercially valued tree species, neatly organized, their forest floors free from the messy organic debris of previous generations.

In a clear cut, the entire stand is removed and the commercial species are hauled away. The remaining jumble of trees, plants and whatever else, is typically burned in what are known as slash piles. As old-growths were clear-cut and the land replanted to make way for even-age industrial forests, the stock of many unwanted species was being depleted without being replaced. Neither the Forest Service nor the timber industry was concerned. One of the species unvalued and unwanted by the timber industry was *Taxus brevifolia*.

By contrast, and unknown to everyone associated with the forest, *Taxus brevifolia* was becoming a very valuable species as a result of the events inside Monroe Wall's laboratory. Wall's revelation that KB activity was concentrated in a chloroform fraction was turning the spotlight on the tree. By March 1966, an interesting juxtaposition had occurred. Perdue and Hartwell, responding to Wall, listed *Taxus brevifolia* as a high priority species; in the forest, it was nothing more than trash.[68]

To get Wall's plant material, Perdue turned back to the Gifford Pinchot National Forest, to where Barclay had first made his collections.

The forest was organized into and administered by eight ranger stations. On 15 March, Perdue was on the phone to Richard Chase, in charge of the Packwood Ranger Station in the Gifford Pinchot National Forest.[69] Perdue requested 100 pounds of bark, 200 pounds of twigs and leaves and 75 pounds of wood, all fresh weight. Who should collect the material would be left to Chase, but Perdue suggested a summer employee, someone who was now unemployed. As to money, Perdue suggested fifty cents per pound fresh weight or one dollar per pound dry weight. Secrecy about the purpose of the collection needed to be maintained to protect the chemists and presumably to protect the programme from unwanted and unwarranted publicity.[70] He needed to know within ten days whether the collection could be made.

The deal was struck with a collector named Bruce Smith. The collection was made sometime in April: 235 pounds – not 375 pounds as originally requested – of plant material arrived in Washington, DC the following month and was promptly sent off to Wall. Perdue spoke to Richard Chase again in July saying that he would be returning to him sometime in the future to fulfil an order for 3,000 pounds. In the meantime, he asked Chase to arrange for a further 200 pounds of bark.[71] By the middle of December, Wall had received 137 pounds. The new District Ranger, James Hendrix, explained that fulfilling the order was proving difficult because, given the time of the year, drying the bark was proving very slow.[72] We know nothing about the collection in detail, except that Hendrix used another collector, Warren Dahlin.[73]

Aside from producing plant material, the collections in 1966 also revealed the messiness of the operations. They were done at a distance, organized in the offices of the USDA in Maryland on one side of the country, and fulfilled in dense forest on the other, separated by a distance of some 3,000 miles. The collectors were known to the Forest Service personnel but not to the botanists on the cancer programme. The amounts requested were not met exactly and there were delays in shipping because of seasonal conditions.[74]

Dealing with the forest was not simple and straightforward, even at this level of collection. Perdue had to get *Taxus brevifolia* and the individuals associated with the forest to align themselves with his objective. During the collection, these actors were as much part of the cancer programme as were the chemists and the CCNSC staff. To get forestry officials to work for the programme, Perdue revealed that their assistance was required for cancer research. 'I find the word "cancer" magic', wrote Perdue in his programme guide. 'Relatively few people will disregard a request if they understand that this is what our material is used for.'[75]

Perdue had to juggle other aspects of the programme. From his perspective and that of the New Crops Research Branch, the interagency programme with the NCI was not cast in stone. The decision to enter into the interagency programme was, as we have seen, at best ambivalent. But one thing was crystal clear: from the New Crops Research Branch perspective, this was primarily an exercise in pure and applied botany.

The responsibilities of the Branch had evolved since the late nineteenth century and these were non-negotiable. They were applicable to any interagency co-operative programme without exception.[76] The botanical effort involved three stages: pre-procurement, procurement and post-procurement. In the case of the cancer programme, the first two stages were mostly the concern of the Branch, as procurement was done on a random basis. The third stage was in many ways the most involved. It consisted of three main elements: first, a three-way dialogue between the Branch, the chemists and the CCNSC, in evaluating the screening results; secondly, the accumulation and analysis of botanical knowledge leading to publications on the field; and finally, an evaluation of the 'potential for development to crop status in some region of the United States'.[77] It is interesting to note that in his formal application to the USDA for an interagency agreement with the CCNSC, Hartwell had explicitly referred to the responsibility of the New Crops Research Branch in developing those species found to have anti-cancer properties to crop status.[78]

Perdue, therefore, had several allegiances, several networks in which he simultaneously performed. He was attached to the interagency programme; he had a responsibility to American agriculture; and he had a responsibility to botany. Five years into the programme, Perdue informed Hartwell that there was an imbalance between the two agencies.[79] He pointed out that, as far as his branch of the USDA was concerned, the botanists were not getting much out of the programme for themselves. Perdue reminded Hartwell that he was dealing with an equal partner. 'The New Crops Research Branch is considered a research organization rather than a service unit...additional service work can be justified only when it is allied with our official responsibilities and provides research opportunities that enhance the standing of the Branch.' The programme was not fulfilling these criteria. It was not generating publications. 'The success of any program in which we participate', he wrote, 'is measured to a considerable extent by publications produced by that program. The five-year duration of our program without publication of any results is making this effort increasingly vulnerable to criticism against which I have little defense.'

While supplying the programme with plant material for screening, Perdue also had to keep in mind his other responsibilities: to accumulate botanical knowledge and to think about potential cultivation of valuable species. At the start of 1966, as we have seen, it had become clear to Wall, Hartwell and Perdue that there was something in the bark of *Taxus brevifolia* that was active. This revelation prompted Wall to embark on the process of fractionation and isolation, in pursuit of the responsible molecule. Perdue organized supplies of *Taxus brevifolia* but he also set about learning more about the species and the genus as potential anti-cancer plants. For this he needed Wall's co-operation, which he got. Wall was known within the programme as a chemist who gave as much as he took.

The chemists, as much as the botanists, had a responsibility to their profession. Publications were crucial to professional advancement. Perdue and Wall had an understanding based on mutual respect. Wall's requests for plant material were fulfilled whether or not they went through the proper channels, that is, authorized by the CCNSC. 'We do our best to fill any request made by Wall. His requests occasionally go beyond the call of duty but not to an extent that puts us in a difficult position. We cooperate fully with Wall because he cooperates fully with us.'[80] Not every fractionator was treated in this way. With Wall on his side, Perdue began investigating the *Taxus* genus. He was interested in answering two questions: How did activity vary by species across the genus? How did activity vary geographically within *Taxus brevifolia*?

The first question impinged directly on the possibility of cultivating *Taxus*. To answer it, Perdue needed samples of every species of *Taxus*. In October 1966, Perdue let Wall know that he had collected a large lot of *Taxus* samples, including the well-known species *baccata*, *cuspidata*, *floridana* and *media*.[81] Both *baccata* and *cuspidata* were species growing in local nurseries and, because they were of overgrown stock, they were due to be bulldozed in a few months' time. *Media*, a hybrid variety, was actually growing in the nurseries at the USDA itself. Samples of *Taxus floridana* were collected in their habitat in the Florida panhandle. The collector, Sidney McDaniel confirmed the rarity of the species – he could only find three small trees at the site he inspected. *Taxus canadensis* had already been tested and shown to be active.[82] The rarer species, *Taxus globosa*, *Taxus chinesis* and *Taxus hunnewelliana* (a cross between *cuspidata* and *canadensis*) were proving difficult to collect. Eventually samples of all three species, growing at different arboreta and botanical gardens, arrived at Perdue's office.[83]

In March of the following year, 1967, Wall told Perdue that, according to the tests on KB, many of the samples of the different *Taxus* species were active – the actives were being fractionated and tested against the WM rat tumour (results were not yet in).[84] Indeed, of twenty-two samples, only four were outside the range of activity. The news was good but not great. For comparison, Wall also tested the bark of *Taxus brevifolia*, freshly collected in Oregon. This sample had the best activity of all. As for the WM results, we do not know them. More importantly though, by the time he was testing these species, Wall had already isolated the active molecule that he had named taxol. Wall could therefore provide more information than simply KB activity. In September 1967, he reported that both *Taxus cuspidata* and *Taxus baccata* contained taxol. The yields were, however, low compared with *Taxus brevifolia*: for the *cuspidata*, the yield was twenty mg per pound of plant material; for *baccata* it was hardly anything.[85] For comparison, the yield of taxol in *Taxus brevifolia* was between fifty and fifty-five mg per pound of plant material.[86]

To answer the second of Perdue's questions – the variation of activity of *Taxus brevifolia* by location – Perdue turned again to the Forest Service. Barclay, it will be recalled, had collected the original sample in Washington. All the collections up to and including the one in April 1966 were made in the same locality. This made perfect sense in view of the objective of isolating the active molecule. Given that Barclay collected at random, he could just as easily have collected the samples of *Taxus brevifolia* in another part of its range where he was searching at the time – in northern California or Oregon. In October 1966, Perdue contacted Edward Cliff, Chief of the Forest Service.[87] Perdue did not withhold his enthusiasm for *Taxus brevifolia*: it was, he said, 'the most outstanding of the positive returns of the screening of over 11,000 plant samples'.[88] On the basis of past experience with other plants, Perdue informed Cliff that the active agent in the tree was probably there in extremely small amounts. He wanted the assistance of the Forest Service for this stage of the research.

> We wish to obtain a series of small samples of bark as a basis
> for determining the geographical variation in yield of this con-
> stituent. This information will be of great value when large
> quantities of the agent must be isolated for detailed evaluation
> of its activity in other animals and finally in human patients.
> We can obtain a suitable evaluation with about 20 bark samples
> (1 pound dry weight each) from throughout the range of the
> species. Our experience with this plant suggests that collection of
> a 1 pound (sample) will require about 30 minutes labor. Samples
> can be taken from the trunk of the tree or can be removed from
> the larger branches. In each case at least three trees should be
> represented in each sample.

Perdue closed the letter with a request that the interest in *Taxus brevifolia* be kept confidential. Notice that only bark samples were going to be collected. As discussed earlier, bark had become the plant part of choice as early as July 1966 when Wall reported on the activity of the April 1966 collection in the Gifford Pinchot National Forest.

The machinery was put into operation. Within the next few months, the samples from Alaska, Washington, Oregon, California and Idaho began to arrive at the USDA.[89] By March, Wall's laboratory had completed the analysis. The results were interesting but difficult to interpret. Overall, there was a wide variation in KB activity, the Washington and Idaho samples showing the best activity.[90] The Alaskan samples performed poorly in KB, although they were quite active in WM.[91] Samples from two locations in California, in Del Norte and Humboldt counties, were active while the one from Siskiyou county was not. The ecology of the different samples, as recorded with the collections, does not appear to have been dramatically different. The samples from Oregon showed considerable and inexplicable variation – those from Mt Hood were fine while those from Umqua and Umatilla National Forests were poor: KB results varied by a factor of fifty, an unusually high range of results.[92]

Late in 1968, Perdue arranged for further tests on *Taxus*. One of these consisted of collecting samples of all parts of *Taxus brevifolia* from a small number of trees growing in Washington and California. The other consisted of three samples of cultivated *Taxus cuspidata*.[93] The results of the *Taxus brevifolia* exercise were mixed. Though stembark emerged as the most active part of the tree, other parts were not devoid of activity.[94] Needles, in particular, varied considerably in activity; still, more than sixty per cent of the samples showed moderate activity.[95] We do not know the results of the test on *Taxus cuspidata*.

All the answers to Perdue's questions about variability were open to interpretation. Nature was inconsistent. The forest was not standardized. That much was clear. But the very notion of variability had different meanings to the major actors. For Wall, information about the range and variability of activity of *Taxus* and its taxol content was of little importance. What mattered to him was the chemistry of taxol. Working with other species of *Taxus* or samples from various localities was only important within the context of the chemical analysis. This is why Perdue needed to have Wall on his side but was always careful not to overstep the boundary. In asking Wall to undertake the chemical analysis of the 1968 samples, Perdue trod carefully. 'My suggestions offered here will extend somewhat the effort on *Taxus* that we discussed while I was at RTI [Research Triangle Institute]', he wrote to Wall; 'I certainly recognize that you may not be able to prepare as many additional extracts as I have suggested. Please be assured that while I will welcome as much data as we can get, I can live with and will do my best with a lesser amount. I fully appreciate that all this represents a "tall order".'[96]

To Perdue and Hartwell, the information about variability had a strategic purpose. The information about the variation of activity and taxol by species was crucial to issues about the source of supply in the long-run. This thinking was already in evidence by 1967. In a letter to James Hendrix, Ranger of the Packwood District, Perdue remarked that the supply problem was critical: even in the short-term he needed considerable amounts of *Taxus brevifolia* to feed Wall's chemical work.[97] Several months later, he also remarked that if the active substance in the cultivated varieties tested by Wall turned out to be taxol, then they would have 'no difficulty in obtaining supplies for many of the plants included in the test are readily available from commercial sources'.[98]

The supply issue, in both the short and long term, was addressed by both Perdue and Hartwell in a 1969 publication. Speaking primarily to botanists, the authors emphasized the variability in activity of *Taxus brevifolia* bark from different locations, and the variability by plant part.[99] Perdue and Hartwell saw taxol in a wide context. They made it very clear that the future of taxol was not with *Taxus brevifolia* bark, as its yield was so low. Taxol, they argued, was present in all *Taxus* species. Should there be a future for taxol as a drug, they maintained, then 'an intensive selection and breeding program could be directed toward development of faster-growing higher-yielding types'.[100]

In the short term, the information about variability was extremely useful in collections for chemical analysis. That bark consistently turned out to be the most active part of *Taxus brevifolia*, regardless of location, was sufficient to warrant its collection exclusively. In March 1967, Perdue wrote to the Forest Service to express his thanks for their co-operation in supplying samples for the analysis of the geographic variation of activity.[101] The programme, he wrote, was now in need of substantially more material, at least a ton of it. Now that he knew more about the variation in the activity of *Taxus brevifolia*, Perdue could pick the best locations. In April and May 1967, Perdue was in contact with the appropriate District Rangers for selected National Forests in Idaho, California, Oregon and Washington, to arrange for this big collection. Perdue explained to the Forest Service that he guided his requests to four different locations, first, to avoid 'putting all my eggs in one basket', and second, to limit '*the resultant destruction of trees at any one location*' (our emphasis).[102] We will return to this point shortly.

Perdue arranged for almost 3,000 pounds of bark to be collected. He used the same District Rangers he had already contacted in the sample exercise. As they were familiar with local conditions, these rangers put Perdue in touch with the local collectors. It is clear from the surviving correspondence that collectors had some knowledge of the yew tree and that the rangers had asked around until they had found someone with this knowledge. The ranger that Perdue contacted in the Nez Perce National Forest in Idaho recommended a collector named Richard Gribble who had been working for a logging firm but was presently laid off.[103] In the case of the collector of bark in Oregon, we know that he, Lester Lewis, was a retired Forest Service carpenter, who knew of yew because he cut it for archery billets.[104] The collection in California took longer to set up and it showed the potential pitfalls in collecting from a distance. The request for the test sample of bark that Perdue had arranged through Edward Cliff, the Chief of the Forest Service in 1966 had gone directly to the Pacific Southwest Forest and Range Experiment Station in Arcata. Kenneth Boe, the Project Leader, sent the sample directly to Perdue.[105] Naturally, Perdue turned to Boe for assistance in this larger collection on 23 March 1967. Boe was at the Experiment Station and not attached to any particular National Forest. His help was, therefore, quite limited. He did, however, pass Perdue on to someone else in Gasquet, in the extreme north-west corner of the state. There the request went through several other people until, finally, two months after Perdue first went in search of *Taxus brevifolia* bark in California, a collector was found. Gertrude Heachock of Crescent City agreed to supply 500 pounds at $1.50 per pound dry weight.[106] With the exception of one consignment from Washington that arrived late, the collection went very smoothly. Nearly 2,500 pounds of bark arrived at the USDA and promptly went off to Wall's laboratory at the Research Triangle Institute.

There is little doubt that Perdue viewed going to the forest for material as expedient and necessary for this part of the programme. The future supplies of taxol lay not in the forest but in the field. Yet events were conspiring to make the association between taxol and the bark of *Taxus brevifolia* far more durable than Perdue and Hartwell probably hoped it would be. The durability of the association was reinforced by two things: first, notwithstanding the long-range possibilities of using cultivated *Taxus* species, the material going into Wall's laboratory, the practice, in other words, was *Taxus brevifolia* bark from the forests of the Pacific Northwest. Secondly, there were publications from Wall's laboratory. Wall and Wani first made their work on *Taxus* public at the annual meeting of the American Chemical Society in April 1967. In that paper, they referred only to the fact that they had discovered considerable cytotoxicity in the extract and an unusually broad spectrum of antitumour activity in fractions of the species *Taxus brevifolia*. No mention was made of any other species. Wall and Wani were speaking to chemists. The point was reinforced several years later. In 1971, Wall and his co-workers published the results of their work following on from their paper at the American Chemical Society meeting four years earlier. In their communication to the Editor of the *Journal of the American Chemical Society* on the isolation of taxol, Wall and his co-workers referred solely to the stembark and to *Taxus brevifolia*.[107] By making taxol the focus of the article, the relative language about *Taxus brevifolia* had now become absolute. To anyone reading the article – and it became the key article about taxol – the molecule was unequivocally associated with *Taxus brevifolia* and its stembark.

As the collections of *Taxus brevifolia* bark increased in volume and frequency, more information accumulated about the species, beyond that which was available in print. This information came from the collectors themselves. Botanical knowledge of *Taxus brevifolia* was extremely limited. Its range was known in general terms. The descriptions of the tree as they appeared in the botanical literature were clear and, as far as they went, helpful in identifying it. Having said that, finding the tree in the forest was another matter. This is where local knowledge was indispensable. And, as this information flowed into the USDA offices, the stock of *Taxus brevifolia* knowledge grew.

In his *A Natural History of Western Trees*, Donald Peattie wrote lovingly of *Taxus brevifolia* and remarked on the difficulty of finding it. The reason is quite simple. *Taxus brevifolia* is an understory tree, living in dense conifer forests, dominated by the giants of the Pacific Northwest, the Douglas fir, western hemlock, western cedar and so forth. The 1966 sample collection provided valuable information of the habitat of *Taxus brevifolia*, largely confirming Peattie's remarks. That is to say, it could be found in dense forest but also in the open, in those areas where selective logging had already taken the valuable species.[108] Another piece of information to emerge from the collection was that *Taxus brevifolia* mostly grew in solitary places, although there were places where it grew in small clumps. From a vantage point beside one yew, it might not be possible to see another one. But perhaps the most important insight, and one which would haunt the programme in decades to come, was the one that Perdue knew only too well.

Taxus brevifolia is a very slow growing tree. An average tree of diameter 9 inches and height 30 feet is 125 years old. The bark is extremely thin, between 1/8 and 1/4 of an inch thick. Such a tree would yield between 3 and 5 pounds of bark. What Perdue knew in 1967 was that collecting bark meant killing trees, whether they were felled first and then stripped or stripped while standing. Considering that only the collector knew how many trees were stripped to meet the contract with the USDA and as this information was not recorded, the extent of the destruction of *Taxus brevifolia* was not known.

At this time much less was known about the tree as a living species than about the chemistry of one compound present in its bark. With the publication of taxol's structure in 1971, Wall and his co-workers, as we have seen, handed the molecule on to the CCNSC for further work. This point needs to be emphasized. By handing the molecule to the CCNSC, Wall was delivering an object devoid of the context of its development. As long as Wall was dealing with Hartwell and Perdue, the associations between the molecule and its source and between the uncertainties of the forest and the alternative of cultivation were alive and visible. Once the focus shifted to the molecule and placed it in the practice of chemical evaluation within the NCI, then these associations were erased. The objective of the programme from the perspective of the CCNSC was to get drugs to the clinic.

As soon as Wall had a process for isolating taxol, his job, in a sense, was over. The molecule was handed over to another part of the CCNSC to take the process forward. Given his background and training, Wall was actually closer to this section of the CCNSC than he was to Hartwell. Robert Engle headed this part of the CCNSC, the Chemical and Drug Procurement Section of the Drug Development Branch. Wall was in contact with Engle by April 1968, informing him of some of the properties of taxol, particularly its low yield.[109] By the end of January of the following year, Engle had received a package of information on taxol, containing everything that Wall's laboratory had discovered about the molecule until that date. At the same time, Engle also learned that Wall had a large quantity – approximately 2,600 pounds – of *Taxus brevifolia* on hand.[110] Because this was Government property and because, in the eyes of the CCNSC, Wall was finished with *Taxus brevifolia* (if not taxol), Engle asked him to release the material.[111] He wanted it to be extracted and partitioned between chloroform and water by Wall's methods but by another contractor, Aerojet General Corporation of Sacramento. Wall complied with the request.

After acquainting himself first with the crude extract, then the fractions, the crystalline pure compound and finally the structure itself, Wall clearly felt close to the molecule. He asked after it, concerned about its future, worried that it was in good hands, hoping, as if it were a child, that it would achieve its true potential. In April 1970, Wall informed Engle that his laboratory had successfully completed the total structure of taxol.[112] Unfortunately, as Wall reported next month, the cleaved products of taxol, both of which were chemically simpler than taxol, had appreciably less KB activity than taxol itself. As a chemist, Wall did not see much hope for a synthetic version of the molecule. Yet the vinca alkaloids, he remarked, were present at a much lower yield in

Catharanthus roseus than taxol in *Taxus brevifolia*.[113] Wall was making the point that taxol's 'low yield and complex structure should not be regarded as a barrier.' At the same time, considering how much taxol would be needed for pharmacological and antitumour evaluation (Wall estimated from five to ten grams), Wall could not devote the time to make this amount.[114]

Wall was expecting the Drug Development Branch of the CCNSC to move with taxol. His enthusiasm for taxol, first communicated to the CCNSC in 1964 and reinforced to Engle in 1970, did not elicit the kind of action Wall expected and wanted.[115] The CCNSC responded to his queries that no decision had been taken on taxol.[116] Harry Wood, the Chief of the Drug Development Branch, gave an ambiguous message concerning taxol. 'Should we decide to do more development work on this material', he wrote to Wall, 'I will be in touch with you. There are so few active compounds coming out of the natural products program that when a good one does come along like camptothecin and taxol I think it is well worth the effort to give it every consideration.'[117] It was a non-committal answer. As far as the CCNSC was concerned, taxol showed only modest activity in the *in vivo* screens.[118]

Wall did not give up. Again in mid-1971, he asked for guidance concerning taxol, whether he should be putting more effort into the purification process or concentrate on other matters.[119] There appears to have been no response to this question, but a year later, Wall received a request from Engle for fifteen grams of taxol for development work.[120] Wall could not fulfil such an order. It took another year, that is until 1973, for an arrangement to be made to produce the amount of taxol that was needed. Monsanto Research Laboratory in Dayton, Ohio, received the contract to isolate taxol from the crude extract – twenty-eight kilograms – that had been prepared by the Aerojet Corporation back in 1969.[121] Wall did have 815 milligrams of taxol on hand and this he handed over to John Douros at the Natural Products Section of the Division of Cancer Treatment at the end of February 1974.[122]

Douros wanted Wall's sample of taxol to test it against two tumour models recently introduced into the evaluation procedure.[123] These tumour models, LL (Lewis lung) and B16 (melanoma), representing slow-growing solid tumours, departed from the dominance of the leukaemia models of previous years. The testing was done in April 1974, repeated in September and then again in June 1975. The results were mixed. The April test gave impressive results, meeting the NCI criteria for development several times over; but the repeat test in September failed to satisfy even the minimum requirements. The June 1975 results were not as good as the first results in the previous year but the criteria for further development had finally been met.[124]

Yet, these mixed results, together with taxol's modest activity in the leukaemia models, conjoined to keep the molecule on the margin. The dominance of the leukaemia models reflected a wider dominance within parts of the NCI of the leukaemia research culture, a culture which had produced clinically-effective drugs, both within and outside the NCI. Because of its marginal antileukaemic status, taxol did not attract a voice in 1975.

Hartwell, it will be recalled, retired as head of the Natural Products Section of the Division of Cancer Treatment in 1975 and was succeeded in this post by John Douros. At the end of March 1976, Douros asked Perdue the cost of 4,000 pounds of *Taxus brevifolia*.[125] In answering Douros, Perdue took the opportunity to inform him of the supply situation. 'I think we can get the required amount, but for the future the supply situation is dismal', he wrote. But all was not lost. He brought Douros into the picture, referring to information that we can only assume had been forgotten or ignored. 'Taxol occurs in other species of *Taxus*, most of which are very easy to cultivate. If this drug has any real prospects for the future, we should get *Taxus* under cultivation. Several species are readily available from nurseries, though they can be fairly expensive.'[126] With this, Perdue, once again, reminded his NCI colleagues that there were two objectives of the cancer programme: (i) to get plants exhibiting anti-cancer properties to the clinic as drugs, and (ii) to get those plants to crop status. There was an alternative to the forest.

Notes

1 Wall and Wani, 'Camptothecin', p. 2.
2 Perdue and Hartwell, 'The search for plant sources', p. 43.
3 Perdue and Hartwell, 'The search for plant sources', p. 44.
4 Gentry and Hadley, 'Listening to my mind', pp. 183–184.
5 Barclay, 'Special Assignments, 1960–1976', SPJ3.
6 The party consisted of Barclay plus Kurt Blum, Ray Barbee and Steve Koch. Blum spotted the tree. According to him, there was no a priori reason for sampling *Taxus brevifolia*. The collection was guided solely by the strategy of collecting everything. Identification was made on site or back at the USDA, comparing the sample with herbarium specimens – personal communication, Kurt Blum, 3 June 1998. See also *Taxus brevifolia*, active files, SPJ1. B-1645 stood for the 1645th plant sample collected by Barclay.
7 Plant material for analysis, Perdue to Wall, 9 January 1963, PER1.
8 See Hartzell, *The Yew Tree*, pp. 132–149 and pp. 164–171 for different uses of yew.
9 Tyler, 'Note on the occurrence'.
10 Fitzgerald, Hartwell and Leiter, 'Distribution of tumor-damaging lignans'.
11 Fitzgerald, Hartwell and Leiter, 'Distribution of tumor-damaging lignans', p. 85.
12 Morelli, 'Costituenti'.

13 Hartzell, *The Yew Tree*.
14 Miller, 'A brief survey', p. 426.
15 See Miller, 'A brief survey' for a short chronological chemical history of *Taxus* alkaloids. The state of research into *Taxus* alkaloids as of mid-1960s can be found in Lythgoe, 'The *Taxus* alkaloids'.
16 The information is derived from Perdue and Hartwell, 'The search for plant sources', p. 43.
17 Statz and Coon, 'Preparation of plant extracts'.
18 The following is based on Suffness and Wall, 'Discovery and development'.
19 *Taxus brevifolia*, active files, SPJ1. The test was done at Microbiological Associates in Bethesda, Maryland.
20 Suffness and Wall, 'Discovery and development', p. 5.
21 *Taxus brevifolia*, active files, SPJ1.
22 Perdue and Hartwell, 'The search for plant sources', p. 43.
23 Hartwell to Perdue, 21 July 1964, PER1.
24 Arthur Barclay, Herbarium labels, 1962–1964, SPJ1.
25 Wall maintains that he asked Hartwell to assign him plants that showed preliminary KB activity – see, for example, in Suffness and Wall, 'Discovery and development', p. 5. The confirmed actives assigned to Wall were certainly KB active, but so were those assigned to Kupchan and to the Pfizer Laboratories, two of the chemical subcontractors at the time. According to Perdue, Hartwell distributed the confirmed actives in a manner to keep the workload equal among the chemists – interview with Perdue, October 1995. The allocation of confirmed actives is in Hartwell to Perdue, 8 September 1964, WLL2.
26 Perdue to Wall, 6 November 1962, WLL1.
27 Wall to Perdue, 1 October 1963, WLL1.
28 Wall to Perdue, 18 October 1963, WLL1.
29 Plant suppliers meeting, CCNSC, 21 November 1963, PER1.
30 Wall, Wani and Taylor, 'Isolation and chemical characterization', p. 1011.
31 Suffness and Wall, 'Discovery and development', pp. 5–6.
32 Perdue and Hartwell, 'The search for plant sources', p. 45.
33 Wall to Hartwell, 20 January 1966, WLL1.
34 Research Triangle Institute, Progress Report no. 18, 20 May 1966, p. 20.
35 Wall to Hartwell, 19 April 1966, WLL1, wherein he asked Hartwell to use his influence in convincing the screeners to treat B670549 as a special priority.
36 Research Triangle Institute, Progress Report no. 18, 20 May 1966, p. 20. The KB cell culture was also called 9KB by some researchers.
37 Research Triangle Institute, Progress Report no. 20, 21 November 1966, pp. 8–10.
38 Wall reported this fact to Hartwell in his progress report – Research Triangle Institute, Progress Report no. 17, 21 December 1965.
39 Hartwell to Wall, 5 January 1966, WLL1.
40 *Taxus brevifolia* collection list, 1962–1968, PER5.
41 Wall to Hartwell, 26 July 1966, WLL1.
42 Hartwell to Perdue, 11 August 1966, PER1.
43 Hartwell to Wall, 29 September 1966, in which he remarks 'That was good news about the crystalline product from *Taxus*.'
44 Wall to Abbott, 13 March 1967, WLL1.
45 Research Triangle Institute, Progress Report no. 21, 26 June 1967, p. 30.
46 Research Triangle Institute, Progress Report no. 21, 26 June 1967, p. 4.

47 Wall and Wani, 'Camptothecin and taxol', p. 757.
48 Interview with Wall, 15 September 1997.
49 Wall and Wani, 'Camptothecin and taxol', p. 757
50 See the discussion in Chapter 5.
51 Suffness and Wall, 'Discovery and development', p. 6.
52 Wall to Abbott, 19 September 1967, WLL1.
53 Research Triangle Institute, Progress Report no. 25, 10 July 1968, p. 3.
54 Wall to Engle, 31 January 1969, WLL1.
55 Engle to Wall, 12 February 1969, WLL1.
56 Wall to Engle, 6 April, 1970, WLL1. The structure was reproduced in the forthcoming report from the laboratory. See, Research Triangle Institute, Progress Report no. 33, 20 July 1970, pp. 2–4.
57 Lythgoe, Nakanishi and Uyeo, 'Taxane'. Also interview with Basil Lythgoe, 7 May 1998.
58 Wani et al., 'Plant antitumor agents'.
59 Miller, 'A brief survey'.
60 This is true for the principal accounts of taxol written by some of the main players; for example, Suffness and Wall, 'Discovery and development'; Wall and Wani, 'Camptothecin and taxol'; and Wall and Wani, 'Paclitaxel'; as well as press statements from Bristol-Myers Squibb showing the chronology of taxol's development.
61 A rough estimate, based on Hartwell and Abbott, 'Antineoplastic principles', p. 120.
62 For the early history of the Forest Service, see Williams, *Americans and Their Forests*.
63 Tuchmann et al., *The Northwest Forest Plan*, p. 14.
64 For an excellent discussion of practices on National Forests since 1945, see Hirt, *A Conspiracy of Optimism*. See also Hays, *Beauty*, p. 395.
65 On clear-cutting and the Forest service, see Clary, *Timber*, pp. 180–188.
66 Farnham and Mohai, 'National forest timber', p. 274.
67 The term is introduced here as a shorthand way of referring to this kind of forest ecosystem. For a fuller discussion of old-growth and the politics behind it, see Chapters 4 and 6.
68 The entry can be found in *Taxus brevifolia*, active files, SPJ1. The description of *Taxus brevifolia* as a trash species would be made many times over the following decades.
69 The letters, memos and notes are in UDA1.
70 Perdue, it will be recalled from the previous chapter, was intent on the point about secrecy. The press pounced on any hint of a cure for cancer no matter how premature. As it turned out, in Perdue's letter of confirmation to Bruce Smith, the collector, a memo from Perdue to Hartwell was mistakenly included. The lengthy memo provided details of the revelations of yew bark. Chase tried to put Smith off the scent by convincing him that the memo had nothing to do with his yew collection – Chase to Perdue, 18 May 1966, UDA1.
71 Perdue to Czemerys, 1 September 1966, UDA1.
72 Hendrix to Perdue, 29 November 1966, UDA1.
73 Perdue to Hendrix, 13 April 1967, UDA1.
74 One reason why the amounts received were short of the requested amount was that requested amounts were stated in dry weight. By the time the shipment arrived back East, it could have dried even more, thus reducing the weight.

75 USDA Program Guide, SPJ3.
76 These were laid down in a document prepared by Quentin Jones and Bernice Schubert of the USDA and attached to a letter from H.L. Hyland, Head of the Plant Introduction Section of the New Crops Research Branch, to Hartwell, 2 July 1959, PER2.
77 Procurement for screening programme, memo from Jones and Schubert to Erlanson, 30 June 1959, attached to above.
78 Hartwell to Shaw, 25 April 1960, PER2.
79 Perdue to Hartwell, 30 September 1965, PER1.
80 USDA Program Guide, SPJ3.
81 Perdue to Wall, 7 September 1966, PER1 and Perdue to Wall, 10 October 1966, WLL1.
82 Perdue to Wall, 7 September 1966, UDA1.
83 Copies of memos and letters pertaining to the samples of these species are in UDA1.
84 Wall to Perdue, 17 March 1967, WLL1.
85 Wall to Abbott, 19 September 1967, WLL1. In this letter, Wall did not provide a quantitative estimate of the yield of taxol from *Taxus baccata*. A recent publication states that the yield was, in fact, 0.0008 per cent – Suffness and Wall, 'Discovery and development', p. 9.
86 Wall to Abbott, 19 September 1967, WLL1.
87 For aspects of Cliff's career in the Forest Service, see Clary, *Timber*, pp. 147–194.
88 Perdue to Cliff, 1 September 1966, UDA1.
89 Spetzman to Liming, 1 December 1966, UDA1. Knowledge about the range of *Taxus brevifolia* was well established. See for example a description and map of the range of the tree in Little, 'Important forest trees', pp. 801–802.
90 Wall to Abbott, 13 March 1967, WLL1.
91 Wall to Perdue, 17 March 1967, WLL1.
92 Wall to Perdue, 17 March 1967, WLL1.
93 Perdue to Wall, 8 November 1968, WLL1.
94 Perdue to Wall, 8 November 1968, WLL1.
95 Suffness and Wall, 'Discovery and development', p. 10.
96 Perdue to Wall, 8 November 1968, WLL1.
97 Perdue to Hendrix, 13 April 1967, UDA1.
98 Perdue to Hendrix, 22 May 1967, UDA1.
99 Perdue and Hartwell, 'The search for plant sources'.
100 Perdue and Hartwell, 'The search for plant sources', p. 48.
101 Perdue to Liming, 21 March 1967, UDA1.
102 Perdue to Liming, 7 July 1967, UDA1.
103 Idaho collection, October 1966, UDA1.
104 Memo to files, Bernard Douglass, Special Products Forester, 17 May 1967, UDA1.
105 Boe to Perdue, 25 October 1966, UDA1.
106 Perdue to Heachock, 9 May 1967, UDA1.
107 Wani et al., 'Plant antitumor agents'. One of the footnotes to the text does mention that taxol had been isolated from *Taxus cuspidata* and *Taxus baccata* but no figures on yields were given.
108 1966 collection information, UDA1.
109 Wall to Engle, 26 April 1968, WLL1.
110 Engle to Wall, 12 February 1969, WLL1.

111 The issue of the ownership of plant materials and their constituents came up early in the history of the programme. It was discussed at length at the Plant Suppliers meeting on 23 October 1964. The point that chemists invested a great deal of time and effort in received considerable attention. The chemists not only felt '. . . a strong scientific interests in the results of the work-up of large quantities of the plants, especially as regards unexpected constituents or the search for such in the mother liquors, but [had] a need for challenging problems whose solution could be carried out under grant or contract'. The point was a good one but conflicted with the fact that all the materials and constituents thereof were Government property. In the end, there was no resolution to the problem in a general sense. Each case would be treated individually. See Minutes, Plant Suppliers Meeting, Bethesda, 23 October 1964, WLL1.

112 Wall to Engle, 6 April 1970, WLL2.

113 Wall to Engle, 5 May 1970, WLL2.

114 Wall to Engle, 5 May 1979, WLL2.

115 In a letter to Engle in February, Wall referred to taxol as a 'very active substance'. Wall to Engle, 19 February 1970, WLL2.

116 Wood to Wall, 3 November 1970, WLL2.

117 Wood to Wall, 1 December 1970, WLL2.

118 Suffness and Wall, 'Discovery and development', p. 12.

119 Wall to Wood, 14 June 1971, WLL2.

120 Wall to Engle, 18 September 1972, WLL2.

121 Engle to Wall, 9 May 1973, WLL2.

122 Wall to Douros, 22 February 1974, WLL2. Douros had joined the Natural Products Section in 1972, working under Hartwell. He became Hartwell's successor as Head in 1975, upon the latter's retirement. The CCNSC and all work in chemotherapy was subsumed within the newly created Division of Cancer Treatment in 1972.

123 Douros to Wall, 5 December 1973, WLL2.

124 Suffness and Wall, 'Discovery and development', pp. 12–13.

125 Douros to Perdue, 31 March 1976, PER2.

126 Perdue to Douros, 22 April 1976, PER2.

3

Act II: 1976–1983

Between 1976 and 1983, taxol went through the developmental procedure established for all compounds at the NCI, from the screening against a panel of murine tumours to the filing of an application to begin human trials. There was no more than a four per cent chance of making it through this part of the system.

The end result for taxol was success, and those who worked with it and advocated its further development were rewarded, but the path was unpredictable. As taxol wound its way through the NCI drug development programme, its attributes as an anti-cancer agent emerged more clearly, but its identity as such an object was still in the making. This was not, however, its only identity. In other hands, it had other attributes. Taxol, as it turned out, had a unique mechanism of action. When they found this out, cell biologists swarmed to get the compound to use as a new research tool, allowing them to explore aspects of cellular activity previously closed to them. To a burgeoning concern for the welfare of *Taxus brevifolia* from a few activists in the Pacific Northwest, the revelation that the tree contained a compound capable of killing tumours provided them with a voice of protest against what they perceived as the wilful and ignorant destruction of living organisms. Chemists, for their part, saw taxol as a challenge in elucidating the structure of one of the most complex natural compounds they had ever seen and for finding ways of making it in the laboratory.

Not only were its attributes changing, but the contexts in which taxol existed and was shaped also changed. The forest was becoming a site of political struggle focused on the impending disappearance of old-growth habitat where *Taxus brevifolia* was growing. The NCI-USDA plant screening programme was brought to an end, leaving the former with responsibilities in an area in which it had no experience. Personnel changes continued to erode memories of practices. France appeared as a new site for taxol research.

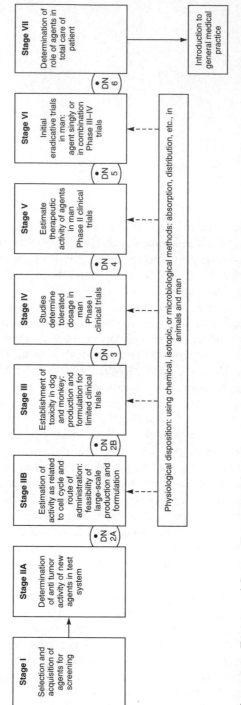
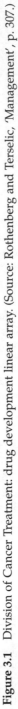

Figure 3.1 Division of Cancer Treatment: drug development linear array. (Source: Rothenberg and Terselic, 'Management', p. 307.)

In the 1970s the NCI adopted the B16 melanoma tumour system in the belief that it would be useful in selecting compounds active against slow-growing human tumours.[1] It was first used for special testing in 1972 and then for routine testing in 1975.[2] The potential of B16 was shown by the case of the drug DTIC that was selected experimentally by L1210 and B16 and proved to be clinically effective against human melanoma.[3] The decision to include a tumour system of this type was based on the need to do something about a troublesome fact. The main screens, the L1210 and P388, were good predictors of clinical effectiveness; but the compounds that reached the clinic, having been initially selected by these screens, were effective only against the fastest growing tumours and ineffective against the slow-growing tumours. Chemotherapy, in terms of the number of chemical agents available in the clinic, was most successful against fast-growing tumours.[4] Unfortunately, the vast majority of deaths from cancer were from slow-growing tumours.

As we have seen, taxol met the criteria of activity against B16, as defined by the NCI, in 1975. Yet nothing happened. Considering how important B16 activity was in principle, it is surprising that taxol did not go forward in the development process at this time. The B16 tumour system was fairly new at the time and this may explain, in part, why taxol remained in limbo. Experimental researchers may have been unwilling to stake too much, including their own reputations, on its results. Part of the explanation must also lie in aspects of the chemotherapy culture of the NCI. According to Matthew Suffness, the NCI staff did not show much interest in a compound that had marginal activity against leukaemia models, regardless of any other demonstrated activity.[5] The leukaemia paradigm was certainly deeply rooted at the NCI, in terms of the history of chemotherapy and the choice of tumour systems, as we have already shown.

To get a compound from the laboratory to the clinic, the NCI operated a system of procedures known as the linear array. It was a complex management tool designed to improve the efficiency of the entire operation leading to the clinical introduction of an anti-cancer drug.[6] Figure 3.1 shows a simplified version of the linear array. It had evolved rather than been designed and was firmly in place when taxol was shown to be active against B16.

The function of the linear array was to advance a compound from the point where it was screened against the NCI experimental tumour system to the point at which an Investigational New Drug Application (INDA) could be filed with the Food and Drug Administration (hereafter FDA), to initiate trials on human subjects. This developmental process consisted of three research programmes and three decision points. The first research programme was the screening of a compound against the tumour system. The decision as to whether a compound met the criteria of advancement on the basis of its screening results was taken by a committee called the Decision Network Committee, consisting of about thirty NCI scientists and oncologists. If a compound met the criteria, it was said to have passed the first of three decision points, DN2A. The compound could then be entered for studies on formulation, schedule and route dependency, and the feasibility of large-scale production. The results of this stage were discussed at the next decision point and those compounds chosen for advancement were said to have passed DN2B. The next research programme focused on toxicology using animals as subjects. Results came before the Decision Network Committee and those compounds meeting the criteria were said to have passed DN3. At this point, the compound had accumulated all of the results necessary to have an INDA filed with the FDA.

Very few compounds made it through the linear array. Of 10,000 compounds tested annually for activity, 250 compounds were screened against the tumour panel, of which approximately ten passed DN2A and were selected as development candidates.[7] Approximately eight of these passed DN2B and five of these passed DN3 leading to an INDA filing. The probability of a compound getting from the first test for activity to an INDA filing was, therefore, no more than one in 2,000. The cost of getting a plant-derived compound successfully from the acquisition of the plant to DN3 was put at $390,000 in the late 1970s.[8]

John Douros was with Natural Products Branch of the NCI's Division of Cancer Treatment when taxol was tested against B16. He was a microbiologist by training having spent his professional career in industry before moving to the NCI. Between 1972, the date of his appointment, and 1975 when he succeeded Jonathan Hartwell as Chief, he was primarily concerned with the fermentation side of the natural products programme. In October 1976, Matthew Suffness joined Douros as Head of the Plant and Animal Products Section of the Natural Products Branch. Suffness was trained as a pharmaceutical chemist, working under Morris Kupchan at the University of Wisconsin.[9] He was, therefore, well acquainted with the chemical side of the plant screening programme. After several years in a university position, he went to the NCI where his experience with plant chemistry complemented Douros's expertise.

Suffness recounted that one of the first things he did in his new position was to review the plant screening data, particularly the most recent results in the B16 screen.[10] As he noticed, taxol had met the criteria for development on the basis of its activity against B16. He was encouraged by Monroe Wall to press ahead with taxol: Wall's own interests in the molecule were, as we have seen, frequently communicated to NCI staff (without much luck) after he and his colleagues published taxol's structure in 1971.[11] On reviewing the data and encouraged by Wall's conviction about taxol, the Decision Network Committee looked again at taxol and, on 18 April 1977, it passed DN2A, two years after having shown activity against B16.[12] It now entered the programme of formulation studies, the first stage of investigation.

Within a few days, Suffness contacted Fred Boettner at Polysciences in Warrington, Pennsylvania telling him that he needed ten grams of taxol for the advanced studies. Polysciences was a small industrial chemical supplier. It had just successfully bid for an NCI contract for the scaled-up isolation of taxol and other natural products. In winning the contract, Polysciences became the NCI's main contractor for the large-scale isolation of taxol. The Monsanto Research Corporation in Dayton, Ohio also had a contract with the NCI for scaled-up isolation of natural products but their procedure for isolating taxol was largely unsuccessful.[13] In 1974, chemists at Monsanto managed to isolate only 6.11 grams of taxol from a sample of 2,418 grams crude extract, part of the larger consignment of 28.34 kilograms of crude extract that had been prepared by Aerojet General in 1969. This gave a yield of taxol well below what Wall himself had managed in the laboratory.[14] Monsanto was, therefore, at a disadvantage and the contract went to Polysciences. Monsanto arranged for the remaining amount of crude extract to be sent to Polysciences. Boettner took delivery of 25.6 kilograms of crude extract on 26 April 1977.[15] These 'two drums of tar', as Boettner referred to the material, contained the concentrated extract of the bark that had been collected in Washington, California and Oregon in 1967 and 1968.[16]

Fred Boettner had been hired as chief chemist by David Halpern, Polysciences' President, a year earlier in 1976, in anticipation of getting the NCI contract.[17] Boettner had just left the chemical company Rohm and Hass, also located in the Philadelphia area, after more than thirty years service. He spent most of the first year with Polysciences as its production manager. The isolation of the ten grams of taxol was Boettner's first big job.

Boettner's isolation and purification procedure derived from Wall's published process, together with information supplied to him by both Douros and Suffness, and his own experience and creativity.[18] The whole procedure took even longer than Boettner expected. The isolation, together with the analysis of the product, took many months to complete. The ten grams of taxol absorbed more than 1,000 person-hours of laboratory and production time, and cost more than $35,000;

the yield was eighty-two per cent more than that achieved by Monsanto with the same crude extract.[19] The work was assigned on 22 April 1977 and completed on 6 September 1977.[20]

While Boettner was isolating taxol at Polysciences, Suffness had to plan for the various investigations of taxol that lay ahead. This meant translating the amount of taxol demanded by the various investigations into a weight of plant material. Suffness was not at the NCI when the collections and screening had been done in the late 1960s. He made no assumptions about the nature of this plant material, only that it came from the *Taxus* genus. Sometime in May or June, he asked Monroe Wall for the screening data of the most active species in the genus. In reply, Suffness received the data for various samples of *Taxus brevifolia* and *Taxus cuspidata*. The data showed Suffness what Perdue, Hartwell and Wall had learned of the chemistry of both species: that the variation within and between the species was considerable. In reviewing the data, Suffness came to the conclusion that for both *Taxus brevifolia* and *Taxus cuspidata*, stembark was the most active part of the plant: roots were also active, but less than bark, and twigs were inactive. Activity of the needles varied considerably, sometimes better than bark and other times much poorer. In communicating the data and his reading of them to Perdue, Suffness concluded that 'although it will be more expensive to collect stem bark I think we should try to get it if available since there will be a large saving in processing costs over other plant parts.'[21]

Suffness was certainly correct in concluding that stembark was the best source of taxol. Its average activity, as measured by the KB readings, was higher than other parts of the plant and the variation was lower. But there were two aspects of the conclusion that were problematical. One was that, on the basis of the data in front of him, *Taxus cuspidata* (Japanese yew) appeared just as good a source of taxol as did *Taxus brevifolia* and available in commercial nurseries. Yet no mention of this was made in further communiqués. Secondly, by talking about processing costs, Suffness was redefining the supply issue in economic terms, an argument that had not been made previously. At the time of writing, there were no comparative data on processing costs by plant parts.

If thinking about taxol exclusively in terms of the stembark of *Taxus brevifolia* needed reinforcing, then Suffness was doing a good job of it. He estimated that the next stages in the linear array would require 600 grams of taxol.[22] Suffness calculated that a new collection of 7,000 pounds of bark would need to be undertaken.[23] Sometime in July, Suffness contacted Perdue giving him the order for the collection.[24] And it was back to the forest, after a gap of ten years since the collections of 1966 and 1967 but on a far greater scale.

In the space of ten years, much had changed and the return to the forest this time would reveal a change in milieu. Gearing up for the collection began in June when staff at the Medicinal Plant Resource Laboratory at the USDA first heard of the renewed interest in *Taxus brevifolia*.[25] Richard Spjut, who had been hired as a botanist in 1972, prepared a background paper on *Taxus brevifolia* in July 1977.[26] This was the first such report on *Taxus brevifolia* written for internal use. It brought together in one place most of what was known about the tree from well-known published sources together with information on occurrence and habitat culled from past collections and personal communications from recent observers in Oregon and Idaho. The report reflected just how poor was the information about *Taxus brevifolia*. The information about its occurrence in its range of habitat, for example, was based on sightings, rather than any kind of inventory. Much more valuable to the collection plans were other facts that Spjut produced. He reiterated that *Taxus brevifolia* was not regarded as having commercial value but that the Forest Service regularly issued permits to locals to cut down the trees for use as fence posts. The price of the permit was twenty cents per tree. Spjut also repeated the fact that the bark could be removed easily from the stem during the spring and summer months when the sap was running.

One of the people Spjut turned to for information about *Taxus brevifolia* was Chuck Edson, a plant supplier from Corvallis, with whom Spjut had been in touch for several years concerning the possibility of collecting plants in the area.[27] Acting on Perdue's suggestion, Spjut asked Edson in early in July to prepare a comprehensive report on *Taxus brevifolia* in Oregon.[28] That report arrived on Perdue's desk about a month later.

In drawing up the report, Edson's main question was whether and how a collection of 7,000 pounds of bark could be handled.[29] His best estimate was that between 2,000 and 3,000 trees would need to have their bark removed to meet the target amount. Edson was in no doubt that such a number of trees could be found in the three National Forests he had surveyed in Oregon. As to the question of how the collection should be made, Edson recommended a broad approach, using as many procedures as possible, including loggers, the Forest Service, fencepost harvesters and plant suppliers, such as himself. Areas that were scheduled to be logged should be targeted as a priority for collection. According to Forest Service sources, many of the trees were wasted during logging operations to harvest other trees. It was important to get into these logging areas before or soon after operations ended because, according to Edson, within the first year after logging, the bark adhered so much to the wood that its removal was impossible.

However the collection was to be made, Edson pointed to two potential problems. One of these, although Edson didn't think it particularly serious, was the possibility of 'contaminating' the collection with bark of other species, inadvertently or intentionally. The second and more serious problem was that no one National Forest district would be able to meet the entire supply. The collection would need to be made from all districts: he recommended what the distribution should be. This was not because of the lack of trees in any one district. Rather it was because of concern about the environmental impact of removing trees from their habitat. Two groups were voicing such concerns. On the one hand, there were the District Rangers who were expressing concern about the possible loss of wildlife cover caused by the removal of *Taxus brevifolia* in their district. In the Ashland District of the Rogue River National Forest in southern Oregon, for example, Edson encountered such a view. The point was that even though *Taxus brevifolia* was considered a 'trash' tree and his district had enough trees to meet the collection need, the Timber Sales Officer did not want to have the whole collection taken from his patch. Edson did not personally meet or speak to representatives of the second group expressing concern. His information came solely from Forest Service personnel. They advised Edson that there were groups in their vicinity who might react to the proposed collection. One of these was called 'Save the Yew Foundation' and the other 'Hoedads'. That was about all he could find out, except that Jerry Rust, a Commissioner of Lane County, Eugene, Oregon, was a representative of one or both of these groups. Edson was warned 'not to stir them up'.[30] We will return to the environmental issue later.

At the beginning of August, before receiving Edson's report, Perdue prepared an open letter to Forest Service personnel in the Pacific Northwest informing them of the renewed interest in *Taxus brevifolia*.[31] Perdue played his 'cancer' card again. The letter explained why taxol and *Taxus brevifolia* were both back in the picture after years of silence. He emphasized the urgent need for 7,000 pounds of bark, requesting information about areas abundant in *Taxus brevifolia* and inviting bids to supply bark in amounts of at least 500 pounds. The deadline for delivery was set at 31 August 1978, just over a year later.

Spjut, it turned out, was making his own inquiries about *Taxus brevifolia* in Oregon, Washington and Montana, using Forest Service personnel as his informants.[32] His information, mostly anecdotal, added little to what was already known. He concluded that the procurement of 7,000 pounds of bark could be accomplished from Forest Service lands in Oregon and Washington. The only question was how to do the practical work: whether to let the Forest Service do it and transfer funds to them, or to ask for bids from small outfits.

Just before Perdue's letter was ready to be sent, Matthew Suffness produced new estimates of his need, based on new information from the NCI investigators as well as estimates from Boettner on the amount of taxol he would be able to isolate from the crude extract. This resulted in a revised figure of 5,000 pounds of bark.[33] Perdue received the information just before his departure to Seattle to meet forestry officials in Washington and Oregon.[34] Also scheduled was a meeting with Edson in Corvallis and a remarkable tree in the Ashland District. Spjut's ideas about using the Forest Service to do the collecting turned out to be impossible as Federal regulations prevented the USDA receiving funds from the NCI and transferring them to the Forest Service.[35]

Because of budgetary difficulties, Perdue did not get around to the matter of the collection until the end of October. Perdue wrote a new letter, enclosing with it specifications for collecting yew bark.[36] Both the letter and the enclosure were sent to all the appropriate Forest Service personnel for their approval before sending the specifications to potential collectors. The letter outlined taxol's preclinical profile. It also repeated a point that Perdue had made in other communiqués to the Forest Service as well as to the NCI; namely, that going to the forest was a short-term expediency. As he put it: 'Our best source for the present is bark of the Pacific yew, *Taxus brevifolia*; however, it does occur in ornamental varieties of Chinese, Japanese and English yews. If taxol becomes a useful drug, ultimately we should be able to grow one of these as a source.'[37] The invitations to potential suppliers to submit bids were not sent out until the end of January 1978.

Perdue decided to take the advice he had received from Edson and Spjut. The letter of invitation was sent to a large number of individuals whose names had been supplied by Forest Service officials. Other invitations to bid were sent to District Rangers who were asked to pass on the enclosures to reliable individuals. Perdue heeded Edson's advice about taking bark over a wide area; he had already followed such a policy in the last collection in 1967. Each District Ranger was informed that the procurement was being organized to avoid collecting too much bark in any one area.[38] In one important respect, however, Perdue did something he had never done before with taxol. Included in the specifications was a fact sheet about taxol, informing potential suppliers that they were collecting *Taxus brevifolia* because it was the best source of this potential anti-cancer compound. With this, Perdue made taxol and *Taxus brevifolia* and their association with cancer public knowledge.[39]

Perdue had already received 1,000 pounds of bark from Robert Warner, an Oregon fencepost maker he had contacted in July. He needed collections amounting to 4,000 pounds. Bids were accepted in lots of 500–4,000 pounds. Several invitees complained that there was not enough time given to complete the collection. Perdue agreed to have it changed: 15 June 1978 was the deadline for bids and 31 August 1978 for delivery of bark.

Perdue knew that, however efficiently the procurement proceeded, it was inherently flawed.[40] One reason was that being a Federal agency, the USDA could not advertise for suppliers in the way commercial firms could. Everything was done at a distance. The Forest Service was happy to help within the terms of their own operations but they were not going to do the collections themselves. They could only supply names. Another reason was that the collections were not supervised locally. They were simply made, bagged up and sent to the Medicinal Plant Resources Laboratory at the USDA in Beltsville, on the outskirts of Washington, DC. The supplier with the lowest bid was offered the contract. There was no quality control. Upward of thirty suppliers responded with a bid, ranging from $1.60 to $30.00 per pound.[41]

The contract for this collection went to Vern Struck and his partner Gene Williams from Medford, in southern Oregon.[42] They supplied the Medicinal Plant Resources Laboratory with at least 4,000 pounds of bark.[43] Struck and Williams heard about the bid from Forest Service personnel when they sought permits to cut yew to make fenceposts. In the event, they were denied the permits. Instead, they contacted officials from the Bureau of Land Management from whom they received permission to cut trees on property under the agency's management. The work was hard. The cut logs had to be dragged out of the forest as the Bureau of Land Management did not allow them to drive their vehicles in. Struck and Williams hired three more workers and a specialist peeler to help them. With a yield of about three pounds of bark per tree, the 4,000-pound delivery meant cutting down more than 1,000 *Taxus brevifolia* in this one corner of the state. Their shipments reached the Medicinal Plant Resources Laboratory by the deadline of late August.

Robert Perdue, as we saw in Chapter 1, was reassigned to other duties as Chief of the Plant Taxonomy Laboratory, on 7 May 1978. Arthur Barclay assumed full responsibility for the plant procurement project which remained in the Medicinal Plant Resources Laboratory. Perdue's last involvement with *Taxus brevifolia* was in January 1978 just before he left for a plant exploration trip. When he returned in May, he was informed of the changes that had taken place. As a coincidence, Barclay, the first collector of *Taxus brevifolia*, also took delivery of the largest collection to date. During the summer of 1978, bark began to arrive at the USDA in substantial quantities. By the end of the summer, the total delivery, at 8,524 pounds, was double what had originally been ordered.[44] As it turned out, this was the last time that Barclay would have anything to do with taxol and *Taxus brevifolia*. Barclay left the service in 1980 because of illness.

Perdue's frequent suggestions to think about supply in the long-term by using the cultivated varieties available in large numbers commercially in the United States fell on deaf ears. With his departure in 1978, the possibilities of using a cultivated and renewable rather than wild resource received a setback. There is no evidence that Barclay attempted to revive it. Certainly no initiative in this direction came from the NCI. They were stuck on *Taxus brevifolia* bark and seemed oblivious to the political changes occurring around them.

The forest in 1977 was different from how it had been a decade earlier. It had become a site of political change defined in local as well as national terms. Barclay was made aware of changes in the local milieu when he received several telephone calls from Jerry Rust, the Lane County Commissioner to whom Edson had drawn attention in his August 1977 report on *Taxus brevifolia*.[45] Rust identified himself as the leader of the 'Save the Yew Foundation' and voiced serious concern about the plight of the yew in the forthcoming procurement. He suggested that the procurement should focus on areas scheduled to be logged and already felled trees.

Rust had run for Lane County Commissioner in 1976. One of his main campaign themes was the 'lunacy of waste' and one of his main examples was yew trees.[46] To make the point, he made campaign buttons from yew trees that were taken from slash-piles in western Oregon. According to Hal Hartzell, Rust's friend and colleague, they were first made aware of the fate of *Taxus brevifolia* while working on slash-piling in the summer of 1974 on a contract for Hoedads, a reforestation workers' co-operative in western Oregon.[47] Slash-piling was a crucial part of logging. The slash, the debris left over from a cut, was stacked into piles about four or five feet high and covered with sheets of black plastic. The slash-piles are made in the summer and burned in the winter. The main reason for slash-piling is to reduce the amount of wood debris left on the forest floor in order to reduce the risk of forest fires and to make replanting easier. Hartzell and Rust both noticed that many yew logs were left on the forest floor to be burned in a slash-pile: many were more than 500 years old.[48] As Hartzell wrote: 'For us, the yew became a real and tangible symbol for the lunacy of waste.'[49]

By the time of the 1977 collection, Rust's and Hartzell's attachment to *Taxus brevifolia*, expressed through the name 'Save the Yew Foundation', was adding a new and potentially countervailing meaning to the species. To the timber industry and Forest Service's labelling of *Taxus brevifolia* as a trash species, together with the NCI's utilitarian meaning of

Taxus brevifolia as a source of a particular compound, was now added a non-instrumental meaning as the living thing for itself. The insistence on thinking about *Taxus brevifolia* as a living species was underlined by Rust when he implored Barclay to peel bark only from felled trees and those that were growing in timber units scheduled for logging.

Barclay's options were, however, constrained. As Edson reported, it was impossible to peel bark from *Taxus brevifolia* later than two to four weeks after it had been felled.[50] This was a small window of opportunity. To use dead trees as a source for bark depended on good timing on the part of the collector. The same held true for land scheduled to be clear cut. Access to it also depended on the goodwill of the forest officials.

Rust's challenge to Barclay was, apparently, one of several he made to Forest Service officials and the senate of the State of Oregon.[51] While Rust focused specifically and purposefully on *Taxus brevifolia* as a species requiring protection, the issue of environmental impact was raised by others who were in touch with the USDA. Edson, for example, was keenly aware of the need to think in terms of environmental impact in sourcing *Taxus brevifolia* for taxol.[52] He hoped that bark from trees long felled would prove active, therefore alleviating the need at this level of collection for felling live trees. The possibility of doing this, as we have seen, never materialized because of the difficulty of removing the bark. V.H. Madis, head of Madis Laboratories, with whom Polysciences had a contract for large-scale extraction and isolation, also referred to the possible environmental problems associated with peeling bark. He inquired into the likelihood of twigs and needles as a source for taxol.[53]

Both Edson and Madis's concerns about environmental impact should be seen in the wider context of the raising of an environmental consciousness in the United States during the 1960s, shifting ideologies and practices from what Samuel Hays has termed, 'conservation to environmentalism'.[54] There were various aspects to this shift. In part, it was reflected in and stirred up by the publication of several key books that drew the attention of Americans to the negative and ignored elements of the post-war economic boom. For example, Rachel Carson pointed to pollution by agrochemicals; and Raymond Dasman to the destruction of the forests of California. The government passed several key acts designed to provide a framework for protecting the environment. The most important of these were: the National Environmental Policy Act of 1969; the Endangered Species Act of 1973; the National Forest Management Act of 1976; and the Federal Land Policy and Management Act of 1976. Finally, citizen participation action groups were formed to channel protest. The year 1967 saw the founding of the

Environmental Defense Fund; Friends of the Earth was organized in 1969; and the first 'Earth Day' was celebrated on 22 April 1970.

The environmental movement of the 1960s and 1970s ventured into many sites and came into conflict with many different individuals and interests. The forest was no exception. The passage of the National Forest Management Act, directed at the Forest Service, and the Federal Land Policy and Management Act, directed at the Bureau of Land Management, was largely a response to protests against clearcutting practices in Montana and West Virginia. Through these actions, both grassroots and policy, the forest became a site of political conflict. At the same time, and from another direction, the forests of the Pacific Northwest became subjected to a radical scientific analysis, while they were being destroyed.

The 1978 collection occurred in a different context from the one a decade before. Though the forest yielded more than 8,000 pounds of yew bark, there was clear evidence that life was getting more complicated. Partly this was the result of procuring such a large quantity of material; but it was equally the result of changing perceptions of the forest and how it should be managed. Yet it is important not to make too much of the environmental opposition for, at that time, it was very small and diffused. It would take the analysis of old-growth forests together with the speed at which they were disappearing to politicize the forest to the extent that it could not be taken for granted. That would not happen until the following decade.

Back in Warrington, Pennsylvania, Fred Boettner was isolating taxol from the remaining volume of crude extract that he had inherited from Monsanto. Once he had completed his isolation of the first ten grams of taxol and delivered it to the NCI in September 1977, Boettner set straight to work to isolate the rest of the extract. He did it quickly but the results, in terms of the yield of taxol, were not as good as the previous work. The yield had fallen from 0.52 per cent to 0.41 per cent.[55] The remaining volume of crude extract – 24 kilograms – produced only 100 grams of taxol. The NCI took delivery of this batch on 18 March 1978.

The first scaled-up industrially manufactured taxol arrived at the NCI fifteen years after Barclay collected the first sample of *Taxus brevifolia* bark. Once it was in the hands of the NCI in sufficient and secure amounts, taxol could begin to circulate to other sites of research. This was normal practice for all potential anti-cancer compounds. Occupying a central position in cancer research, the NCI subcontracted laboratories to find out about the compounds that it had helped develop, although it also had a Laboratory of Chemical Pharmacology in the Division of Cancer Treatment that did some of this work.

One of the first extramural researchers to receive taxol was Susan Horwitz, a molecular pharmacologist at the Albert Einstein College of Medicine in New York. By the time she received her first consignments of taxol in June and October 1977, Horwitz was already familiar with the biochemistry of natural products, particularly those that had shown cytotoxic and/or antitumour activity. Her chief interest was in investigating the mechanism of biological activity of these compounds. By 1977, she had already worked with colchicine, podophyllotoxin, camptothecin, vinblastine, and bruceantin, and was engaged in a study of steganacin.[56] She was, therefore, familiar with the plant programme and with its chief contract chemists, Monroe Wall and Morris Kupchan.

The biological activity of most antitumour compounds resides in their ability to interact with and cause irreparable damage to DNA or to inhibit specific enzymes.[57] There is, however, a group of compounds that repress tumour growth by inhibiting mitosis or cell division. These compounds are typically referred to as antimitotic.[58] Most are natural products derived from plants.[59]

The systematic investigation of antimitotic compounds began in the 1930s with colchicine in the pathology laboratory at the University of Brussels, headed by Albert Dustin.[60] This was the first plant compound known to have such effects on cells. While it was clear that colchicine inhibited mitosis, the precise mechanism of action remained unknown. This state of affairs continued until the 1960s when key discoveries about the nature of mitosis were made. One of these was the discovery of microtubules, tube-like organelles (structural and functional units) in the cell. With the help of the electron microscope and a new fixation agent, microtubules were first observed during mitosis. During the process of cell division, microtubules begin to form at both ends of the cell as well as from the cell's chromosomes. The microtubules create a kind of skeleton within the cell, rather like scaffolding in a building. As the microtubules first elongate and then shorten, they pull with them to each pole of the cell the separated chromosomes. At the same time, the cell walls begin to converge and the microtubules at the centre of the convergence start to disassemble. The cell splits and the microtubules disappear in a process termed depolymerization.

This was all known by the end of the 1960s.[61] What was also known was that colchicine inhibited mitosis by binding to the microtubules themselves and disrupting their formation. Colchicine did this by binding tightly and specifically to a protein, named tubulin, the protein from which microtubules were made.[62] The process by which tubulin is turned into microtubules is called polymerization; the binding of colchicine to tubulin inhibits polymerization leading to the arrest of cell division. These insights resulted in colchicine becoming a standard item in cell biology laboratories by the 1960s. It was indispensable in the study of cellular motion for the simple reason that if in the presence of colchicine a particular function seemed to be disrupted, the chances were that microtubules were involved at some stage. Colchicine also became the standard by which the mitotic effects of other compounds could be evaluated. By the end of the 1960s, it was well known among cell biologists that the vinca alkaloids and podophyllotoxin behaved similarly to colchicine.[63] The link between plant-derived anti-cancer drugs, mitotic arrest and microtubule disruption was firmly made: the plant-derived anti-cancer drugs worked by stopping cell division, which they did by inhibiting the formation of microtubules from tubulin.

In 1972, Morris Kupchan and co-workers at the University of Virginia, under contract from the NCI, isolated a compound they called maytansine from various species of the plant *Maytenus*, growing in East Africa.[64] At the time, this was the hottest compound at the NCI. In 1975, just three years after its isolation, an INDA was filed for maytansine as a clinical candidate.[65] That same year, Kupchan, together with another chemist and two biologists, announced that maytansine was an antimitotic compound, inhibiting the polymerization of tubulin, as did colchicine and vincristine.[66] The following year, a group at the NCI supported these conclusions and reported that maytansine bound to tubulin at the same site as did vincristine.[67] Though the yield of maytansine from the plant material was very low – 0.0002 per cent – the treatment dose was in terms of milligrams.[68] Maytansine was entered for Phase I trials in 1975 and Phase II trials in 1977.[69] It was the only compound discovered in the plant screening programme in Phase II trials at the time.[70] There was great excitement about its possibilities.

Horwitz's work with plant compounds during the 1970s needs to be seen against the background of the huge interest in and potential of maytansine at the same time as the flurry of activity in understanding microtubules and their cellular function. Her work on podophyllotoxin beginning in 1975 focused on the effect of this compound on microtubule assembly in HeLa cells.[71] It is not surprising therefore that she should have been invited to investigate the mechanism of action of taxol in 1977.[72] She was not, however, the only researcher concerned with this problem. David Fuchs, a researcher in the Laboratory of Chemical Pharmacology in the Division of Cancer Treatment at the NCI, began to work with taxol in June 1977 just two months after it had been accepted for development at Stage 2A.[73] He soon teamed up with Randall Johnson, also of the Division of Cancer Treatment and together they published the first study of taxol's mechanism of action. Fuchs and Johnson chose to investigate taxol's cellular effects by inoculating mice that had previously been injected with P388 leukaemia. What they discovered was that taxol was indeed an antimitotic compound but that it was 'less efficient than other mitotic spindle poisons in producing mitotic arrest'.[74] The comparison was made with maytansine and the vinca alkaloids.

In the context of its time of publication, the message of the report was ambiguous. On the one hand, it added a significant piece of information to taxol's profile. Fuchs and Johnson had shown taxol to arrest mitosis and had thereby revealed another natural product with this unusual property. On the other hand, because it seemed to act like maytansine and the vinca alkaloids but without their potency, it was not such a hot compound. What was hot and what was not mattered at the NCI. The competition for resources was acute. Cases had to be made for compounds to pass through the various stages of the decision network. It was not simply a matter of objectively weighing technical data. It was also a matter of persuading members of the Decision Network Committee that they should put their trust in a particular compound and in the compound's sponsor – it was common practice for the Committee to appoint a member of staff to act as the compound's advocate, 'to provide the impetus for sustained development of the drug'.[75] Being no better than maytansine and the vinca alkaloids did taxol no good. Moreover, because they were voices from within the NCI, Fuchs and Johnson gave institutional weight to their conclusions.

In a climate of competing claims for fixed resources, it would not have been surprising if taxol had been dropped from further development. But this did not happen, although the reason for it is not known. At any rate, Susan Horwitz and her workers were considering taxol's mechanism of action at about the same time as Fuchs and Johnson were. Moreover, almost coincidentally with Fuchs and Johnson submitting their report for publication, Horwitz and colleagues were announcing at an annual symposium on molecular and cellular biology some preliminary results from their research. They too observed mitotic arrest in the presence of taxol and were able to suggest that it occurred in the metaphase, that is, the stage of cell division when the microtubules are elongated. But they went one step further than Fuchs and Johnson. They reported that in the presence of taxol microtubules could not be induced to depolymerize.[76]

This was a remarkable find because it suggested taxol did not behave like the other antimitotic compounds that inhibited polymerization.[77] Having worked, at one time or another, with most of the other antimitotic plant compounds, Horwitz realized she had a winner on her hands. There is no exaggerating the importance of this find. Taxol worked in a quite different way from the other antimitotic compounds, by promoting not inhibiting polymerization. It had, therefore, a unique mechanism of action and might be the first in a new range of compounds with this property. This was far more important than its level of activity relative to other compounds. If it were to be first in a new range, other compounds might be found with greater activity. This is precisely what Robert Perdue and Jonathan Hartwell wanted from the plant screening programme – the identification of compounds with new structures and mechanisms of action. Their insistence on this point had finally borne fruit.

In April 1978, one month after the preliminary results were announced at the symposium, Susan Horwitz asked the NCI for a twenty-five-milligram supply of taxol; in June she asked for a further 100 milligrams.[78] With this amount, Horwitz's team returned to dig deeper into the cell's behaviour when it was treated with taxol. They were able to reproduce their earlier results and, at the same time, confidently proclaim that they had found an antimitotic compound with a unique mechanism of action. In the laboratory at the Albert Einstein College of Medicine they were able to show that cells treated with taxol looked and behaved differently from cells treated with other antimitotic compounds. Taxol promoted microtubule assembly, the opposite of other antimitotic compounds. Indeed, it seemed to act in a similar way to tubulin itself as, in the presence of taxol, the critical concentration of tubulin necessary for microtubule assembly was substantially decreased. Once again, the microtubules did not depolymerize when bathed in cold water, as they were expected to do. In other words, taxol was stabilizing the microtubules, paralysing the polymerization–depolymerization process. Division of the cell could not occur. The group published these remarkable results in *Nature* early in 1979.[79]

Fuchs and Johnson's article appeared late in 1978; Horwitz and her colleagues published theirs five months later. It is important to understand that the two groups were writing for different scientific audiences. Put simply, the former was written for cancer researchers while the latter was aimed at biologists. The titles of the two pieces make this point quite explicitly: Fuchs and Johnson refer to taxol as an anti-cancer agent, first and foremost, while Horwitz and colleagues refer to microtubule assembly.

There are moments in science when a particular piece of knowledge has enormous ramifications within a particular practice. This was the case with taxol at this time.[80] Cell biologists swarmed to taxol as they realized that they had a new biochemical tool on their hands to study cell dynamics, to complement the depolymerizing agents such as colchicine.[81] The NCI was flooded with requests for taxol. The number of individual requests increased in the following fashion: 40 in 1979; 78 in 1980; 154 in 1981; and 219 in 1982.[82] Publications also mushroomed. Before the paper by Horwitz and colleagues, only three articles had been published in which taxol was even mentioned. In 1980 and 1981, the number of publications dealing with taxol and microtubules reached seven and grew to 62 during 1982 and 1983.[83] Not only did cell biology benefit from the appearance of taxol, so did physiology. Soon after Horwitz's paper, Steve Heidemann and Peter Gallas of Michigan State University showed that taxol's microtubule activity *in vitro* was similar *in vivo*.[84]

For all the excitement in the cell biology community, taxol's unique mechanism of action was not a decisive factor in its progression through the linear array. Mechanism of action was not one of the stops along the way. Indeed, in general, how a compound worked was of less interest than whether it worked. For example, the INDA for indicine-*N*-oxide, an antitumour compound isolated in 1976, was filed in 1978 but its mechanism of action was still unclear many years later.[85] This was as true of antitumour compounds as it was for other drugs. The introduction of the sulpha drugs in the 1930s and penicillin after World War II happened long before it was understood why these compounds were effective in specific therapeutic areas. On the other hand, it was certainly easier to make a case for a compound that was attracting a great deal of interest in the scientific community, many of whom were receiving grants from the NCI. Given that the decision to go ahead with or drop a compound often rested on the amount of interest it attracted, or its novel structure or activity, anything that set it apart from the pack could be crucial.[86] In this sense, and as others have argued, Horwitz's paper was critical.[87]

Yet as far as the NCI was concerned, if a compound was not highly active in at least one tumour model, it had little chance of progressing, whatever its mechanism of action.[88] As we have seen, it was the B16 melanoma results that brought taxol from a marginal position to that of a potential development candidate. In 1976, in addition to the B16 melanoma, the NCI also introduced new antitumour models that, it was hoped, would more accurately predict responses in human cancers. These models, called xenografts, were human tumours implanted into specially bred mice whose thymus gland was non-functional – such mice were referred to as athymic or nude, because the genetic defect that caused athymia also caused hairlessness. This deficiency also caused immunosuppression: in principle, therefore, the mice would not reject a transplanted human tumour. Experiments in the transplantation of human tumours into non-athymic mice had been going on since the 1960s but without much success. A chance mutation of a mouse from inbred stock in 1965 in the Viral Laboratory of the Ruchill Hospital in Glasgow had aroused interest at the Institute of Animal Genetics in Edinburgh because of the animal's hairlessness. Investigation of the phenomenon led to the conclusion that the mouse had a recessive gene responsible for its lack of hair.[89] Though the mouse died, selective breeding produced nude animals that formed the basis of a nude stock. Further investigation of the nude mouse in 1967 at the University of Strathclyde in Glasgow showed that it lacked a thymus and that, by implication, its immune system was highly defective.[90] One year later, a group in Denmark showed experimentally that it was possible to transplant human tumours into the nude mouse.[91]

The road from an experimental demonstration of xenografts in athymic mice to their incorporation within a large-scale screening programme was tortuous. The absence of an immune system was a two-edged sword: it meant that the mouse would not reject human tissue, but it also meant that the animal was prone to widespread infections. The degree and extent of sterilization needed to keep the animals pathogen-free was considerable and this had a marked impact on the costs of producing and maintaining a stock of experimental animals.[92] These were problems on the supply side. Other issues and problems concerned the question of the behaviour of the xenograft compared with that of the tumour in a human. Two important issues were metastases and the kinetics of growth. Metastatic behaviour in the xenograft seemed erratic.[93] Tumours did not seem to grow as slowly in the athymic mouse as they did in humans.[94] Despite these problems, the NCI launched into a full-scale programme to ensure an adequate supply of mice and to select the 'best' tumours to be implanted.[95] The concern that many compounds selected on the basis of earlier screens did not show clinical activity while the chemotherapy of human solid tumours lagged far behind that of leukaemias and lymphomas, overrode that of the problems in xenografts.

The tumours were chosen for implantation on the basis that they represented the major types of cancer then in evidence in the United States. The tumours included a colon tumour from a forty-four-year-old woman, called CX-1; a lung carcinoma from a forty-eight-year-old man, called LX-1; and a primary breast tumour from a twenty-nine-year-old woman, called MX-1.[96] One of the questions that interested researchers in the Division of Cancer Treatment and the Drug Evaluation Branch was the relationship between activity in a murine tumour model and in a human xenograft model. Because taxol had shown activity in B16, it was chosen as a compound to be tested in the new xenograft models.[97]

The test against the colon xenograft, CX-1, was conducted in November 1978 and showed that taxol inhibited tumour growth but did not cause regression. These results were obtained in 1980.[98] The test against the lung xenograft, LX-1, took place in January 1979 with results very similar to that of the CX-1 test: these were confirmed in August 1980. These results were not impressive but in a sense that did not matter, for in November 1978 and confirmed one month later, taxol showed the ability to cause considerable regression in the mammary xenograft, MX-1.

By the beginning of 1979 and on the basis of its activity in the NCI screens, taxol had met the criteria for further development. It is important to understand that the status of a compound at the NCI was based on the interpretation of the screening data. Taxol had an activity profile less impressive than many compounds – maytansine and ellipticine, for example – but more impressive than a few others – thalicarpine, for example.[99] Some of these compounds had already progressed to clinical trials, whether they were more or less active than taxol.[100] The point is that what earmarked a compound for special notice was particular, rather than general activity.[101] On that basis, a case could be made that it might be selective, hopefully, against a particular cancer type. This was precisely the case with taxol. The activity against B16 melanoma and against MX-1 had two messages, both of which the NCI was receptive to in the late 1970s, when seen in the context of the reorganization of the model systems to screen for slow-growing tumours and the shift away from the dominant leukaemia paradigm. These were: (i) that taxol showed activity against two difficult tumours, and (ii) that these were the slow-growing varieties that the NCI was specifically trying to target. For once, taxol's strengths were timely.

Activity looked good but a potentially devastating problem had arisen. Coincidentally, as news of taxol's unique mechanism of action was coming out of Susan Horwitz's laboratory in New York, taxol was experiencing difficult formulation problems. As discussed earlier, the decision network consisted of certain critical stages in the process of drug development. Formulation was one of these critical stages. Whatever a compound's experimental activity, if it could not be added to a medium to be administered clinically, then it was dropped as a development candidate. Taxol was virtually insoluble in water.[102] In other aqueous solutions and organic solvents the solubility was not much better, and even when it was in solution taxol easily precipitated out. There were two exceptions to this profile. One was a formulation based on polyethylene glycol. Unfortunately, in this formulation, taxol was both more toxic and less active against B16 than the compound alone. When these facts were presented to the decision network in August 1979, there was a strong possibility that taxol would go no further.[103] Another formulation was tried, based on polyoxyethylated castor oil (Cremophor EL). This appeared to work and, in June 1980, it proved to be active against B16.[104] The Cremophor formulation was presented to the decision network for the intravenous administration of taxol in human trials. In October 1980, taxol passed Decision Network stage 2B and was sent for toxicology studies.

The substantial interest shown by cell biologists in taxol as a biochemical tool resulted, as we have seen, in a rush for samples of the new compound. Though the number of such requests was large and growing, it did not translate into an overwhelming demand. Figures suggest that in the wake of Horwitz's publication of the mechanism of action of taxol, demand for the compound for 1979 was twenty-five grams or less than a quarter of the total manufacture from Polysciences.[105] Formulation studies took the lion's share.

Fred Boettner, it will be recalled, received a delivery of more than 8,500 pounds of bark at the end of the summer of 1978, representing the collection that was put out to tender in January of that year. In November 1979, Boettner sent 145 grams of taxol to the NCI.[106] As Boettner pointed out to the NCI, the yield from this batch of bark was less than one-third what he expected. Boettner suggested that the large amount of woody material in two big collections was to blame. What he did not know was that the bark had been stripped by machine.[107] It was a crude operation. Nearly ninety per cent of the delivery contained more wood than bark.[108]

This experience demonstrated, once again, the precarious nature of collecting from afar. There is no doubt that collecting *Taxus brevifolia* presented problems, which increased with the size of the collections. Despite Boettner's setback with the 1978 collection, the scale-up procedure was working. It was possible to convert large amounts of bark into taxol. Bark was also the most active part of the tree. The data to support this assertion were reviewed again in 1980.[109] But the data also revealed, and not for the first time, that the needles were consistently active.

By 1980, formulation problems were using up taxol at a far greater rate than predicted. These, together with the increased demand for taxol from cell biologists and the lower than expected yield from the previous collection, meant that a further collection would be needed. It was time to return to the forest. To satisfy toxicology studies and the scientific community, the collection would need to be about 20,000 pounds.[110] This produced anxiety at the USDA.

James Duke, the head of the Economic Botany Laboratory, voiced this concern. What bothered him was not logistical problems but the issue of renewability.[111] He felt that procuring seeds might make for a renewable resource. Suffness informed him that *Taxus brevifolia* seeds had never been screened for activity but that seeds from *Taxus baccata* were marginally active.[112] Nothing more was heard about seeds as an alternative to bark. Suffness, however, did not ignore the ambiguous data for the activity of needles. He asked Duke to procure 200 pounds of needles in the summer of 1980. The amount was collected in Oregon several months later. Boettner received the delivery soon thereafter and, within a little time, was able to report back to Suffness on the results. Suffness, in turn, reported back to Duke that 'the content of taxol [in *Taxus* needles] is only 1/2–1/3 that of the stem bark'.[113] Once again, Suffness appealed to an economic argument: 'Since the cost is the same for plant material and since it will require two to three times as much plant material as well as a large increase in materials costs in the pilot plant, we do not want to get leaves [needles] unless we are unable to get stem bark.'[114] No mention was made of renewability. Needles were dropped from further consideration.

On 15 December 1980, the USDA asked for bids to supply *Taxus brevifolia* bark in lots from 500 to 10,000 pounds by September 1981.[115] The invitation to bid was sent directly to thirteen individuals in Oregon and Washington. Many of those on the list had already done business with the USDA in collecting material. The strategy for accepting bids was based on the need to spread out the collection, to avoid concentrating on any one area, and to choose those areas where 'yew is so abundant that the local forest office grants permission to cut it for fence posts and/or firewood'.[116] Only two bids were accepted. One of them was from Robert Warner, a collector who was in the fencepost business and had done some collecting in the summer of 1977. Though Warner's price was slightly above the minimum, he clearly impressed the USDA because of his local knowledge. He understood the need to collect widely. At the same time, he was able to report that the west coast of southern Oregon had an abundant supply of *Taxus brevifolia*: he was confident that he could collect the entire amount.[117] We have no detailed information on this collection. All we know is that part of it, about 3,000 pounds, was completed by autumn 1981.[118] The collectors contracted directly with the NCI even though they delivered the material to the USDA. Fred Boettner took delivery in October 1981. In order to speed up the isolation work, the bark was sent off to Dr Madis Laboratories, a large facility in New Jersey for the extraction of medicinal plants, and a subcontractor for Polysciences. The 3,366 pounds of *Taxus brevifolia* bark returned in January 1982 as 890 pounds of extract. The isolation process was highly successful this time, modifying the technology and achieving better yields in less time. In June of 1982, the NCI received 234 grams of taxol; in October they received the remaining thirty grams. All together, Boettner had managed to get a yield of 0.017 per cent.[119]

The same month as he sent pure taxol to the NCI, Boettner received just under 16,000 pounds of *Taxus brevifolia* bark, the single largest delivery to date.[120] This represented collections made in late spring and summer of 1982, using the same two collectors as in the previous year. Boettner received no instructions as to what to do with the collection. It was to sit on the factory floor for almost one year.[121]

As it turned out, much happened in the time gap between the delivery of the bark to Polysciences in October 1981 and the delivery of the smaller production of taxol to the NCI in October 1982. One momentous event occurred on 2 October 1981 when the Board of Scientific Counselors of the Division of Cancer Treatment brought an end to the NCI–USDA plant screening programme. The USDA would, therefore, no longer be involved in any kind of plant procurement for the NCI and would not even be asked to complete the outstanding part of the present collection.

The termination of the interagency agreement had two major implications. First, it meant that plants were no longer to be screened as potential anti-cancer agents. Second, those plants that were already in the process of evaluation would continue their way through the linear array of the Division of Cancer Treatment, but the NCI alone would be responsible for the procuring of the material as and when it was necessary. In this, they had no experience whatsoever.

Another important event that took place in the intervening period was that John Douros left his position as the Chief of the NCI's Natural Products Branch in 1982 and took up a new position at Bristol-Myers, the pharmaceutical and general health care company, in Syracuse, New York. Soon after he got there, he requested one gram of taxol for Bristol Laboratories.[122] Matthew Suffness was promoted to Douros's position.

The final significant event in this period took place in June 1982 when toxicology studies were completed. The results of this stage were good for taxol. Toxicity in laboratory animals depended critically on schedule and dosage and on the Cremophor vehicle.[123] When the toxicology results were presented to the Decision Network 3 meeting in November 1982, it was decided then that various schedules and dosages would be tried in the clinical setting.[124] Taxol passed Decision Network 3 in November, approving taxol for an INDA, the granting of which would initiate clinical trials.

These were all events with immediate effects, but two other events occurred that went largely unnoticed at the time but would have profound ramifications in the future. They both happened in 1981. These were the publication of research in France on the semi-synthesis of taxol from renewable parts of *Taxus baccata*; and the first serious report on the ecology of the old-growth forest in the Pacific Northwest.

Pierre Potier headed the Institut de Chimie des Substances Naturelles (ICSN) of the Centre National de la Recherche Scientifique (CNRS).[125] He had extensive experience in the field of natural products chemistry. He was also interested in potential anti-cancer agents and had been working on the synthesis of other antimitotic compounds. In 1979, as a result of the excitement generated by Susan Horwitz's publication of taxol's unique mechanism of action, he decided to look at taxol himself. He identified the main problem with taxol as a potential drug as one of yield, stimulating his curiosity about possible alternative sources.[126] His research centre was situated in a park (also owned by CNRS) full of *Taxus baccata*, but, as Potier knew from Wall and Wani's 1971 publication, taxol was present in this species only in minute quantities. Potier thought it was possible he could find another substance in *Taxus baccata* needles that might act as a precursor for the synthesis of taxol and new compounds related to taxol that might have anti-cancer properties. In 1980, ICSN signed a collaborative agreement with the chemical and pharmaceutical company Rhône-Poulenc, to explore the chemistry of taxoids, to build structure–activity relationships, and to seek new and patentable anti-cancer compounds.[127]

An important difference between the research carried out in the United States and at Potier's laboratory was that while the Americans looked at the cytotoxic and antitumour activity of extracts from plants they collected using various *in vitro* and *in vivo* screens, the French group looked at the activity of the extracts on tubulin itself, because they had identified that as the biological target. Potier's group developed an assay to measure the inhibition of polymerization or depolymerization of tubulin, based on Shelanski's method.[128] This approach shortened the time for pharmacological testing on *in vivo* and *in vitro* preparations, and required fewer animal experiments: animal screens were used only for the compounds that had successfully passed the tubulin test. Potier's group used this technique on an extract made from the needles of *Taxus baccata*. The extract was found to have some activity on inhibiting the depolymerization of tubulin. Using the tubulin assay to guide the fractionation, the researchers isolated the major constituent of the extract, 10-deacetylbaccatin III (10-DAB) (see Figure 3.2) as well as a number of other compounds. 10-DAB was present in substantial concentration and easy to isolate. The yield was much higher than that of taxol: 0.5–1.0 grams per kilogram of fresh needles, compared with (their own) yield of 100–150 milligrams of taxol from a kilogram of dried bark.[129]

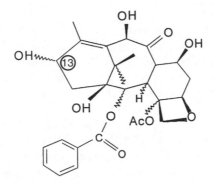

Figure 3.2 10-DAB (10-deacetylbaccatin III).

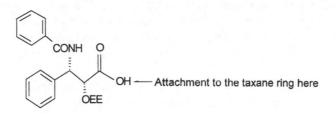

Figure 3.3 Side chain of taxol protected as in the Potier–Greene semi-synthesis.

They reported these results in an important paper in 1981.[130] Some of the chemical properties of 10-DAB were already known, as the compound had previously been isolated from *Taxus wallichiana*, a species growing in the Himalayan region.[131] The interesting point about 10-DAB is that it had the familiar taxane ring structure, but it lacked a side chain at the carbon 13 position (C-13).[132] Potier's group knew from Wall and Wani's work that both taxol's nucleus and its side chain were essential for the compound's antitumour activity.[133] The side chain, they thought, could be made synthetically and attached to this compound to produce taxol (see Figure 3.3).[134] Meanwhile, another CNRS research unit, that of Andrew Greene at Grenoble, had been working on other biologically active natural products. Pierre Potier proposed a collaborative project in which his group would isolate 10-DAB, and deal with any problems posed by the molecule's shape for attaching the side chain, while Greene's group would synthesize the side chain, and together they would combine both parts to form taxol. This was precisely what the two groups set out to do, although it would be several years before they were successful.[135]

The point of the 1981 article for the future of taxol is that it used a renewable resource as its starting material, even though that would not become significant until later. Potier claims that he chose to examine *Taxus baccata* needles because they were available on site and in large amounts – *Taxus brevifolia* bark, by contrast, had to be harvested in the wild.[136] The renewability of needles was not viewed as important until 1988, when growing requirements of the clinical trials increased the demand for bark, and concern about saving *Taxus brevifolia* began to surface.

Chemists in the United States, including Bob Holton[137] (now at Florida State University), David Kingston[138] (at Virginia Polytechnic Institute) and Paul Wender[139] (at Stanford University) had also started to work on taxol in the early 1980s. At this point none of them was looking for a semi-synthetic route to taxol, or any other way of making it that addressed supply issues. For them, taxol was primarily a complex and therefore interesting chemical, and even though Kingston and Wender, in particular, expressed a general hope that the knowledge they generated might contribute in some way to the treatment of cancer, they did not have a specific practical goal in their work on taxol in the early 1980s.

They all received funding from the NIH, including the NCI, but all report it as being somewhat sporadic in the early and mid 1980s, although all were in regular contact with Matthew Suffness. Kingston was mainly concerned with studying the activity–structure relationship, while both Holton and Wender attempted total syntheses, not as a practical way of making taxol but in order to generate chemical knowledge.[140] Bob Holton, for example, said that he had no interest in semi-synthesis, which, in his view, was not an interesting challenge chemically, until his attention was grabbed by Andrew Greene's work. He did not believe that taxol would ever become an anti-cancer drug until he heard, in 1989, that the NCI were about to seek a CRADA (Cooperative Research and Development Agreement) partner.[141] He started working on a semi-synthesis in 1988, because by then it was feared that demand would exceed supply and that a practical route was needed.

The other event of 1981 that would have enormous consequences for the rest of the decade and beyond was the publication in February of that year of a study of the old-growth forests of the Pacific Northwest.[142] Written by Jerry Franklin, of the Pacific Northwest Forest and Range Experiment Station in Corvallis, Oregon, together with seven other scientists, the report set out to answer a number of questions posed in February 1977 to a work session sponsored by the Forest Service.[143] The questions were basic ones about the nature of an old-growth forest. The fact that they were being asked in 1977 may be surprising, but very little was known about these kinds of forests. Though the questions were specific, the reason for an interest in old-growth forests was not purely academic. As the authors pointed out at the very beginning of their report, at the time of writing, almost all remaining old-growth forests were on Federal lands. Only a small proportion, five per cent, was in protected areas. If current practices continued, the ninety-five per cent would be eliminated within half a century. 'The end of the unreserved old-growth forests is in sight', the authors chillingly wrote.[144]

This was no ordinary publication. It differed radically from the usual technical literature on forests which highlighted specific, and most often, commercially valuable species. It focused, instead, on the ecology of a specific kind of forest. By adopting an ecosystem approach, Franklin and his colleagues were able to think of the forest in its entirety. And this meant focusing on dead and decaying, as well as living features.[145] They concluded that there were four structural components to the forest on which the distinctive compositional and functional characteristics strictly depended, and which were unique to old-growth forests. These components were: live old-growth trees (Douglas fir, western hemlock, Sitka spruce, for example); standing dead trees, known as snags; down dead logs on the ground; and down dead logs in the streams.[146] Almost half of the report was taken up by a discussion of the composition and function of snags and down dead logs. As the authors put it in a direct challenge to the received wisdom: 'Old-growth forests provide highly specialized habitats and are neither decadent, unproductive ecosystems nor biological deserts . . . An old-growth forest is much more than simply a collection of large trees. The dead, organic component is as important as the highly individualistic, large trees . . . To a large degree, success in managing forests for old-growth attributes will depend on learning to manage the dead, organic material as cleverly as the live trees.'[147] The report did not proffer a simple definition of old-growth. Such definitions, and there were many of them, already existed and typically referred to tree size or age.[148] The authors resisted a simple definition because it was the complexity of the forest ecosystem that was the key to understanding it. Old-growth was a process, the characteristics of which begin to emerge after a period of between 175 and 250 years under natural conditions. The characteristics were those that the report discussed.

The Franklin report was as much about managing forests as it was about developing an ecological definition of old-growth forests. It laid the ground for what has become known as 'New Forestry', that is, managing younger forests by recreating certain old-growth characteristics.[149] It also had another crucial implication. In effect, it authorized the ecologist to speak for the forest and put ecological metaphors at the disposal of public discourse.[150]

Back in Warrington, Pennsylvania, meanwhile, Fred Boettner took delivery of almost 16,000 pounds of *Taxus brevifolia* bark in October 1982. Nothing was done to this shipment until July of the following year, when Boettner was instructed to work-up one half of the collection.[151] The procedure to extract and then isolate the taxol was the same as it had been for the previous large batch. The first substantial output of taxol was not delivered to the NCI until October 1984, two years after taking delivery of the collection.

With toxicology studies completed in 1982, there was no demand for supplies of taxol apart from the biological research done extramurally. But while the number of requests for this kind of work was substantial – almost one per day – each request was still in milligram amounts and the annual total did not amount to more than seven grams.[152] The main pressure at the NCI was bureaucratic, in preparing the INDA. The clinical brochure, the heart of the INDA, was completed in September 1983 and submitted to the FDA for approval. Dale Shoemaker, the Executive Secretary of the Decision Network Committee, informed the committee's members that the FDA had given approval to initiate clinical trials of taxol on 6 April 1984.

At this point, taxol had been more than twenty years in the making. It had gone through considerable development and passed through many hands. Many of those who had been a part of its biography were no longer associated with it. Gone, too, was the interagency organization in which it was born and through which it revealed its characteristics and its lurking problems. The network had been cut, and with it many of the uncertainties, the instabilities and the difficulties were buried and forgotten.[153] In particular, the association between taxol and *Taxus brevifolia* bark had been made to seem natural, at least in the minds of the NCI administrators. All suggestions and considerations about long-term supply through cultivation of bioactive *Taxus* species evaporated. What remained constant and was reinforced several times was that the forest was the source of taxol.

But the forest and *Taxus brevifolia* were not constant. They were changing. First, a voice of authority with powerful metaphors and the backing of science was emerging to speak for a unique forest ecosystem, located in the Pacific Northwest, and rapidly disappearing.[154] Second, within that unique forest, a voice was being raised for *Taxus brevifolia*. We have already met Jerry Rust, the Lane County Commissioner, and his friend Hal Hartzell. Rust ran for Governor of Oregon in 1982 but lost in the Democratic primary.[155] The yew, in the form of campaign buttons, was used to symbolize the Rust's chief concern, the destruction of the state's resources. Nearly one-quarter of a million yew campaign buttons were made and distributed. To pay off campaign debts, Rust and Hartzell decided to write a book about the yew tree, addressing, in Hartzell's words, 'the myth, legend, lore, historical and poetical associations . . .' Published in 1983, it was probably the only such full-length treatment of the yew, and certainly the first in recent times.[156] It was also radically different from the kind of literature that existed about trees. Rust and Hartzell's treatment of *Taxus* was in the form of a biography, emphasizing its cultural and historical associations, in direct contrast to the exploitative and utilitarian texts for other species, such as the Douglas fir and the western spruce. Their book emphasized a mythical, magical species residing in a unique ecosystem.

Most of the book concentrated on the cultural history of *Taxus baccata*, but there was a specific chapter set aside for a discussion of *Taxus brevifolia*. The discussion was remarkable. Not only did it give a rich impression of the tree and its habitat, it discussed individual trees with a feeling just short of reverence. What is also remarkable about the discussion is that it begins with an ethnobotany of *Taxus brevifolia* derived from indigenous native culture. The use of yew to make hunting and fishing tools, domestic utensils and in medical therapies is discussed fully. This was not done simply as a background, but to draw a parallel between a vanishing culture and a vanishing species.

Hartzell and Rust made one reference to taxol, without naming the compound as such. They reported that the bark of *Taxus brevifolia* yielded an alkaloid that had significant activity against tumours in laboratory animals. This was but the latest revelation of a remarkable tree. 'It is clear', they wrote, 'that the tradition of utility and awe associated with the yew-tree continues, but it seems that we, as a modern society, are only dimly aware of its full potential value.'[157] The book sold out its entire run of 500 copies. Whoever purchased and read it knew more about *Taxus brevifolia* than most experts, including those at the Forest Service, the Bureau of Land Management and the NCI.

Notes

1 Venditti, 'Relevance of transplantable', p. 246.
2 On B16, see Griswold, 'Consideration'.
3 Luce et al., 'Clinical trials'.
4 Skipper, 'Improvement'; Zubrod, 'Chemical control'; and Suffness, 'New approaches', pp. 91–92.
5 Suffness and Wall, 'Discovery and development', p. 13.
6 A good and detailed description of it can be found in Rothenberg and Treselic, 'Commentary'.
7 These data are taken from Driscoll, 'The preclinical new drug research program', p. 68.
8 DeVita et al., 'The drug development and clinical trials programs', p. 204. Though Driscoll does not put a figure to the overall costs, he states that

toxicology alone cost more than $325,000 per compound. If Driscoll is right, then the true total cost would be much higher than DeVita's quoted figure. See Driscoll, 'The preclinical new drug research program', p. 68.

9 Interview with Suffness, 13 March 1995.

10 Interview with Suffness, 13 March 1995. The same point is made in Suffness and Wall, 'Discovery and development', p. 13.

11 Suffness and Wall, 'Discovery and development', p. 13.

12 Minutes, DN meeting, 18 April 1977, Regulatory Affairs Branch. What is unclear from the published and unpublished accounts about taxol at this time is how taxol came up before the Decision Network Committee. According to Vincent DeVita and his co-authors at the Division of Cancer Treatment of the NCI, each compound being discussed at the Decision Network Committee was represented by an 'advocate' – someone who would put the case for the compound in front of the members. Suffness was not, apparently, taxol's 'advocate', although who was is not known – DeVita et al., 'The drug development and clinical trials program', p. 201 and Dale Shoemaker, personal communication, 13 May 1998.

13 Interview with Boettner, 10 November 1997. Some correspondence between Monsanto and Perdue concerning other plant compounds can be found in PER3. Monsanto's difficulties with taxol were not met with other plants. For their work on *Maytenus buchananii*, a plant with enormous promise in the early 1970s, see Suffness and Douros, 'Drugs of plant origin', pp. 96–99.

14 Monsanto's yield of taxol from bark was 0.0063 per cent compared with Wall's yield of 0.02 per cent, reported in 1971 – Wani et al., 'Plant antitumor agents'. Monsanto's data are in James Ellard, Lynn Lanier and Joseph Satanek, 'Demonstration of a scaled-up process NSC125973, Taxol', 26 April 1977, NPBI/1. Wall's early isolation of taxol yielded only 0.004 per cent – Research Triangle Institute, Progress Report 21, 26 June 1967, p. 30.

15 Polysciences, Preparation Report No. 2, 1 December 1977, p. 1.

16 Interview with Boettner, 10 November 1997.

17 Interview with Boettner, 10 November 1997.

18 Interview with Boettner, 10 November 1997.

19 Polysciences, Preparation Report No. 2, 1 December 1977, pp. 3,10.

20 Polysciences, Preparation Report No. 2, 1 December 1977, p. 10.

21 Suffness to Perdue, 14 June 1977, PER2.

22 POSI, *Taxus*, PER3.

23 Perdue, 'Taxol, the antitumor agent from Pacific yew (*Taxus brevifolia*)', 8 August 1977, PER3.

24 Perdue, 'Taxol, the antitumor agent from Pacific yew (*Taxus brevifolia*)', 8 August 1977, PER3.

25 Notes for POSI, Richard Spjut, SPJ2.

26 Richard Spjut, '*Taxus brevifolia*', 14 July 1977, PER3.

27 See for example, Spjut to Hatcher, 3 July 1974, SPJ1, referring to Edson's intention to collect a number of plant species in Oregon for the USDA.

28 Chuck Edson, 'Oregon reconnaissance report: *Taxus brevifolia*', p. 1, SPJ1 and Edson to Spjut, 19 July 1977, SPJ2.

29 Information in this and the following paragraphs is based on Edson's report.

30 Chuck Edson, 'Oregon reconnaissance report: *Taxus brevifolia*', p. 5, SPJ1

31 Perdue, 'Taxol, the antitumor agent from the Pacific yew (*Taxus brevifolia*)', SPJ2.

32 Spjut to Perdue, 15 August 1977, PER5.
33 Suffness to Perdue, 12 August 1977, PER2.
34 Perdue, Itinerary, August 1977, PER5.
35 Perdue to Forest Service contacts, 26 October 1977, PER3.
36 Perdue, 'Procurement of yew bark' and 'Specifications for procurement of yew bark (*Taxus brevifolia*)', 26 October 1977, PER3.
37 Perdue, 'Procurement of yew bark', 26 October 1977, PER3.
38 The correspondence with District Rangers is in UDA2.
39 Perdue, 'Information for prospective suppliers of yew bark', 11 January 1978, UDA2. Perdue exaggerated taxol's status as an anti-cancer compound. He stated that the NCI had decided to initiate Phase I clinical trials as soon as an adequate supply of taxol was available. No doubt this was designed to get the operations moving quickly. In fact, Phase I clinical trials did not begin until April 1984.
40 He made the following points in Perdue to Suffness, 12 December 1977, PER5.
41 All correspondence concerning the bid is in UDA2.
42 Their bid is in UDA2.
43 The following is based on an article published in the *Mail Tribune*, the local paper of Medford, Oregon, entitled 'Two local men help in cancer fight', dated August 1978. It may be the first newspaper article referring to taxol and the bark of the Pacific yew.
44 There is no information available that would help document the decisions leading to a change in amount ordered.
45 The following is based on Barclay to Rust, 22 March 1978, UDA2.
46 Hartzell and Rust, *Yew*, p. 8.
47 Hartzell has written the history of Hoedads in *Birth of a Cooperative*. In his reconnaissance report, Chuck Edson mentioned the existence of this venture but had nothing to say about it.
48 Hartzell and Rust, *Yew*, p. 7.
49 Hartzell and Rust, *Yew*, p. 7.
50 Edson to Perdue, 5 October 1977, PER5.
51 Barclay to Rust, 22 March 1978, UDA2.
52 Edson to Spjut, 24 July 1977, SPJ2.
53 Madis to Perdue, 29 August 1977, PER3.
54 Hays, *Beauty*.
55 Calculated from Polysciences, Preparation Report no. 2, 1 December 1977 and Preparation Report no. 4, 29 March 1978.
56 For examples of her published work on these compounds, see the following: podophyllotoxin – Horwitz and Loike, 'A comparison'; camptothecin – Horwitz and Horwitz, 'Effects of camptothecin'; bruceantin – Liao, Kupchan and Horwitz, 'Mode of action'; and steganacin – Schiff, Kende and Horwitz, 'Steganacin'. Bruceantin was isolated from *Brucea antidysenterica*, a plant growing in Ethiopia. Steganacin was isolated from the plant *Steganotaenia araliacea*. Both plants were collected in the NCI-USDA programme and both compounds were isolated by Morris Kupchan.
57 Hamel, 'Antimitotic drugs'.
58 They are also, sometimes, called mitotic or microtubule poisons.
59 Hamel, 'Antimitotic drugs', p. 141.
60 This research is discussed in greater detail in Goodman, 'Plants, cells and bodies', pp. 19–20.

61 A more detailed discussion is in Goodman, 'Plants, cells and bodies', pp. 30–33. A good review of the state of knowledge at the end of the 1960s can be found in Olmsted and Borisy, 'Microtubules'.

62 See Wilson et al., 'Pharmacological and biochemical properties' for a good discussion of microtubules, tubulin and colchicine.

63 See Wilson et al., 'Interaction of drugs'.

64 Kupchan et al., 'Maytansine'.

65 Suffness and Douros, 'Drugs of plant origin', p. 123.

66 Remillard et al., 'Antimitotic activity'.

67 Mandelbaum-Shavit, Wolpert-DeFilippes and Johns, 'Binding of maytansine'.

68 Suffness and Douros, 'Drugs of plant origin', p. 94.

69 Suffness and Cordell, 'Antitumor alkaloids', pp. 154–155.

70 Suffness and Douros, 'Drugs of plant origin', p. 123.

71 Loike and Horwitz, 'The effects of podophyllotoxin'.

72 Interview with Horwitz, 28 August 1996. See also, Max, 'Action woman'.

73 David Fuchs, 'Preclinical testing of taxol: an antineoplastic, metaphase-arresting agent isolated from *Taxus brevifolia*', 11 March 1978, PER3.

74 Fuchs and Johnson, 'Cytological evidence', p. 1219.

75 DeVita et al., 'The drug development and clinical trials programs', p. 201. This was the practice in the pharmaceutical industry.

76 Schiff et al., 'Effects of taxol'.

77 In an interview with *Taxane Journal*, Horwitz recounts that her graduate student, Peter Schiff, was amazed when, with the aid of an electron microscope, he saw that the taxol-treated cell was 'loaded with microtubules': he expected the very opposite. See Max, 'Action woman', p. 16.

78 NCI, Taxol shipments (non-screener investigators).

79 Schiff, Fant and Horwitz, 'Promotion of microtubule assembly'.

80 One of the first to position taxol as a biochemical tool was Horwitz and her co-workers. See, Horwitz et al., 'Taxol: a new probe'.

81 For an overview of taxol in cell biology research, see Vallee, 'The use of taxol'.

82 NCI, Taxol shipments (non-screener investigators).

83 MEDLINE.

84 Heidemann and Gallas, 'The effect of taxol'. Also, personal communication with Heidemann, 7 October 1997.

85 Suffness and Cordell, 'Antitumor alkaloids', pp. 32, 36.

86 An article written by several members of staff of the Division of Cancer Treatment was hard-pressed to find 'rational' explanations for why some compounds were dropped from further investigation. The authors found the whole process by which decisions on compounds were taken disturbing. Lack of interest seemed to account for the lack of progress as much or more than anything else. See Von Hoff et al., 'Whatever happened to NSC—?'.

87 For example: Suffness and Wall, 'Discovery and development', p. 14; Wall and Wani, 'Camptothecin and taxol', p. 759; Wall and Wani, 'Paclitaxel', p. 27; and Persinos, 'The Pacific yew and cancer', p. 339.

88 See Suffness, 'The discovery and development of antitumor drugs', p. 116.

89 Flanagan, 'Nude'.

90 Pantelouris, 'Absence of thymus'.

91 Rygaard and Paulsen, 'Heterotransplantation'.

92 Giovanella and Stehlin, 'Heterotransplantation of human malignant tumors'.

93 Goldin et al., 'Historical development', p. 216 and Giovanella et al., 'Metastases'.
94 Goldin et al., 'Historical development', p. 216.
95 Suffness and Wall, 'Discovery and development', pp. 15–16.
96 Venditti, Wesley and Plowman, 'Current NCI preclinical antitumor'.
97 Suffness and Wall, 'Discovery and development', p. 16.
98 All of the following test data are from NCI, Division of Cancer Treatment, Developmental Therapeutics Program, Screening Data Summary.
99 Suffness and Cordell, 'Antitumor alkaloids'.
100 Suffness and Douros, 'Drugs of plant origin', p. 123.
101 See the activity in the tumour panel of a number of compounds in Goldin and Venditti, 'Progress report on the screening program', pp. 169–171.
102 Information on formulation is based on Adams et al., 'Taxol', pp. 141–143.
103 Regulatory Affairs Branch, NCI, Review of DN2A agents, Taxol, 1 August 1979.
104 Suffness and Wall, 'Discovery and development', p. 21.
105 NCI, Taxol shipments (non-screener investigators).
106 Polysciences, Preparation Report 9, 27 November 1979. Boettner first estimated that he would be able to isolate between 300 and 350 grams of taxol from this collection.
107 Bid from Strunck and Williams, May 1978, UDA2.
108 Polysciences, Preparation Report 9, 27 November 1979, p. 2. See also Boettner to Suffness, 12 March 1979, PER2.
109 Suffness to Hatcher, 11 July 1980, PER4.
110 Boettner to Suffness, 12 March 1979, PER2 and Suffness to Hatcher, 11 July 1980, PER4.
111 Suffness to Hatcher, 11 July 1980, PER4.
112 Suffness to Hatcher, 11 July 1980, PER4 and Boettner to Suffness, 4 May 1979, PER2.
113 Suffness to Hatcher, 19 November 1980, PER4.
114 Suffness to Hatcher, 19 November 1980, PER4. In this same memo, Suffness reinforced the need for peeling the *Taxus brevifolia* bark by hand as 'the machine peeled stuff was 80–90% wood with bark attached and gave a poor yield of taxol.' Fred Boettner had made the original complaint about the state of the material he had received at Polysciences.
115 Hatcher, invitation to bid, 15 December 1980, NPBII.
116 Hatcher, invitation to bid, 15 December 1980, NPBII.
117 Warner bid, 31 December 1980, NPBII.
118 *Taxus* collections, SPJ1.
119 Polysciences, Preparation Report no. 22, 12 October 1982.
120 Taxus collections, SPJ1.
121 Polysciences, Preparation Report no. 36, 22 February 1985.
122 NCI, Taxol shipments (non-screener investigators).
123 Minutes, Decision Network 3 meeting, 23 November 1982.
124 Suffness and Wall, 'Discovery and development', p. 17.
125 The CNRS is the state's major organization for the funding of science and the employer of scientists.
126 Interview with Potier, 2 December 1996.
127 Bissery and Lavelle, 'The taxoids', p. 178.
128 Shelanski, Gaskin and Cantor, 'Microtubule assembly'.

129 Sénilh et al., 'Hémisynthèse', p. 1039 quote 100 milligrams while Bissery and Lavelle, 'The taxoids', p. 178 quote 150 milligrams.

130 Chauvière et al., 'Analyse structurale'.

131 McLaughlin et al., '19-hydroxybaccatin III', p. 317 and Powell, Miller and Smith, 'Cephalomannine'.

132 Organic chemists number the carbon atoms, according to specific conventions, to distinguish their positions in a complex molecule.

133 Wani et al., 'Plant antitumor agents'.

134 Kingston, Hawkins and Ovington, 'New taxanes', pp. 467–469. 10-DAB was present in a number of *Taxus* species, including *Taxus brevifolia*.

135 The key publications were: Sénilh et al., 'Hémisynthèse'; Guéritte-Voegelein et al., 'Chemical studies'; Denis et al., 'A highly efficient'; and Denis et al., 'An efficient', covering the period 1984–1988. A more detailed review of the work of this group can be found in Chapter 4.

136 Interview with Potier, 2 December 1996. In 1984 and in 1986, the French team highlighted their method of semi-synthesis in the context of the slow growth of *Taxus brevifolia* and the low yield of taxol from its bark, but not in terms of a threat to the tree's numbers – see Sénilh et al., 'Hémisynthèse', p. 1039 and Guéritte-Voegelein et al., 'Chemical studies', p. 4451.

137 Interview with Holton, 22 May 1998.

138 Interview with Kingston, 29 March 1996.

139 Interview with Wender, 8 April 1996.

140 A total synthesis is one in which the desired molecule is entirely assembled from readily available simple compounds. A partial or semi-synthesis starts from a complex molecule obtained from a natural product (but typically one more widely available and therefore cheaper) and transforms it (usually with only a few steps) into the desired product.

141 Holton said (interview 22 May 1998): 'as an academic natural product synthesiser, we go through this litany with the NIH. You know, this compound has this activity and that activity and the other activity. None of those compounds ever made it, or only a small fraction. I didn't believe taxol would make it. I didn't even know what clinical trials meant. And people would keep saying, 'Oh yes, it's doing this and that and the other in clinical trials', and 'I just ignored that stuff.'

142 Franklin et al., *Ecological Characteristics*. An earlier publication focused on the adaptive characteristics of the temperate rainforest of the Pacific Northwest, concentrating particularly on the conifer dominance of the area. See Waring and Franklin, 'Evergreen coniferous forests'.

143 A sympathetic portrait of Franklin can be found in Dietrich, *The Final Forest*, pp. 97–115.

144 Franklin et al., *Ecological Characteristics*, p. 1. For a recent profoundly moving and beautifully illustrated account of clear-cutting and its landscape effects, see Devall, *Clearcut*. For an equally moving account of an old-growth forest, see Kirk, *The Olympic*. For a biography of an old-growth forest, see Maser, *Forest Primeval*.

145 For an interesting discussion of the emergence of the ecosystem in biological thinking, see Golley, *A History of the Ecosystem Concept* and Hagen, *An Entangled Bank*.

146 Franklin et al., *Ecological Characteristics*, p. 20.

147 Franklin et al., *Ecological Characteristics*, pp. 40–41.

148 Ervin, *Fragile Majesty*, p. 15.

149 For discussions of New Forestry, see Dietrich, *The Final Forest*, pp. 97–112, Gillis, 'The new forestry' and DeBell and Curtis, 'Silviculture and the new forestry'.

150 Willems-Braun, 'Buried epistemologies'.

151 Polysciences, Preparation Report no. 36, 22 February 1985.

152 NCI, Taxol shipments (non-screener investigators).

153 The idea of cutting the network leans heavily on the essay by Strathern, 'Cutting the network'.

154 For the importance of metaphors, see Lakoff and Johnson, *Metaphors*, Maasen, 'Who is afraid?' and Leary, 'Naming and knowing'. On the role of science, especially as it applies to environmental issues and conflicts, see Ozawa, 'Science', Satterfield, 'Voodoo science'. In general, see Nelkin, 'Science controversies' and Franklin, 'Science as culture' and the references therein.

155 This and the following references are from Hartzell, *The Yew Tree*, p. xiii and from interviews with Rust and Hartzell, 1 and 2 April 1996.

156 Hartzell and Rust, *Yew*.

157 Hartzell and Rust, *Yew*, p. 132.

4

Act III: 1984–1989

This chapter covers the period from 1984 to 1989, from the initiation of Phase I clinical trials to the publication of taxol's remarkable activity against refractory ovarian cancer. During this same period, taxol was also becoming increasingly difficult to manage. Supply was the key issue. The amount of bark needed to progress taxol through clinical trials escalated while access to the forest became increasingly difficult as political tensions rose. Collections did not go according to schedule and were fraught with difficulties and setbacks. The planning of clinical trials was erratic: many of the approved trials were postponed indefinitely because of the lack of supplies of taxol. The failure to take a long-term view, to explore comprehensively alternative sources of plant material – such as cultivated species of *Taxus* and renewable parts – all of which had been suggested in the past, came to haunt the natural products programme. Special meetings were convened to find solutions. In desperation, and after more than a quarter of a century of research and development, the NCI turned to the private sector for help. Rather than try to solve the primary and pressing problem of alternative sources of supply, for which there were a number of possible solutions, the NCI decided to hand the entire matter over to the pharmaceutical industry.

The odds of a compound being selected for clinical trials in 1984 was about 1 in 2,000 of those compounds screened for activity; the odds of a compound making it as a commercially available anti-cancer drug was 1 in 10,000.[1] Taxol, therefore, was in a small and privileged group of compounds. By the time of taxol's INDA, only four other plant compounds were in clinical trials; a year later, and into the first stage of taxol's clinical trials, one of the plant compounds had been dropped, leaving only three others in the running.[2]

Until the filing of an INDA, a compound is tested on cell lines and animals only. The granting of an INDA allows the NCI to begin testing a compound on humans. These tests, called clinical trials, are sequenced into phases, each of which evaluates specific criteria of the compound. Phase I evaluates for safety; Phase II for effectiveness; and Phase III for comparison against standard therapies. In general the time needed to complete and the number of patients enrolled in clinical trials increases as the phases progress.

Clinical trials have been around both as an idea and in practice for a long time.[3] These evaluations of a drug did not, however, become part of the regulatory mechanism leading to the commercial availability of a drug until relatively recently. The two main changes in the United States were the 1938 Food, Drug and Cosmetic Act that required drugs to be evaluated for safety and the 1962 Kefauver–Harris Amendments that increased the stringency of the safety requirements and stipulated efficacy as well.[4]

Phase I clinical trials began in April 1984 and were conducted at seven clinical sites. The purpose of a Phase I clinical trial is to establish that a compound is safe, with respect to dosage, for human consumption. The principal goal of this trial is to determine a maximum tolerated dose (MTD). The underlying paradigm is that the greatest chance of a tumour response with a particular compound occurs at the highest possible dose.[5] Patients on the trial begin with an initial dose, determined from previously conducted studies on animals, and then escalated until the MTD is reached.[6] The MTD is defined as the dose at which toxic effects, known as dose-limiting toxicity, occur whose severity limit further escalation.[7] The escalation process may be done with the initial cohort of patients or with new accruals to the trial. Anticancer drugs are toxic and it is their toxicity that correlates with their antitumour activity.[8]

Each compound seeking FDA approval for commercial availability must be tested in this trial. But there is an important difference between antitumour and other types of compounds in the selection of the patients in this trial. While the latter are tested on 'normal volunteers', patients in a Phase I clinical trial for an antitumour compound are selected only if they have 'histologically proven malignant disease, which at the time of the study is no longer amenable to more established forms of treatment'.[9] These terminally ill patients are expected to survive for at least two months to give enough time to observe the effects of the compound. As these patients have some form of cancer, Phase I trials also produce some information about tumour response, although it is accepted that little therapeutic effect is produced at this stage of the testing process.[10]

Seven oncology centres participated in Phase I trials of taxol. They were the Johns Hopkins Oncology Center, the Memorial Sloan–Kettering Cancer Center, the Albert Einstein College of Medicine

Center, the MD Anderson Cancer Center, the University of Wisconsin, the Dana Farber Cancer Center and the Mount Sinai School of Medicine. A total of 101 patients participated in the trial, ranging from the smallest number (10) at the Dana Farber Cancer Center to the largest number (20) at the MD Anderson Cancer Center.[11]

As mentioned before, as antitumour compounds are toxic, physiological reactions in the patients are expected. On 27 December 1984, on his second course of taxol (his first course was administered one month earlier), a fifty-four-year-old man with renal cell carcinoma (a type of kidney cancer) at the Memorial Sloan–Kettering Cancer Center experienced a severe and irreversible drop in blood pressure and died following cardiorespiratory arrest.[12] The patient had no previous record of cardiac disease. All trials were halted and a review of procedures initiated.

By the end of December 1984, Phase I clinical trials had been progressing for several months. Of the 95 patients who had entered into the trials, seven had already experienced some form of cardiovascular toxicity, typically hypotension (low blood pressure) and shortness of breath.[13] Most of these reactions occurred with the second course of taxol and at four of the seven centres. Reactions were observed within minutes of taxol administration.[14] On the basis of this and the single death, modifications were made to the trials, including administration by twenty-four-hour infusions, premedication with several drugs to prevent hypersensitivity and exclusion from trials of patients with potential cardiac risk factors.[15] The trials were resumed.

It was argued that many of the adverse reactions only occurred under specific schedules of administration. Continuous infusion, it was observed, caused the fewest problems. By April 1985, two studies had been completed. In one the dose-limiting toxicity was myelosuppression (suppression of bone marrow activity leading to decreased production of red blood cells, white blood cells or platelets, a not uncommon problem with many toxic compounds) and on the other leukopenia (an abnormal reduction in the number of white blood cells). All of the information about these trials as well as the reaction data from other, ongoing studies, was presented to the Decision Network Committee on 16 April 1985.[16] Taxol passed DN4 at this meeting. Phase II trials could, therefore, begin. Taxol would be given as a continuous intravenous infusion and patients would be pretreated with benadryl, cimetidine and an oral steroid, all used to suppress allergic reactions.

The minutes of the Decision Network Committee do not record the discussions leading to the final decision to proceed to Phase II. According to Matthew Suffness, however, the idea of dropping taxol received substantial support, because the number and extent of the hypersensitivity reactions were considerable and, on the evidence of the death, possibly life-threatening.[17] In addition, in the two completed studies, no objective responses, that is no effect on the patients' tumours, were observed.[18] The overall incidence of hypersensitivity was twelve per cent, although in one or two cases, it went as high as eighteen per cent. These figures were higher than that of other compounds that were formulated with Cremophor, which was known to cause allergic reactions. What was not clear was whether the higher incidence rate was accounted for by the larger amount of Cremophor used in administering taxol.[19] Looking closely at the distribution of the incidence of reactions, it is clear that several variables were at work, including the schedule, the formulation and perhaps the patients selected. In the end, the committee probably decided to go ahead, rather than drop taxol, precisely because its profile was somewhat ambiguous. As we have seen, only a handful of compounds ever got this far.

Phase II clinical trials are on a far bigger scale than Phase I. They consume a considerable amount of the compound under investigation. Collecting more bark was now a matter of urgency. On 10 July 1985, after a short bid period, Robert Warner of Ashland, in southern Oregon, was awarded a contract to supply the NCI with 12,000 pounds of dried *Taxus brevifolia* bark. Warner, a fencepost dealer, had collected *Taxus brevifolia* on several occasions in 1977, 1978, 1980, 1981 and 1982 for the USDA. This was the NCI's first contract for collection since it ended its interagency agreement with the USDA in 1981. Warner's was one of three bids the NCI received, but the prices on the other two were considerably higher than his, at $2.75 per pound of dried bark.[20] He was given a deadline of 8 November to deliver the bark.[21]

The period of the contract was short – four months – but sufficiently long, everyone must have thought, to find and strip the trees, and to dry the bark. Because the bark can only be peeled when the sap is running, the main part of the operation needed to be completed by the end of September, at the latest. Warner was confident that he could supply the bark in the quantity contracted, on the grounds that this part of southern Oregon was rich in *Taxus brevifolia*; he had, on the occasion of an earlier and unsuccessful bid, pointed this out to the USDA. He would need to peel bark from about 4,000 trees. As he had experience with *Taxus brevifolia*, he also saw no problems in getting permits to cut the trees and peel them.

In principle all seemed well. Unfortunately, the forest did not behave as it was expected to. The summer of 1985 turned out to be one of the hottest and driest on record throughout the western States. The Forest Service closed the National Forests to logging and collecting over long periods during the summer. In the end, Warner was unable to meet the commitments in the contract. By the end of September, he had managed to collect only about 5,000 pounds.[22] Gordon Cragg, a newly arrived chemist on the staff of the Natural Products Branch of the NCI argued that Warner's contract should be extended until 31 August 1986, by which time, weather permitting, he would be able to collect the remainder of the contracted supply.[23] Cragg helped smooth the collection by convincing the Butte Falls District Ranger in southern Oregon to set aside a good stand of *Taxus brevifolia* for Warner to peel during the coming summer.[24] Warner made his collection during the summer months and, by early autumn 1986, a year later than expected, the NCI had a new stock of about 11,000 pounds of bark.

This episode showed the unreliability of procuring supplies from the forest and the crucial part it played in the entire taxol programme, principally on the clinical side, but also in all the research areas that had come to rely on the molecule either as its tool – in cell biology – or its object – organic chemistry. Not only was the forest unreliable, the extraction and purification process was equally unstable. Fred Boettner, the chief chemist on the taxol programme at Polysciences, and those who succeeded him in that post, found that yields varied considerably from batch to batch. It was, therefore, impossible to predict the yield from any particular batch. Climate, location, harvesting, storage, shipment, any of these could affect the quality of the raw material.

Nevertheless, as a rule-of-thumb, everyone involved in the taxol programme, apart from those at Polysciences, adopted the yield of 0.01 per cent as standard. The Developmental Chemotherapy Section of the Investigational Drug Branch worked on the rule-of-thumb that a pound of dried *Taxus brevifolia* bark would yield 1.36×30 milligram vials of taxol – vials contained thirty milligrams of taxol; put another way, Warner's collection was expected to translate into 15,000 vials of taxol for clinical use.[25] Unfortunately, that turned out to be rather optimistic. The yield of taxol was twenty-five per cent less than expected at 337 grams, or about 11,000 vials.[26] In terms of the ability to sustain clinical trials, the actual yield meant that there would have to be one fewer trial.

Yield and weather conditions were two elements that could not be controlled and had considerable impact on the planning of clinical trials. A third source of difficulty was the span of time between the delivery of the bark and the delivery of the purified taxol to the NCI. In the case of Warner's collection, the delivery of bark was in September 1986 but the first delivery of bulk taxol did not take place until November 1987, with the remaining part in June 1988.[27] This was in line with previous contracts at Polysciences where the time span between the delivery of bark and taxol averaged fourteen months. Adding to that about four months for formulation, eighteen months would be expected to pass between delivery of bark and the availability of taxol in the clinic.[28] A further nine months could be added to that figure to arrive at the time span between the notice to bid for a contract and delivery of bark, assuming, of course, that the forest behaved perfectly. Even in ideal circumstances, two and a half years would pass between the time that a notice to collect was posted and clinically formulated taxol was available in the clinic.

Phase II clinical trials focus on efficacy. Under normal circumstances, trials are conducted simultaneously at several research centres where the active compound is tested in patients with specific tumours. The number of patients enrolled in Phase II trials typically varies between 700 and 1,000 with a range of thirty-five to fifty patients per trial.[29] Patients are normally given a course of at least six treatments to see if the tumour is responding to the compound.

Very soon after the initiation of Phase II trials, it became clear that the typical pattern would not apply in the case of taxol. On 1 December 1986, Gisele Sarosy, the Senior Investigator in the Developmental Chemotherapy Section of the Investigational Drug Branch, placed on record that the clinical trial programme was facing a severe taxol shortage.[30] The available stock amounted to 1,795 vials, not enough to supply even one Phase II clinical trial (a typical trial used 2,000 vials). The bulk taxol of 410 grams that had been recently delivered to the NCI would be formulated into 10,500 vials, but the next shipment of 6,500 vials was not expected before February 1987 and the remaining shipment outstanding in April. With no further supplies, there was no option but to bring a halt to the Phase II clinical trials of taxol, suspending those in action and postponing those in the planning stage.

The reason for this abnormal state of affairs lay in the asymmetry of bark collections and taxol purification. In the period between the decision to enter taxol into the developmental process in 1977 and the supply crisis in 1986, the collection of bark of *Taxus brevifolia* in the Pacific Northwest and the deliveries of taxol from Polysciences to the NCI were erratic. Major collections were made in 1977 and 1981/2. The taxol isolated from these collections was delivered to the NCI on five occasions between 1978 and 1986.[31] The total amount of taxol produced over this period was 1,600 grams.[32] Formulation and toxicology had consumed about 1,000 grams together, and Phase I and Phase II trials to date a further 600 grams.[33] It was proving difficult to co-ordinate collections, extractions, isolations, formulations and clinical trials in order to move the process along smoothly and efficiently. Decisions were made in response to changes rather than in their anticipation.

Three Phase II clinical trials were accepting patients by 1 December 1986. It had already been decided as far back as January 1985, that is before approval to proceed to Phase II clinical trials, that taxol would be tried out at the same seven centres that participated in the Phase I clinical trials.[34] Accordingly, patients with ovarian cancer at Johns Hopkins; patients with melanoma in research centres belonging to the Eastern Cooperative Oncology Group; and patients with renal cancer at the Albert Einstein College of Medicine were involved in these first Phase II clinical trials.[35] Just over thirty patients had been enrolled. Both ovarian and renal cell carcinoma were selected because there was some evidence of tumour response to taxol in earlier Phase I trials; in addition, melanoma, it will be recalled, responded well to taxol in the B16 murine screen.[36] Trials on breast cancer, which was indicated as a possibility because of taxol's activity in the MX-1 mammary xenograft, were scheduled to accept patients in 1985 but were, in fact, postponed for several years.[37]

Preliminary results on those patients who were already entered and evaluated for responses to taxol by December 1986 were mixed. None of the patients with renal cancer showed any response to taxol. The melanoma responses – only one in fourteen patients – were not great, although not all these patients were yet evaluable. The only promising results were from the Johns Hopkins Oncology Center where, of seven patients entered with refractory ovarian cancer (who had not responded to the standard therapy), two showed partial responses and one a marginal response.[38]

At the end of December 1986, the situation regarding the supply of taxol and the Phase II clinical trials was as follows. The supply of taxol currently on hand and expected by April 1987 was enough to cover the trials currently under way at Johns Hopkins, the Eastern Cooperative Oncology Group and Albert Einstein College of Medicine, and to start those trials previously on hold, namely the MD Anderson Cancer Center, the University of Maryland Cancer Center and the Albert Einstein College of Medicine, on melanoma and ovarian cancer, respectively.[39] There were at least seven Phase II clinical trials and one Phase I clinical trial that were on hold. Whether these would go ahead depended on the outcome of the current trials with ovarian and melanoma patients. Should the latter prove satisfactory, then the programme would need to focus on these diseases with further trials, leaving trials on all the other types of cancers suspended. Gisele Sarosy's notification on 1 December 1986 that there was an impending taxol shortage prompted an emergency meeting, convened by Matthew Suffness and attended by Gisele Sarosy, Gordon Cragg and several other representatives of interested branches of the NCI. The meeting was told that taxol 'could take off as a big drug' and that the Natural Products Branch had just put in a requisition to announce bids for the largest single collection to date – 60,000 pounds of bark, expected to yield 3–3.5 kilograms of taxol.[40] Even so, it was felt that this would prove to be insufficient 'if currently promising results continue in the clinical trials'.[41]

The requisition for 60,000 pounds of *Taxus brevifolia* needs to be seen in its various and simultaneous contexts. Let us first take the forest. This quantity of bark was unprecedented. It represented a collection of bark, in just one season, exceeding by a large margin the total bark collected since 1962. Just how many trees the collection figure represented is unknown, but newspapers at the time were talking about five pounds of bark per tree, or 12,000 trees in total.[42] Even before bids closed on the collection, local newspapers were tracking the story. *The Register-Guard* of Eugene, Oregon, carried an interview with Jerry Rust, the Lane County Commissioner who, with Hal Hartzell, had written the book about the yew tree back in 1983. Rust, according to the report, expressed nervousness about the collection. While supporting the cancer research effort, he was worried that 'it won't take many more ambitious bark-collection efforts to rapidly use up the region's slow-growing yew resource'.[43] His concern was shared by Bob Leonard of the Willamette National Forest. Referring to the possibility of issuing permits to collect 10,000 pounds of bark from his area, Leonard expressed his worries to *The Register-Guard* reporter in the following manner: 'How often can you do that? . . . If in fact they're going to be looking at doing this on a repeated basis, it's going to be necessary to look at some other way of creating the supply bark. I'm not sure it exists in our natural stands at that level.'[44] Gordon Cragg spoke for the NCI. He agreed that asking for this much bark was problematic but that, at the moment, there was no alternative to the forest. There had been attempts at synthesizing the molecule, he said, but without success. Other avenues would need to be explored, but Cragg gave little indication to the reporter what these might be. He concluded that the NCI was aware of the environmental impact and wished to keep it at a minimum. In the foreseeable future, however, the practice of taking bark from the forest would continue.

Various versions of the story were carried in several newspapers nation-wide, including the *Philadelphia Inquirer*, the *Los Angeles Times*, *Newsday* (New York) and the *New York Times*. For the first time, the American public was made aware of the existence of taxol. They were told quite a lot about it: that it was a promising anti-cancer compound, being tested on patients in clinical trials; that it came from a tree growing in the Pacific Northwest; and that there was an environmental concern about the viability of the supply. But there was more to it than that because many of the reports spoke directly about taxol's effectiveness against the dread disease. Cragg spoke about taxol's activity against melanoma while William McGuire, one of the oncologists involved in the Phase II clinical trial with ovarian cancer patients at Johns Hopkins, spoke about taxol's good results against this disease. Bob Holton, an organic chemist at Florida State University, was also solicited for his views about taxol. He referred to its activity against a broad range of cancer types, including colon, lung and breast cancer.[45] Headlines spoke of a tree involved in the war on cancer, of a cancer cure in a common yew.

The request to collect 60,000 pounds of bark was generating voices from spokespersons for the yew tree, from chemists at the NCI and the Florida State University, from an oncologist at Johns Hopkins, and from newspaper reporters. This mix of humans and trees had not occurred previously in taxol's history. The public was being invited into several sites where the performances of the drama of taxol were being played out: in the forest, in the NCI, in a chemistry laboratory in Tallahassee, in the Lane County Offices and in an oncology ward at the Johns Hopkins Oncology Center. A wide network of individuals, tools, instruments and premises were making taxol and Americans were made aware of its existence.

What they did not know was that the 60,000 pound collection was also eliciting financial concerns. At the December 1986 meeting when the announcement of the bids for the 60,000 pound bark collection was made, Matthew Suffness reported that the cost of working-up *Taxus brevifolia* bark into taxol would be $1.5 million, spread over the fiscal years 1988 and 1989.[46] This was a substantial amount for a single compound. Taxol was not the only compound under investigation: it had to compete for funds with others in preclinical and clinical investigation. Money was getting very tight.[47] The available funds had to be devoted exclusively to the collection, extraction and isolation, leaving other important projects – for example, on alternative methods of producing taxol – unfunded.[48] Financial concerns would surface again in the near future.

The unprecedentedly large amount of bark requested raised questions about how it should be collected. It could not be said that the NCI had much experience in this kind of work. After all, this was only the second time, since Robert Warner's collection in 1985/6, that the NCI had directly contracted for bark. The Natural Products Branch was under no illusion that finding 12,000 *Taxus brevifolia* to supply 60,000 pounds of bark would be easy. Gordon Cragg, who was charged to co-ordinate the collection for the Natural Products Branch, understood as much. He wished the collection to be made in multiple lots of 3,000 pounds minimum, to encourage small contractors to put in a bid at the same time as satisfying the Forest Service's demands that excessive amounts not be taken from any one area.[49] Cragg provided the procurement officer with a list of potential contractors – these were contractors and unsuccessful bidders from previous collections – from central and southern Oregon. He also asked that the bids be advertised in a number of local newspapers in southern Oregon and northern California. The deadline for accepting bids was 12 April 1987 and the bark was expected to be delivered to the warehouse of the Natural Products Branch as soon as the harvesting season was over.[50]

To help contractors, Cragg provided a number of specifications together with the forms.[51] *Taxus brevifolia*, he pointed out, was most abundant in areas controlled by the Forest Service and the Bureau of Land Management but was also available on private lands. The bark would need to be hand-peeled, in the spring or summer and then air-dried or, exceptionally, kiln-dried, using a temperature not exceeding 70°C. When it came to describing *Taxus brevifolia*, its appearance, habitat and specific distribution, Cragg could do no better than reproduce parts of Richard Spjut's report on *Taxus brevifolia* prepared a decade earlier in 1977. Despite the interval of time and the considerable changes to taxol's growing identity as an anti-cancer drug, nothing new was known about the tree of its origin. At least, not to those in Bethesda. Finding *Taxus brevifolia* rested, therefore, entirely on local knowledge. This was going to be more difficult than it was ten years earlier, or even since Robert Warner's collection in 1985. The forest had not remained still. Logging operations were clearing away parts of forests where *Taxus brevifolia* grew. In the Pacific Northwest region of the Forest Service, forty-six million-board-feet of timber had been cut between 1977 and 1987: one-third of this amount was cut between 1985 and 1987 alone.[52] How much of this cut was old-growth is not known, but it must have been considerable.[53]

One of those who thought he had the background and qualifications to bid for and carry out the NCI's contract was Patrick Connolly. Connolly grew up in the lumber business in Oregon, working at various times with an import–export company and sawmills.[54] He learned about trees from a commercial perspective. He could tell the difference between a Douglas fir and a Pacific yew, but, while he was employed in the lumber business, the latter meant nothing to him. Though he was somewhat surprised by the interest shown by the NCI in the Pacific yew, Connolly decided to pursue the offer for bids soon after he was made aware of it in early March 1987.

Bidding for the bark collection was not as simple as jotting down a reasonable price on a piece of paper. Though the price was the critical bit of information in deciding the successful applicant, the bid required a full disclosure of the methods of collecting the bark, a list of collecting areas with the quantities to be collected from each area and copies of the permits to collect.[55] To get a bid together required a commitment of time and energy. Connolly threw himself into the preparation, beginning with letters to the Ranger Districts of the National Forests in Oregon and the Nez Perce National Forest in Idaho – he was following the NCI's specifications to guide him to where he could expect to find *Taxus brevifolia*. Through these communications, Connolly learned that each National Forest had its own specifications and guidelines concerning stripping bark from *Taxus brevifolia*.[56] The Umpqua National Forest, for example, imposed a limit on the amount of bark that could be collected in terms of the number of trees, in this case 2,000.[57] The Rogue River National Forest, by comparison, imposed a limit in terms of the weight of bark that could be harvested – in this case, 10,000 pounds.[58] Conditions of being granted a permit varied in other respects as well. In the Umpqua National Forest, the collectors would be able to get bark from trees left standing and those cut during logging operations: in the Rogue River National Forest, by contrast, the collectors would need to strip the bark from living trees, leaving the trunk intact.[59] The reason for the difference is that in Rogue River National Forest, there was a considerable demand for yew as posts, for which the National Forest would issue separate permits.

Connolly's strategy was to subcontract the collection to local individuals who not only knew the area but knew the conditions and requirements of the local National Forest or Bureau of Land Management lands. He asked each of the District Rangers to provide him with a list of names of those who had previously harvested *Taxus brevifolia* for the wood. Connolly expected that paying fencepost makers, for example, for the bark which they would otherwise discard, would act as an incentive for them to come forth and help him with the contract.[60] Thinking simultaneously about yew wood and yew bark, Connolly was also in touch with contacts in Japan who were importing yew logs for manufacture into panelling.[61]

Connolly had a lot going for him right from the beginning. In one communication with the Cottage Grove Ranger Station of the Umpqua National Forest, Connolly learned of Bobby Ray Eller, a resident of Cottage Grove with whom he was in contact on 18 March 1987. Eller was, in many ways, a perfect complement to Connolly. Whereas Connolly knew the lumber business at the commercial end – hence his familiarity with Douglas fir – Eller knew the forest and *Taxus brevifolia*.[62] At the time of their first conversation, Eller was sixty-one and had spent virtually all of his working life in the Oregon forest, cutting firewood and in various other logging jobs. That was not unusual in this part of the state. What was unusual, however, was that Eller had spent the last eight years making a living strictly from selling *Taxus brevifolia*. Eller declined calling himself an expert to the reporter who interviewed him. 'An expert knows: I'm still learnin', he modestly answered. Eller admitted that, although he had sympathy with the environmental arguments concerning the depletion of the resource, he had a special but unemotional attachment to trees. He preferred them to people. 'Me and the trees get along real good. I cut 'em down and they don't talk back.' His wife, it turns out, had been diagnosed with throat cancer several years earlier. This experience of cancer and his familiarity with *Taxus brevifolia* produced in him a combination of emotions that would be repeated by many others during the taxol controversy of the early 1990s. Eller felt the 'magic' of cancer, as Robert Perdue had spoken of it back in the late 1960s. As Eller put it, in describing bark collection: 'In a way, it's a special job. I feel different about this job. I don't know how to describe it. Maybe it'll get some-body well. I don't know. But I'm no hero. It's a job. I'm gettin' paid . . . Some lady called and said she wanted to start an Eller fan club because she thought I was doin' a wonderful thing.' There was nothing sentimental about *Taxus brevifolia*. 'It wouldn't bother me to cut everything – the yew, the firs and all the brush – if it would help her. A tree's a tree. It'll grow back. I don't think anybody loved that tree like I love my wife.'

Eller was confident that with three or four crews of four people each, he could collect 5,000 pounds of bark in three to four weeks.[63] Using chicken-wire to make several levels of drying beds, Eller would be able to satisfy the NCI's specifications on method and timing. Connolly was impressed. He also learned other extremely valuable pieces of infor-mation from Eller, such as the wages paid to the crew, on which he could base a reasonable bid price. Connolly continued to pump Eller for information during the last week of March, preparing himself for the deadline of 12 April.[64]

Connolly decided on a price of $3.58 per pound of dried *Taxus brevi-folia* bark, translating into a total payment to him of $214,800. He met the deadline for the bid without trouble. Connolly, however, was not the kind of person who would sit back and await the results of a decision. He had, after all, put in a single bid for the entire amount of bark, something that Cragg's specifications discouraged. He felt that he needed to explain his reasons for bidding for the entire consignment by pointing out the large advantage in giving a single contract for the entire amount, while showing an environmental concern for the resource.[65] Whether his arguments and/or his price were crucial in tipping the decision his way, we cannot say. It would be difficult, however, to think that the knowledge Connolly displayed about *Taxus brevifolia* in these communications did not impress the staff at the NCI. On 6 May 1987 Connolly learned that he had been successful.[66] Despite the strength of belief in his own arguments, Connolly was still somewhat surprised by his success.[67] Within a few days of receiving notice of the contract, Connolly had gone into partnership with Eller, forming a company in Cottage Grove which, it was intended, would collect eighty per cent of the contracted amount, the remaining proportion being made up of various subcontracts in other parts of Oregon and Idaho.[68] Throughout the month, Connolly contacted various people in the state able to collect bark, building up a substantial network of subcontractors and their workers. He offered $1.47 per pound of dried bark, bagged and delivered to his leased warehouse in Drain, Oregon.

Connolly expected the collection to move swiftly and effortlessly. On many occasions he remarked upon the long-term nature of the venture, referring particularly to the economic benefits that would accrue to southern Oregon, an area that had recently become depressed.[69] Bark did flow into his warehouse rapidly, as he predicted, but the smooth operations soon became bumpy. Sometime in June, Connolly fell out with Eller and their partnership was dissolved on 15 June 1987.[70] The subcontracting system, as envisioned by Connolly, was fine in principle, but messy in practice. Recall that Connolly had set a price of $1.47 per pound for bark bagged and delivered to him by collectors independent of his arrangement with Eller. For those working directly under him (or Eller before he resigned), Connolly paid ninety cents per pound. As it turned out, it became difficult to distinguish between someone collecting on their own, as an independent subcontractor, and someone collecting on behalf of a subcontractor. Disputes over the correct payment boiled over into accusation and counter-accusation.[71] Then there was the problem of matching the NCI's payments, on receipt of bark, to those made by Connolly. Many times, he had to plead with his bankers for an extension of credit.

These matters were difficult enough, but the most serious problem came when the Forest Service closed access to the forest during July and August of 1987 because of acute fire risk.[72] Exactly the same had befallen Robert Warner when he was under contract in 1985 to collect bark. In September, Connolly asked Gordon Cragg of the Natural Products Branch to extend his contract into the following year in order to complete the contract: a new deadline of 6 September 1988 was set.[73] By the time the Forest Service closed the forest, Connolly had managed to provide the NCI with just over 37,000 pounds of *Taxus brevifolia* bark, two-thirds of the contracted amount.

The forest shut-out was a blow, not only to Connolly's finances in the medium term, but also to the NCI's plans for supplying taxol for the few active and the many promised clinical trials. Once again, the forest, the sole source of taxol, demonstrated the extent to which it could not be tamed, could not be relied upon to deliver its supplies.

Connolly waited out the winter until the sap started to run in *Taxus brevifolia*. At the NCI, by contrast, Cragg began his own inquiry into the tree. In February 1988, he got in touch with Charles Bolsinger, Principal Resource Analyst at the Pacific Northwest Research Station of the Forest Service in Portland, asking about *Taxus brevifolia*, particularly about its numbers.[74] Bolsinger gave Cragg descriptions of *Taxus brevifolia* and its habitat that were, in most respects, the same as had appeared in Spjut's guide of 1977. Bolsinger reiterated that the best place to find *Taxus brevifolia* was in the old-growth forests but, he emphasized, it was becoming scarcer because of its destruction through the practices of clear-cutting. As he put it: 'Unless deliberate measures are taken to perpetuate yew on commercial timberland it could eventually disappear from these lands.' Despite the dwindling numbers, Bolsinger felt that, taking into account the presence of *Taxus brevifolia* in areas that were generally not logged, 'it doesn't appear to be a threatened species'. This judgement relied entirely on estimates of the number of *Taxus brevifolia* growing on timberland *outside* (our emphasis) National Forests in western Oregon and western Washington. Nothing was known about the numbers on timberland *inside* (our emphasis) the National Forests.

It is important to explain why Bolsinger could not come up with a more comprehensive inventory.[75] Bolsinger worked in the Forest Inventory and Analysis Branch of the Forest Service. His duties were to provide whatever information was needed on the status and trends of forests in the Pacific Northwest, primarily for policy makers. Bolsinger and his colleagues prepared inventories by enumerating every vascular plant they could. No species was deliberately excluded. There were several counting methods including aerial photographs, ground reports, and sitings. The catch was, however, that Bolsinger and colleagues only inventoried private and state lands. The National Forests did their own inventory, but only enumerated species of timber with commercial value. As *Taxus brevifolia* was not considered a commercial species, it did not appear in any National Forest inventories.

Bolsinger's inventory of *Taxus brevifolia* showed that the population on private and state lands in five areas of the Pacific Northwest was 7.6 million trees.[76] Cragg, apparently, was delighted with the answer, especially as the figure did not include *Taxus brevifolia* in National Forests where, it was believed, there were more and larger trees growing. The reason for Cragg's delight is easy to understand. According to his own calculations, there was no shortage of trees for the purposes of supplying taxol to Phase II trials and he felt confident that expanding the clinical activity was justified.[77]

It was standard practice for the Division of Cancer Treatment to report annually to the FDA on those compounds for which an INDA had been filed. The first annual report on taxol was issued in March 1986. The second annual report, dated March 1987, provided the first preliminary indication of taxol's effectiveness. It reported that partial responses to taxol had been seen in patients with melanoma and refractory ovarian cancer, although nothing was seen in the case of renal cancer.[78] Though the number of evaluable patients was fairly small – twenty-four, eleven and twelve in the three diseases, respectively – the results were very encouraging.

The melanoma trial (Eastern Cooperative Oncology Group) had stopped taking patients in February of 1987 and, therefore, its results of three partial responses among twenty-four evaluable patients could only change within this fixed population. The ovarian cancer trial at Johns Hopkins University was still taking patients and with two partial responses in eleven evaluable patients was showing the best results in the current crop of trials. The eyes of the NCI fixed, therefore, on the Hopkins trial. So did others. By October of 1987, Dr William McGuire, one of the physicians involved with this trial, it will be recalled, had already been quoted in the *Philadelphia Inquirer* as saying that two of his twelve patients had shown dramatic improvement with taxol.

A complete response in oncological terms refers to the disappearance of the tumour; cases where the tumour decreases by fifty per cent are called partial responses. The two responses added together and divided by the number of evaluable patients, expressed as a percentage, is called the response rate. A response rate exceeding twenty per cent is considered good enough to warrant further, serious study in that specific disease.[79] The preliminary results of taxol on patients with refractory ovarian cancer at Johns Hopkins reported in the 1987 Annual Report to the FDA suggested a response rate of just under twenty per cent. When, according to McGuire, word got out that taxol was active in ovarian cancer, patient accrual accelerated – the first half of the accrual took well over a year, whereas the second half took just four months.[80]

News about the Hopkins trial reached the public only sporadically, but as the NCI was informed, the Hopkins trial kept producing even better results. By March 1988, the response rate had reached thirty per cent with fifty per cent more patients.[81] By the beginning of April, Cragg was able to record, on the basis of information from the Investigational Drug Branch of the Division of Cancer Treatment, that there was 'intense interest in taxol. People are begging for it.'[82] McGuire and his colleagues first made their results public when they announced taxol's thirty per cent response rate in refractory ovarian cancer at the 24th Annual Meeting of the American Society of Clinical Oncology in May 1988.[83] Even the melanoma response rate was reasonable, although significantly below that for ovarian cancer. Both melanoma and ovarian cancer were examples of 'signal' tumours: to have good response rates in two 'signal' tumours was considered quite an accomplishment.[84]

Whatever delight Cragg may have felt at finding out from Bolsinger that there was a considerable population of *Taxus brevifolia* in the Pacific Northwest was short-lived. Cragg calculated that three kilograms of taxol would satisfy Phase II trials. But these are experiments on a very small number of cancer patients and not therapies. They are once-and-for-all. Therapy, by contrast, is given over long periods and is available, in principle, to all patients with the cancer for which the treatment is indicated. Cragg calculated on the basis of the number of ovarian and melanoma cases presenting annually in the United States alone that, as a therapy, taxol would be consumed at the rate of ninety kilograms per year, equivalent to the destruction of 360,000 trees.

When one remembers that at this point taxol had only been tested in Phase II trials against melanoma, ovarian and renal cancer, then it is easy to understand how the reports from Hopkins and the Eastern Cooperative Oncology Group were simultaneously exciting and frightening. To put it simply, if taxol should prove to be effective against the major cancers of the time – breast, lung, or colon, for example – then the demand for the drug in clinical use would be phenomenal. Whatever the true population of *Taxus brevifolia* in the Pacific Northwest was, it was finite and depleting. Cancer was not.

Something needed to be done to prepare for taxol's success. Alternative sources of supply needed to be encouraged but Bethesda was not where the action was. Cragg, therefore, planned to visit the Pacific Northwest in April 1988. This was the first time that an official involved in the natural product cancer programme had ventured to the source of the molecule since Robert Perdue visited in August 1977.[85] Though Cragg wished to meet Connolly and discuss the collection with him and his colleagues, his chief reason for the trip was to meet with representatives of Weyerhaeuser, the Pacific Northwest's largest timber company.[86] Both Matthew Suffness and Susan Horwitz, of the Albert Einstein College of Medicine, were to meet him at Weyerhaeuser headquarters. Cragg began his visit on 18 April 1988, in central Oregon, meeting with Connolly and a number of associates, friends, officials and 'a representative of a local "Protect the Yew" group'. Among those present were several collectors from whom Cragg learned, first-hand, about the nature of collecting – he also learned about the amount of bark they could strip from a tree, hearing that the yield could reach as much as fifty pounds from a very large tree. He came away from this experience convinced that he could do business in the Northwest, that the NCI network could not only extend to the Pacific, but that it could be sustained easily. As he wrote in his report:[87]

> My overwhelming impression after the project. The project has received ample coverage in the Oregon media, and I feel that Oregonians regard taxol as their own special contribution to the cancer program. NCI will not have any problem soliciting collectors as long as reasonable supplies exist, even if it entails hauling trees from ravine bottoms where they tend to be more prevalent! Even the 'Yew protectionist' reacted favorably, and I assured all present that collections would not be pursued to the detriment of the environment.

The next day took him to Portland where he met with officials of the Forest Service and the Bureau of Land Management. At this meeting, Cragg verified for himself the lack of interest by both the Forest Service and the Bureau of Land Management in *Taxus brevifolia* despite their involvement in collections and their knowledge of taxol's rise in importance since the late 1960s. He did, however, get some assurance from the representatives of the agencies, that in future they would take the species more seriously by restricting its indiscriminate destruction – in clear cuts, for example – and by enumerating its population. The assurances, however, were not without condition: in principle, they were in favour of a *Taxus brevifolia* inventory, but stressed that, in practice, it was expensive. Other matters that came up were such questions as whether taxol occurred throughout the bark or in a particular layer; whether it was in the sap; and to what extent the yield of taxol varied by the location of the tree. The latter question had, as we have seen, been asked several times before and answered on several occasions. The former questions were new and reflected primarily environmental concerns about the method and impact of the present harvesting techniques, attempting to find a non-destructive way of making *Taxus brevifolia* part with its precious molecule. There was much talk about cooperative research projects but finances always got in the way.

On the third day of his visit, Gordon Cragg met with two geneticists employed at the seedling production facilities of Weyerhaeuser. These facilities concentrated on Douglas fir, on improving the genotypes in order to increase the rate at which they grew once the seedlings were transplanted as part of the company's reforestation activities. Discussions had already taken place at an earlier date about the possibility of the mass propagation of *Taxus brevifolia* seedlings. Nicholas Wheeler, one of the geneticists involved in these discussions, had been studying these possibilities. In 1987, Weyerhaeuser began to test *Taxus brevifolia* genetically, starting with sowing 25,000 seeds in the company's greenhouses.[88]

On his fourth and final day, Cragg teamed up with Matthew Suffness and Susan Horwitz to discuss taxol with representatives of the company. These were preliminary discussions, rather than substantive talks, exploring possibilities for mass propagation of *Taxus brevifolia* and the company involving itself in primary extraction and isolation of taxol.

Cragg was pleased with his trip but he was clearly anxious about the supply problem. His concern was not about the practicalities of collecting nor the likelihood of meeting future requirements from the forest. In the latter regard, as we have seen, he was already assured by Charles Bolsinger of the Forest Service that there was more than enough out there for the foreseeable future. Rather, the supply problem had become complicated because the forest had changed and because of the voices that were prepared to speak on its behalf. In the summary of his visit, Cragg noted simply that 'environmental considerations will probably permit only one or two more large collections (60,000 lbs) of dried bark.' He and Matthew Suffness were, however, not prepared to let things run their course, but actively sought to produce activity leading to alternative supplies of taxol. Cragg reiterated his wish for some kind of research association between the Forest Service and Weyerhaeuser when he wrote to Charles Philpot, Station Director of the Pacific Northwest Research Station shortly after returning to Bethesda.[89]

The contact with Weyerhaeuser was the first time that the Natural Products Branch had reached out to a large established private company for help in the crisis looming within the programme. It was a crisis that had not been so much predicted as anticipated by Robert Perdue at the USDA from the late 1960s onwards, a point which he repeatedly made to the NCI and the Forest Service equally. In the meantime, the milieu had changed dramatically. Taxol was in Phase II clinical trials showing remarkable results against refractory ovarian cancer with pent-up demand among the clinical oncology community for more and larger trials; but the forest was no longer a resource to be plundered at will.

The tension between short-term needs and long-term planning was intense and growing. It surfaced in 1988 in many dealings of the Natural Products Branch. At the same time as he enjoined Philpot to join him in working with Weyerhaeuser and others in the search for alternative supplies to those of stripping bark from wild trees, Cragg also announced that the NCI would be asking for another large collection in the following year.[90] Matthew Suffness expressed his extremely worrying concerns about the supply of taxol to John Douros, his former boss at the Natural Products Branch, by then at Bristol-Myers. He was deeply pessimistic about supplies from the forest and predicted that continued collection of bark would 'exhaust the available supplies in the National Forests within the next two to three years'.[91] He also mentioned to Douros the facilities at Weyerhaeuser and their interest, in principle, in growing *Taxus brevifolia*. Meanwhile, Patrick Connolly had not yet completed his contract which had been put on hold because of the fire risk in the previous summer. Little is known about this part of the collection, but it was completed on time and successfully by August 1988.[92]

The difficulties in co-ordinating the demand for taxol for clinical trials with the collection of bark, its extraction and purification, together with the finances necessary to cover costs, escalated in 1988. Connolly's collection would not appear as taxol for some time. The first batch of bulk drug was expected early in 1989, with formulation into 13,500 vials being completed approximately three months later.[93] The rest of the formulated taxol was not expected to be ready until late 1990 and 1991 at the earliest. Ultimately it depended on funding. To complete the transformation of Connolly's collection into taxol required almost $750,000, an amount that would need to be found in the following fiscal year.[94]

Funds were not the only problem, however. Yield was another, which despite variations, doggedly stuck at an average of 0.01 per cent.[95] How to increase it would become a main preoccupation over the next few years. That and alternative supply sources were long-term concerns. More immediately, however, there was yet another issue; namely, that the amounts of taxol necessary for clinical trials stretched the extraction and purification capacity of Polysciences, the current contractor. That it was a long and complicated process was taken for granted, but with collections of 60,000 pounds (and even bigger collections anticipated), the present arrangements meant very long waiting times. The relative lack of isolation facilities for natural products in the United States was an acknowledged shortcoming.[96] In order to get the job done, the NCI needed to look elsewhere for capacity, as Polysciences would not or could not expand any further.[97] After soliciting help from several quarters, their searches finally took them to Hauser Chemical Research, a company based in Boulder, Colorado, founded in 1983 and with experience in extracting compounds from natural products.[98] Gordon Cragg had made a site visit to the facilities to inspect them in anticipation of Hauser applying for an NCI contract for the isolation of antitumour agents from natural sources in January 1987.[99] At that time, the topic of taxol was discussed. Hauser received its first Master

Agreement in December 1987 and an order under this agreement to perform the extraction from *Taxus brevifolia* bark in October 1988.[100] Hauser's first responsibility was to obtain the crude extract from 25,000 pounds of Connolly's collection. This was completed successfully in February 1989.[101] Hauser received its first contract to isolate pure crystalline taxol from crude extract in February 1989.[102] Sharing work with Polysciences was a short-term solution. The disadvantage of this arrangement lay in further complicated planning.[103]

The long gap between collection and formulation, complicated by budgetary planning, put acute pressure on the planning of clinical trials and, therefore, importantly, on collecting the clinical information necessary for an approval application. But the programme could not stand still and planning for trials needed to be done on the assumption that funding would be forthcoming. In any case, the cost of collecting bark was the least expensive part of the process of getting taxol; at the very least, collections would go ahead, even though lack of funding might hold up extraction and purification of taxol.[104]

So great was the interest in taxol and so complex the planning details that the small group most familiar with taxol decided that it would be in everyone's best interest to institutionalize the flow of taxol information, in the form of a regular monthly meeting. The first meeting of what would be called the 'Taxol Working Group' was planned for 23 June 1988.[105] The crisis of supply dominated the discussions. The meeting was told again of the current low level of taxol supply. Only two new trials – a Phase I combination trial of cisplatin and taxol and a larger Phase II trial on advanced ovarian cancer patients – would go ahead, but all other trials would remain on hold. Indeed, so tight was future planning that serious consideration was given to pursuing clinical development in ovarian cancer alone.

Three other matters were raised at the June meeting. The first was the announcement that it was necessary to collect a further 60,000 pounds of bark and that this would be scheduled for the following summer. Bids would be asked for in the usual manner in due course. The Forest Service was given due notice of this intention, as was the Bureau of Land Management and the Investigational Drug Branch of the NCI.[106] The second matter was that of money. The meeting was told that, even though the Board of Scientific Counselors of the Division of Cancer Treatment had approved $700,000 for taxol development, the funding, once again, would not be made available because of budget cuts. Finally and perhaps most strikingly, a discussion took place on how to facilitate collaboration with a pharmaceutical company. Several companies were mentioned: Bristol-Myers, Upjohn, Lyphomed, Unimed and Adria.

It seems that at certain times the impetus to contact pharmaceutical companies came from the NCI while at other times it was the companies themselves who initiated the contact. A memo dated 6 July 1988 from Matthew Suffness to John Douros, who was then at Bristol-Myers but was about to leave the company, retaining his contact with them as a consultant, makes it clear that Suffness was anxious to enlist industrial support. He said 'I did speak with Dr Julius Vida' (of Bristol-Myers) 'but a push from you might help.'[107] But then many companies were asking about taxol in the latter part of 1988, in part, no doubt, because of the announcement of taxol's activity in ovarian cancer presented at the American Society of Clinical Oncology meeting in May of that year. These included those companies mentioned above as well as Lederle, Schering, Merck, Sharpe and Dohme, Sterling Pharmaceuticals and Rhône-Poulenc.[108]

Though a pharmaceutical company would inevitably be involved in the commercial end of taxol's development, as would happen with any drug developed at the NCI, at this stage the role of such a company was not finalized. Indeed, there were at least three roles discussed or foreseen. One was that of a licensee. Robert Wittes's discussions about taxol with Schering-Plough was in this vein.[109] Another was that of joining with Weyerhaeuser in pursuing mass propagation and, as we have seen, extraction and purification of taxol. This is the point that Suffness tried to impress on Douros in discussing the future of taxol.[110] Weyerhaeuser, Suffness told Douros, was interested in growing *Taxus brevifolia* through mass propagation, but what would seal their interest would be a partnership with a pharmaceutical company. There was a lot in it for a pharmaceutical company. As Suffness stated: 'Since the only good, clean source of Taxol is *T. brevifolia* which only grows in the Pacific Northwest a joint project with Weyerhaeuser could lock up the supply from a practical viewpoint. In view of the current exciting results in ovarian cancer this is well worth pursuing.' Suffness was not alone in pushing Weyerhaeuser together with a pharmaceutical company. Each inquiry from a pharmaceutical company regarding taxol that came Cragg's way was told of Weyerhaeuser's interest and pointed in their direction for further discussions.[111] The third way in which pharmaceutical industry participation was envisioned was by the injection of cash. Suffness was frank about the problem of money. He told Douros that 'even at the current level of clinical trials, taxol is expensive for us and we would not be able to put enough money behind it to produce enough for broad trials. This is a case where industrial support is needed to fully develop the drug.' This same point was made by Cragg to the Forest Service in a letter in which he also informed them that, because of budgetary constraints, the research projects they discussed at their meeting in Portland in the spring, could not be financed by the NCI.[112]

The July meeting of the Taxol Working Group had little new to report, but the next meeting in August was more eventful.[113] For one thing, Gisele Sarosy, the Senior Investigator in the Investigational Drug Branch, confirmed that the results of the Phase II clinical trial on ovarian cancer patients at Johns Hopkins were striking: to date, the trial was showing a thirty per cent response rate. While this must have been welcomed with delight, it also focused subsequent discussions on to supply and finances. It looked as though whatever funding was available would be devoted entirely to collecting bark and extracting and purifying taxol: development work and alternative strategies, such as those envisioned by the Forest Service, would have to be shelved.[114]

The supply issue came up in discussions about alternative methods of making taxol. Michael Hawkins, Chief of the Investigational Drug Branch, reacted to the problem by suggesting that the NCI seek to cooperate with a biotechnology company to produce taxol through genetic engineering methods (as with interleukin-2). This proposal had merit in that, while taxol itself could not be patented, the envisioned synthetic process could. On the other hand, the technical difficulties were great. Nevertheless, Hawkins was asked to pursue the idea by contacting the appropriate people at Agrocetus, the Wisconsin-based biotechnology company. Cragg, on the other hand, argued that the most feasible way of producing taxol was mass propagation, using technology developed by Weyerhaeuser. Four- to seven-year-old saplings, he maintained, contained as much as fifty per cent of the taxol content of adult trees. He could not envision, in the foreseeable future at least, another method that might yield a solution to the supply problem. The taxol molecule had not yet been totally synthesized, and tissue culture methods, another possibility, had not yet been applied to the commercial production of any drug, let alone taxol. Cragg made no mention of semi-synthesis. Matthew Suffness also seems to have ruled out not only total synthesis but also semi-synthesis. In his memo to Douros in July, mentioned above, he said: '... the likelihood of a practical total synthesis in the future seems close to zero. Semi-synthesis is likewise not meaningful because the genus *Taxus* is the only source of the taxane ring system.'[115]

In fact an article describing a semi-synthetic route to taxol from renewable parts of the (more abundant) *Taxus baccata* had been received by the *Journal of the American Chemical Society* in April 1988 from Pierre Potier's group in Paris and Andrew Greene's group in Grenoble, France, while a French patent application had been made at the same time.[116] The NCI did not greet the French semi-synthesis with overwhelming enthusiasm as a solution to the supply problem.[117] The following year, *The Journal of the National Cancer Institute* reported the Potier–Greene synthesis without mentioning their names, first quoting their work as 'a 1988 article in the *Journal of the American Chemical Society*', describing taxol as 'quite possibly the number one target of synthetic organic chemists', and then referring to 'French researchers [who]...have identified a precursor of taxol in the needles of ... *Taxus baccata*...which they can then convert to taxol in a four-step procedure', without indicating that the authors of the article and the 'French researchers' were one and the same.[118] But it was not long after the Potier–Greene synthesis that NCI funding for taxol chemistry projects began to take off. Paul Wender at Stanford says he put in a research proposal in 1989, was told it was 'too modest' and was encouraged to scale up his programme.[119] According to him, the NCI then put out requests for grant applications for alternative routes to taxol, and he was asked to chair one of the groups reviewing the applications.[120] David Kingston at Virginia Polytechnic Institute also reports that the NCI began to pump funds into taxol chemistry and actively to seek bids from researchers in the area. 'Funding mushroomed around 1990,' he said.[121] By mid-1991, a review by Charles Swindell at Bryn Mawr was able to report on some thirty groups' work on the synthesis of taxol.[122]

In 1988 *Chemical and Engineering News* reported that the NCI was supporting several research studies towards a total synthesis of taxol, and that Bob Holton alone had funds totalling almost one million dollars.[123] Some of these projects were undertaken to generate new chemical knowledge, but some of them aimed at the goal of a commercially viable route to taxol, although it seemed a total synthesis would take some thirty to fifty chemical steps and generate such low overall yields that it would not be suitable for making commodity amounts.

Bob Holton's recollection is somewhat different from that of Wender and of Kingston: he does not remember an active seeking by the NCI of research proposals aimed at a practical process, but rather that in about 1988:[124]

> The NCI never said a thing. But I was aware that the NCI had gotten to a point where they thought the drug was commercializable and needed a partner, and were putting out feelers. People at the NCI were very very high on taxol, particularly Matthew Suffness who had been an advocate for taxol since the beginning. I started thinking about how you might put the side chain on, particularly since Andy Greene showed me how hard it was. The issue was putting the side chain on at 13. I mean they had worked out a reasonable protection scheme.[125]

The focusing of attention on a practical route to taxol may or may not have been stimulated in individual chemists' cases by the NCI, but two other trends would certainly have influenced them. First of all, between 1980 and 1986 several Acts were passed by Congress – Bayh-Dole, Stevenson-Wydler, the Federal Transfer of Technology Act – whose purpose was to stimulate the commercial exploitation of publicly funded research (with a focus on the vast programmes of expenditure of the Department of Defense and the NIH).[126] These Acts, together with the attendant publicity, would have encouraged public sector researchers to patent and think of new ways to make money out of their work. Secondly, articles about taxol and the supply problem were beginning to appear in scientific journals, and would have given a more precise focus to natural product chemists interested in commercializing research output.

There were three main issues to tackle in devising a semi-synthetic route to taxol. These were: first, the reactivity of the four hydroxyl (–OH) groups of 10-DAB and the need to attach a side chain to only one of them; second, obtaining the correct stereoisomerism of the molecule;[127] and third, the difficulty of accessing the site at which the side chain was to be attached, owing to the shape of the molecule. For Greene, Potier and their colleagues' semi-synthesis, the side chain was made separately, and then attached to the 10-DAB.

A complex molecule, such as taxol, has several centres of asymmetry. Alternative forms, or isomers, differ rather like left and right hands. Biologically active molecules are often less active, or not active at all, in one of their stereoisomeric forms. This means that the synthesis of a compound is complicated by the need not only to attach the right groups to the right parts of the molecule's skeleton, but also to achieve the desired orientation in space. In the case of taxol, the side chain itself had to be attached to the skeleton and also have the required orientation.

When Potier and Greene made taxol by semi-synthesis in 1988, the key was to make an acid form of the side chain react with a particular hydroxy (or –OH group) in order to attach the side chain. However, 10-DAB has four –OH groups, and in principle an acid form of the side chain could react with any of them.[128] In fact two of the –OH groups are more reactive than the one in the desired position (C-13). This is because the –OH group at C-13 on 10-DAB is obscured by other parts of the molecule – in three dimensions, 10-DAB is cup- or dome-shaped, with the –OH group at C-13 tucked underneath the concave face of the molecule. This makes it difficult to attach the side chain as it has to approach the molecule from underneath the dome (see Figure 4.1).

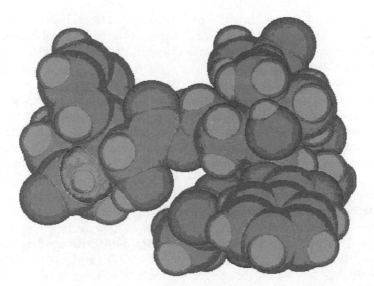

Figure 4.1 Three-dimensional representation of taxol, as produced on a computer screen.

To prevent the side chain from attaching to either of the two more reactive –OH groups in 10-DAB, they can be blocked by a reaction that is easy to reverse once the side chain has been attached in the right place. This is a normal procedure with complex molecules. In the Potier–Greene semi-synthesis, there is an additional –OH group on the side chain, and it, too, had to be protected.

When Holton decided to make taxol semi-synthetically he tried to find a molecule that would act as a surrogate for the side chain while it was being attached, which was smaller and more compact than the side chain itself. It would then be transformed into the side chain afterwards. He wanted something that would fold up, and a β-lactam, which has a ring structure, seemed to fit the bill. It gave a very high yield, and he took out a patent on it in 1990.[129] Several other research groups have also reported methods using β-lactams as precursors of the taxol side chain, including those of Ojima, Georg, Farina and Palomo.[130] Holton also patented a modified method in which less concentrated reagents were used, making the process easier to scale up.[131] A whole plethora of semi-synthetic processes then began to appear.

In the meantime, however, it was back to reality and the forest. Cragg felt that there were an additional 120,000 pounds of bark out there. The next collection would take place in spring 1989. Formulated taxol from this collection would be available sometime in 1991. Cragg also reported that he would try and put some pressure on Bruce Chabner, director of the Division of Cancer Treatment, to make available funds that were awarded to the pharmaceutical development of taxol and subsequently frozen.

The tenor of the meeting, at least to the extent that it can be reconstructed from the minutes, suggests that the taxol supply problem was putting the NCI into a situation that was difficult and possibly unprecedented. The Taxol Working Group was clearly trying to find a solution or solutions to solve the supply problem at the same time as the financial commitments to maintain clinical trials grew. A pharmaceutical company partnership, of whatever kind, was proposed as one among other options. Behind the scenes, though, events were taking place that would constrain choices of action and funnel decisions in one direction.

The key player in the behind-the-scenes actions during this period, that is 1988, was Weyerhaeuser. In July, Matthew Suffness briefed his colleagues in the Division of Cancer Treatment on developments at Weyerhaeuser.[132] The taxol project was scheduled to go before the vice-president in charge of research and development for the approval of funds for research on the biology and growth of *Taxus brevifolia*, and the development of processing methods and technology.[133] The company was taking a broad approach to taxol production, entertaining seriously each possible method. One such approach, the production of taxol by tissue culture, pioneered by Alice Christen of the USDA Southern Regional Research Laboratories in New Orleans, was being pursued by Weyerhaeuser in co-operation with her. Suffness remarked that the company's strategy was to cover all the possibilities, giving them the opportunity to license any emerging technology.[134]

Weyerhaeuser, according to Suffness, was interested in taxol as a 'wedge to start a major push internally towards high value products (including fine chemicals) from trees as opposed to only producing boards and pulp which is their main business now'. They hoped for some encouragement from the NCI but were not dependent upon it. Suffness maintained that the firm's move to taxol would be part of a major corporate strategy towards diversification.[135] Though he gave no indication why Weyerhaeuser might be interested in this change of direction, an important part of the reason lay in the changing politics of the forest, a topic to which we will return shortly.

Suffness was clearly impressed by Weyerhaeuser's plans. He also revealed, importantly, that they had been in talks with Bristol-Myers, discussing an exclusive sales agreement in which 'Bristol will buy taxol (or equivalent raw material) only from Weyerhaeuser and conversely Weyerhaeuser will not sell to anyone but Bristol'. Suffness would not have been surprised that Weyerhaeuser and Bristol-Myers were talking as, a few weeks earlier, he had been in touch with John Douros at Bristol-Myers, and had asked him to push in that direction.[136] This followed quickly upon a meeting, held in July 1988, between Suffness and Julius Vida, vice-president of Licensing for the Science and Technology Group of Bristol-Myers.[137]

Though Suffness's brief focused on Weyerhaeuser and, less directly, on Bristol-Myers, it also confirmed that the NCI's long involvement with taxol was nearing an end. The NCI was aiming at 'getting out of the expense of producing taxol.' As he wrote in an earlier memo: 'If a marriage can be arranged between Weyerhaeuser and Bristol or another large pharmaceutical company, the long term supply situation on taxol could be resolved.'[138] But, he emphasized, this was in the long term. In the short to medium term he expected that the NCI would continue to collect bark, extract, isolate and formulate taxol.

Taking all this into account, it would seem that by the time of their next meeting, in September 1988, the Taxol Working Group had cast a wide net in search of the solution to the problem of supply. Biotechnology companies, pharmaceutical companies, Weyerhaeuser, and several different kinds of technologies were mentioned as possible solutions. But it was the lack of funds within the NCI that was the main stumbling block in thinking through the possibilities.[139] The meeting was told that two million dollars was needed to complete the extraction and purification of taxol from Connolly's collection and that of the forthcoming 60,000 pound collection. Unfortunately, the Developmental Therapeutics Program had only one-tenth of this amount available for the large-scale isolation of natural products, and a portion of it had already been committed to another promising product, bryostatin.[140]

The bulk of the discussion, however, focused on how to get a pharmaceutical company to collaborate. Why this issue received so much attention at this time is unclear. Certainly there were ongoing discussions with pharmaceutical companies, but as we have seen other possibilities were also discussed. Perhaps it was the looming financial crisis that focused attention on a more universal, rather than a piecemeal solution to the supply problem. Discussions between Weyerhaeuser and Bristol-Myers offered indications that such a universal solution was feasible. At any rate, events at the meeting moved rapidly and concentrated not on the question as to whether an NCI collaboration with a pharmaceutical company was in everyone's best interest, but on the nature of such a collaboration.

Several proposals for the shape of the collaboration were put forward, including one where the NCI would designate the partner and another where the designation would be open to competition. It is clear that whatever option they decided to take, the Taxol Working Group were thinking in terms, not of collaboration, in the sense of a partnership in which each party would get some tangible benefit, but rather of a hand-over of taxol (and its problems) to a pharmaceutical company. These are the crucial words recorded in the minutes.

> The NCI may be able to offer the following concerning taxol:
> 1) current supply (both formulated and bulk); 2) a drug of true orphan stature; 3) the only source of drug for at least 2 years; and, 4) a proprietary IND. Alternatively, the drug company may be expected to provide: 1) funds for the isolation of collected raw material; 2) funds for obtaining future supplies of taxol; and, 3) a large proportion of the funds needed for clinical trials of taxol.

Robert Lanman, the NIH legal advisor, was approached for advice as to which mechanism should be adopted. The memo to Lanman spelled out, as clearly as possible, what the Division of Cancer Treatment wanted from a pharmaceutical company.[141] Its main objective was to provide resources to process the *Taxus brevifolia* bark already collected and in the planning stage for the following year, in return for the exclusive rights to data from the key Phase III trials – discussions about the latter for ovarian cancer were already under way with the clinical oncologists at Johns Hopkins University. Money, to the tune of two million dollars, was the reason put forth for this needed collaboration. There was no patent on taxol but it did classify as an orphan agent.[142] Sarosy emphasized that time was of the essence. If it were legally possible to avoid an open competition and, instead, simply choose a partner through negotiation, so much the better.

By the time of the December meeting of the Taxol Working Group, the memo to Lanman had done the rounds and a representative of the Division of Cancer Prevention and Control, rather than a legal representative, attended to inform the members of the kind of mechanism that would meet their needs.[143] The representative, Dr Barney Lepovetsky, outlined a mechanism for collaboration with the private sector, called a CRADA – Cooperative Research and Development Agreement. This grew directly out of the newly enacted Federal Technology Transfer Act of 1986, designed to facilitate the transfer of commercially promising knowledge from federal agencies to private industry.[144] Because of the relative novelty of the CRADA, several of its features had not been fully settled and were, therefore, open to modification.[145] The questioning of Dr Lepovetsky also suggested that the guidelines were flexible, partly because each cooperative venture had features unique to it. In the case of taxol, the fact that subcontractors were used to collect and process the raw material, meant that the nature of the cooperation extended beyond the two-party scheme defined by the CRADA.

Dr Lepovetsky described the CRADA as a mechanism that did not require a competitive bid. All that had to happen was for a representative from NIH to contact a representative from industry interested in the terms of the CRADA. The NCI Director and an equivalent senior person at the prospective company would then negotiate towards a final agreement. Lepovetsky thought the whole process would take four months to conclude. The lack of a patent on taxol was not a problem. Unpatentable products, Lepovetsky maintained, had been licensed previously and, in any case, the NCI would be giving the pharmaceutical company exclusive rights to the taxol supply. The meeting agreed to pursue the CRADA and asked Dale Shoemaker from the Regulatory Affairs Branch and Paul Davignon from the Pharmaceutical Resources Branch to initiate the process. A draft of the proposed CRADA was ready by the middle of January 1989.[146] This contained the essential features that the Taxol Working Group wished to see in a collaborative agreement. In one respect, however, the draft CRADA departed from Lepovetsky's suggestions: instead of choosing a partner, the writers felt it was in everyone's best interest to make the application to be the taxol CRADA partner competitive.[147] An announcement to the effect that the NCI was seeking a pharmaceutical company as a partner to develop taxol would appear in the *Federal Register* when the final form of the CRADA document was approved at the highest level.

At virtually the same moment as the draft CRADA was circulated, bids were opened for the next 60,000 pound collection of *Taxus brevifolia* bark, scheduled for the coming summer: the deadline for accepting bids was 21 February 1989.[148] John Destito was one of several individuals who bid for the contract. The NCI received his bid on 16 February 1989. At a price of $2.74 per pound of dried bark, Destito's was by far the lowest bid in this, or for any of the previous competitions for collection.[149] After some delay, Destito received his contract on 17 April 1989.

Destito was a former gun-shop owner in Walla Walla, Washington State. In 1988, he set up a company, Advanced Molecular Technologies, based in Bellevue, Washington (near Seattle), with a small but highly experienced scientific staff to produce and supply a variety of natural, biologically active products to the research community and the pharmaceutical industry.[150] Destito's bid for the *Taxus brevifolia* collection contract was unusual in the context of the objectives of his company. Furthermore, he had had no previous experience in the forest business. Destito's bid price of $2.74 was a guess, but as it was the lowest bid, he got the contract.[151]

Destito may have lacked forest experience, but his bid did not come out of the blue. By the end of 1988, Destito had already made contact with several people at Weyerhaeuser and at the Natural Products Branch of the NCI including, particularly, its Chief, Matthew Suffness. He had asked Suffness about the likely market for bioactive compounds as he had asked others who would have this knowledge.[152] From his contacts at Weyerhaeuser, Destito had also learned about the NCI's taxol programme. By late 1988, Destito had already had preliminary discussions with several people at Weyerhaeuser about the possibility of a joint venture with the company, in which Weyerhaeuser or another party would provide *Taxus* raw materials to Advanced Molecular Technologies from which it would extract and purify taxol.[153]

The contact with Suffness was particularly important and could not have come at a better time. In the last quarter of 1988, Suffness's relationships with his superiors became difficult, and his days in the Natural Products Branch became numbered. Suffness began to look around for other openings including the possibility of working for Advanced Molecular Technologies.[154] For personal reasons, Suffness did not pursue employment with Advanced Molecular Technologies, but his tenure at the Natural Products Branch did come to an end. Suffness moved to a position of equal seniority in the Grants and Contracts Operations Branch effective from 1989.[155] Though he never lost touch with taxol, this change of employment meant that after more than a decade of being so closely associated with its performance, Suffness watched events from the sidelines. Gordon Cragg replaced Suffness as Chief of the Natural Products Branch.

The departure of Suffness was, in terms of connections with the Natural Products Branch, a set-back for Destito. Suffness was a player, to be sure, but Destito's strategy was not to focus on any one individual, but rather to map out all the connections and networks in which taxol existed. His lack of background in the forest business was not an impediment. His efforts at networking covered not just the community at the NCI, but the timber community, pharmaceutical companies, biotechnology companies, and so forth, right across the country and abroad. 'He wove himself into all sorts of characters concerned with taxol' is how one colleague has described Destito.[156] In this way, his bid and his company were a break in the whole history of *Taxus brevifolia* collections.

Destito may have been surprised at winning the collection contract, but he was not the only one. Patrick Connolly, who had collected the previous 60,000 pounds at a bid price of $3.58 per pound, filed a protest, on the grounds of Destito's experience and 'unrealistically low' price.[157] He maintained that these two features would jeopardize the entire collection and, by implication, all of the NCI's planning for clinical trials. The General Accounting Office who handled the matter found against the protest and supported the NCI's award of the contract to Destito.

The protest held up the award of the contract to Destito and accounts for the long lag between the deadline for bids – 21 February 1989 – and the award of the contract – 17 April 1989. Another week passed while Forest Service and Bureau of Land Management officials were notified that Destito was the NCI's official collector. Destito did not get the go-ahead to start collecting until 22 April 1989, two months after the deadline and into the season when the sap was running.[158]

On the basis of inquiries with Forest Service and Bureau of Land Management officials, Destito felt he could collect all the necessary bark in Washington, Oregon and Idaho: he also notified the NCI of the possibility of collecting on private lands owned by the region's timber companies, particularly Weyerhaeuser and the Simpson Timber Company.[159] In order to advertise his presence and his newly created part as a player in the Pacific Northwest forest business, Destito sent an open letter, on 1 June 1989, to anyone connected, in whatever manner, to the timber industry. In this letter, he informed the timber community of his contract with the NCI and linked his and the NCI's fate with them. As he stated it: 'It is essential for Advanced Molecular Technologies to gain the support, enthusiasm, and co-operation of the Northwest Timber Industry. The fate of the development of this "cancer wonder drug" rests in the hands of the logging industry!'[160] He reinforced and played on this network of fate further on in the letter when he appealed for the soul of the region by triangulating cancer, *Taxus brevifolia* and the timber industry. This is how it read.

> In the name of *'cancer research'*, we are making the plea to all individuals, companies, and associations that represent the timber industry in the Pacific Northwest and the West Coast to stand up and lend their assistance to their fellow man and the National Cancer Institute in this worthy cause. If there are any yew trees in the areas that have been logged, are being logged now, or will be logged in the future, please salvage their useful-ness in the fight against cancer by keeping the tree and branches intact and placed in a pile at the landings or slash piles. Please keep in mind that *Taxol is derived from the bark of the tree*, there-fore caution should be taken to preserve as much of the tree as possible.

Given the time of the year he was starting, however, it would have been difficult, if not impossible, to collect the 60,000 pounds of bark in one season, as required by the contract. According to Destito, by the time all the paths were cleared to allow for his collection, it was the end of July.[161] By then, however, the season was coming to an end. Instead of stopping the collection because of the increasing difficulty of stripping the bark by hand, Destito decided to stockpile the trees and strip them in the winter. By the beginning of September, Destito had managed to collect only 8,000 pounds of dried bark, less than fifteen per cent of the amount he should have had.[162] For the third time, since Robert Warner's contract in 1984, the collection had not gone according to plan. This time it was bureaucracy, rather than the forest, that was to blame. The collection would resume in 1990, by which time, Destito and taxol were in a new and uncertain position.

On 1 August 1989, the *Federal Register* carried the announcement of the CRADA for taxol.[163] It called for pharmaceutical companies who were interested in developing 'taxol to a marketable status to meet the needs of the public and with the best terms for the Government', to respond by 15 September.[164] The announcement carried the latest results of the Johns Hopkins trial on advanced ovarian cancer, quoting a response rate of thirty per cent, without mentioning any other trials.[165] Indeed, shortly after the appearance of the taxol CRADA announcement, the results of the Johns Hopkins trial were published amidst a flurry of media interest.[166] Not surprisingly, the news release was far more up-beat than the scientific communication.[167] William McGuire spoke for the oncology team, the cancer patients and taxol. 'Thirty percent sounds low, but it is really quite remarkable for this type of cancer. There is no other drug that has produced this kind of response in drug refractory ovarian cancer... There were patients treated who were two to three weeks from death who are still alive today because of taxol.' Taxol, according to the news release, was 'the first promising new drug introduced for ovarian cancer since 1975'.

By the end of the summer of 1989, taxol had finally emerged from clinical trials as a potent molecule in the treatment of what was commonly known as the 'silent killer'.[168] Through the announcement of the CRADA and the Johns Hopkins trial results, taxol came under public gaze to an extent rarely accorded a specific anti-cancer compound. How taxol and all its human and non-human accompaniments fared in this new light would be revealed in the next few years.

Before we embark on this part of taxol's long and twisting history, one other element needs to be put in place, the politics of the forest. As mentioned earlier, Matthew Suffness informed his colleagues at the NCI at the end of July 1988 that Weyerhaeuser was considering a change in corporate strategy away from its traditional concentration on lumber to a more diversified portfolio including forest by-products. *Taxus brevifolia* and taxol were viewed as a wedge in this process of corporate realignment. Weyerhaeuser's plans need to be viewed in the context of important changes that had been and were occurring in the forests of the Pacific Northwest.

The late 1980s were a complicated time for the forest, and all those whose livelihoods and positions depended upon it. These complications will be examined in Chapter 6, but for now two critical events need mentioning. The first of these was the formation of the Old-Growth Definition Task Group of the Forest Service.[169] This group, chaired by Jerry Franklin, was charged with developing an interim definition of old-growth for use in forest management decisions. It produced its report, in the form of an extended workable definition of old-growth, in order to standardize current and future discussions and research activities.[170] In accordance with the pioneering work that Franklin and his colleagues had undertaken in the late 1970s and early 1980s, the authors of the report adopted a strictly ecological definition of old-growth, at the same time as providing a straightforward quantitative standard by which to assess whether any particular forest qualified as old-growth.[171] The definition was important for two principal reasons. First, it established that ecological characteristics were the basis of definitions of place. In the case of old-growth, the age of the stand – one of the most widely used definitions – was but one among several other features. The presence of snags and logs was firmly established as being part of the definition. Secondly, it was a workable definition in that it allowed anyone with access to a tape measure to construct arguments about old-growth forests.[172] This would become crucially important in the following years.

The publication of Franklin's report was a major development in the discourse of Pacific Northwest forests. It did not, however, produce much media interest. The second major event, by contrast, was hardly ever outside media gaze. Yet it, too, directly affected the discourse as well as the practices of the forest.

Environmental concerns about the decline of the great forests of the Pacific Northwest were, as we have seen, growing considerably through the 1980s. Surprisingly, while the debates continued to traverse this large and contentious political terrain, administrative and legalistic activities became focused on a single species within the old-growth forests. The species, the northern spotted owl, first emerged out of the legislative achievements of the 1970s when, in accordance with the National Forest Management Act, the Forest Service designated it as a Management Indicator Species.[173] This designation interconnected, for the first time, the fate of the spotted owl with that of its habitat, the old-growth forest.[174]

The interconnection continued to be reinforced through the 1980s through legal challenges to federal agencies, culminating in the eventual listing of the spotted owl as a threatened species. The first challenge came in 1987 when both Green World, a tiny environmental group in Massachusetts and the larger and more influential Sierra Club Defense Fund, representing a host of small groups, petitioned the Fish and Wildlife Service to list the owl as an endangered species under the Endangered Species Act.[175] An endangered species was defined under the act as one in imminent danger of extinction: a threatened species, a less restrictive designation, was one that was likely to be endangered in the future. The Fish and Wildlife Service declined the petition, on the grounds of insufficient evidence to decide the case, but in November 1988, US District Court Judge Thomas Zilly threw the case back to the Fish and Wildlife Service, arguing that its decision was 'arbitrary and capricious' and that it should think again.[176] After a review of its procedures and the attention to the evidence on the spotted owl that was available to it but apparently ignored in the previous decision, the Fish and Wildlife Service found in April 1989 that the spotted owl was threatened and a notice in the *Federal Register* of 23 June 1989 was posted to that effect.[177]

A listing of a species as either endangered or threatened needs to be followed by a ruling that sets aside critical habitat, a specific area or a range of areas protected from human activity.[178] Yet the Fish and Wildlife Service made no indication of critical habitat at this time, although further legal challenges in the next few years managed to extract a directive. Even though the agency did not initially legislate critical habitat, previous legal challenges had already shown that the spotted owl was a surrogate for a much wider debate about the fate of the forests. In 1988 and 1989, both the Portland Audubon Society and the Seattle Audubon Society had successfully challenged the Bureau of Land Management and the Forest Service with injunctions to prevent timber sales in spotted owl habitats.[179]

The Pacific Northwest forest was becoming a contentious place with conflicting claims over its fate. It was the last place in the United States where old-growth stands could be found; little of it remained. The field of action in federal forests of companies such as Weyerhaeuser, who had been given carte blanche over its timber resources since World War II, was now being constrained. The amount of timber sold by the Forest Service and the Bureau of Land Management began to decline for the first time in more than forty years.[180]

Notes

1 Driscoll, 'The preclinical new drug research program', pp. 68, 75.
2 The other compounds were maytansine (INDA – 1975), bruceantin

(INDA – 1977), indicine-*N*-oxide (INDA – 1978) and homoharringtonine (INDA – 1981). Maytansine was dropped in 1984 after it showed little activity in Phase II trials. This information is compiled from Suffness and Douros, 'Current status', p. 12 and Suffness and Douros, 'Drugs of plant origin', p. 39.

3 The best and most recent discussion of the history of the clinical trial can be found in Marks, *The Progress of Experiment*. See also Bull, 'The historical development' and Lilienfeld, '*Ceteris paribus*'.

4 On drug regulation, see Temin, *Taking your Medicine* and Lasagna, 'Congress'. For Phase II clinical trials in oncology, see Muggia, McGuire and Rozencweig, 'Rationale, design, and methodology'.

5 Daugherty et al., 'Perceptions of cancer patients'.

6 Woolley and Schein, 'Clinical pharmacology', pp. 183–186.

7 Holmes et al., 'Current status', p. 33.

8 Woolley and Schein, 'Clinical pharmacology', p. 195.

9 Woolley and Schein, 'Clinical pharmacology', p. 193.

10 Estey et al., 'Therapeutic response' and Daugherty et al., 'Perceptions of cancer patients'. Phase I clinical trials of antitumour compounds raise a host of difficult ethical issues. The accrual of patients to these trials pivots on informed consent. Though the trial is not designed to produce therapeutic benefit, it appears that this, rather than sheer altruism, is the principal reason why patients sign up. There is also some degree of ambiguity in the extent to which there is therapeutic intent. This is not the place to discuss these issues. The literature on this is vast and growing. A reasonable place to start is Daugherty et al., 'Perceptions of cancer patients'. See also: Cassileth et al., 'Attitudes toward clinical trials'; Lipsett, 'On the nature and ethics'; and Capron and Strong, 'Ethics of Phase I clinical trials'.

11 Lassus to Head, Developmental Chemotherapy Section, 31 January 1985, NPBI/1.

12 Lassus to Phase I investigators using taxol, 10 January 1985, NPBI/1.

13 Lassus to Phase I investigators using taxol, 10 January 1985, NPBI/1.

14 Lassus to Head, Developmental Chemotherapy Section, 31 January 1985, NPBI/1.

15 Lassus to Head, Developmental Chemotherapy Section, 31 January 1985, NPBI/1 and Arbuck and Blaylock, 'Taxol: clinical results', pp. 381–384.

16 Decision Network Minutes, 16 April 1985, Regulatory Affairs Branch, NCI.

17 Suffness and Wall, 'Discovery and development', p. 18.

18 See Sarosy to Wittes, 4 February 1987, NPBI/2.

19 Lassus to Head, Developmental Chemotherapy Section, 31 January 1985, NPBI/1.

20 Cragg to Cooper, 1 July 1985, NPB(S).

21 Cragg to Cooper, 20 September 1985, NPB(S).

22 This and the previous information can be found in Cragg to Cooper, 20 September 1985, NPB(S).

23 Cragg to Cooper, 20 September 1985, NPB(S).

24 Cragg to Reavis, 20 September 1985 and Cragg to Randall, 4 April 1986, both in NPB(S).

25 Sarosy to file, 1 December 1986, NPBI/2.

26 Purification contracts 1977–1990, NPBII.

27 Purification contracts 1977–1990, NPBII.

28 Sarosy to file, 13 May 1988, NPBI/2.

29 Holmes et al., 'Current status'.
30 Sarosy to file, 1 December 1986, NPBI/2.
31 Polysciences, Preparation Reports, various, 1978–1986.
32 Polysciences, Preparation Reports, various, 1978–1986.
33 Calculated from various sources, including 'Taxol supply status as of December 2, 1986', NPBI/2.
34 Lassus to Head, IDB, 31 January 1985, NPBI/1.
35 Sarosy to file, 1 December 1986, NPBI/2.
36 See Sarosy to Wittes, 4 February 1987, in which partial responses in ovarian cancer and melanoma are mentioned. See also: Einzig et al., 'Phase II trial'; Donehower et al., 'Phase I trial'; and Wiernik et al., 'Phase I trial'.
37 Holmes et al., 'Current status', p. 33.
38 Sarosy to file, 1 December 1986, NPBI/2.
39 Sarosy to file, 1 December 1986, NPBI/2.
40 Suffness to New, 9 December 1988, NPB(S).
41 Suffness to New, 9 December 1988, NPB(S).
42 See, for example, Brooks, 'Tree holds hope in cancer war', 4 October 1987.
43 Strycker, 'Cancer cure', 7 April 1987.
44 Strycker, 'Cancer cure', 7 April 1987.
45 Matthew Suffness took Holton to task about his remarks to the press. As he put it: 'I do not know whether you were misquoted or not but I wish to clarify for you that to date taxol has only showed some hints of response in humans and enough data are not yet available to make claims for effectiveness in any type of human cancer.' (Suffness to Holton, 20 October 1987, NPBII). Whether Suffness reprimanded others on the subject of taxol's activity is not known.
46 Suffness to New, 9 December 1986, NPB(S).
47 The Board of Scientific Counselors of the Division of Cancer Treatment, for example, approved $500,000 for the fiscal year 1988 for taxol research but the money was not forthcoming. Leland-Jones, Cragg and Sarosy to Wittes, 29 August 1988, NPBI/1.
48 See, for example, Cragg to Philpot, 12 September 1988, in which he tells Charles Philpot, Station Director of the Pacific Northwest Research Station of the Forest Service, that none of the funding requests, apart for those for collection, extraction and isolation, were approved. Philpot had previously put a number of research projects, concerning alternative methods of producing taxol, such as tissue culture, to Cragg.
49 Cragg to Koontz, 3 December 1986, NPB(S).
50 Strycker, 'Cancer cure', 7 April 1987.
51 Cragg to Koontz, 3 December 1986, NPB(S).
52 Pacific Northwest Research Station, 'Timber cut and sold, 1909–1997'.
53 See Norse, *Ancient Forests*, pp. 243–252 and Bolsinger and Waddell, 'Area of old-growth forests', p. 3.
54 All personal details come from an interview with Patrick Connolly, 17 April 1997.
55 Connolly to Wamsley, 18 March 1987, CON.
56 This knowledge was not exclusive to Connolly. In March 1987, a firm called Second Growth Forest Management Inc. wrote to the Contracting Office of the NIH to get clarification on a few issues raised by the bid specifications. In their letter, the firm referred to the fact that permits were difficult to get, speculating that it might not be possible to meet the

60,000 pounds from National Forest land. Mt Hood National Forest, they said, would not be issuing any permits. The letter also raised other issues, such as the absence of a market for yew bark, apart from the NCI which, if demand dropped, was not obliged, under conditions of the contract, to purchase the entire 60,000 pounds. The subjective nature of the word dry was also questioned. Cragg answered these issues in a memo. It is not known whether the firm put in a bid. See Viscardi to Cooper, 13 March 1987, NPBII.

57 Umpqua National Forest, Yew wood bark, 10 March 1987, CON.
58 Schlotter to Connolly, 20 March 1987, CON.
59 Schlotter to Connolly, 20 March 1987, CON and Umpqua National Forest, Yew wood bark, 10 March 1987, CON.
60 See, for example, Connolly to Tim Cummins of C&B Logging Co. in Tiller, Oregon, where he makes this argument: 20 March 1987, CON.
61 Connolly to Koyama, 30 March 1987, CON.
62 The following details are derived from Strycker, 'Cutting trees'.
63 Connolly to Eller, 18 March 1987 and notes on conversation with Eller on 20 March 1987, CON.
64 Connolly to Eller, 18 March 1987 and 23 March 1987, CON.
65 Connolly to Cooper, 18 April 1987, NPBII and Connolly to Cooper, 29 April 1987, CON. In both these letters, Connolly spoke about a 'reasonable harvest at the lowest cost'. He knew that stripping bark from a tree killed it and referred to massive debarking as 'genecide' *sic*. He also informed the NCI that there was variation in the means by which a contractor could get bark out of the forest.
66 Connolly notes, 6 May 1987, CON.
67 Interview with Connolly, 17 April 1997.
68 News release, 7 May 1987, CON.
69 See for example, news release, 7 May 1987, and Connolly to Hickok, 11 May 1987, CON.
70 Connolly to Eller, 18 June 1987, CON.
71 There are many examples of tension and dispute in Connolly's communications with collectors and subcontractors in CON.
72 Interview with Connolly, 17 April 1997.
73 Cragg to Cooper, 13 October 1987, NPB(S).
74 The following is based on Bolsinger to Cragg, 22 February 1988, NPBI/1.
75 The following is based on an interview with Bolsinger, 17 April 1997.
76 Bolsinger to Cragg, 22 February 1988, NPBI/1. The count also produced a sampling error overall of ±4.9 million. This large error seems to have been overlooked.
77 Cragg estimated that each Phase II trial consumed seventy-five grams of taxol, isolated from 1,500 pounds of bark or, assuming five pounds of bark per tree, 300 trees. Forty Phase II trials was considered a reasonable number to test the effectiveness of a potential drug in disease sites, consuming 3,000 grams of taxol, or the equivalent of 60,000 pounds of bark or 12,000 trees – figures are from NPBI/2. These are the figures Cragg produced for a two-page description of taxol that he distributed to Forest Service and Bureau of Land Management officials during 1988 (see NPBI/1).
78 Annual Report to the Food and Drug Administration, Taxol, March 1987.
79 Interview with William McGuire, 26 March 1996.
80 Interview with William McGuire, 26 March 1996. McGuire finally had to

close the trial even though there was no shortage of patients who were volunteering.

81 Taxol: clinical studies, 23 June 1988, NPBI/1.

82 Cragg, notes on conversation with Brian Leyland-Jones, 13 April 1988, in NPBI/2.

83 Rowinsky et al., 'Phase II study of taxol', p. 136.

84 A 'signal' tumour was a tumour selected by the NCI to be tested, as a panel of tumours, in Phase II trials. The panel of signal tumours has changed over the years, but they are chosen on the basis that they are either very common in the population of cancer patients – colon and lung tumours – or they resist standard therapy – breast and ovarian tumours – or they are easy to evaluate – malignant melanoma. See, Muggia et al., 'Rationale, design, and methodology', p. 200.

85 The following is based on Cragg, 'Trip report, Oregon and Washington, April 17–22, 1988' in FRD2.

86 Personal communication, Gordon Cragg, 14 July 1998.

87 Cragg, 'Trip report, Oregon and Washington, April 17–22, 1988' in FRD2.

88 Wheeler et al., 'Genetic variation'.

89 Cragg to Philpot, 23 May 1988, NPBI/1.

90 Cragg to Philpot, 23 May 1988, NPBI/1.

91 Suffness to Douros, 6 July 1988, FRD4.

92 Cragg to Purchasing Agent, DCT, 24 August 1988, NPBII.

93 Memo, Taxol drug supply, 13 May 1988 and Sarosy to Cragg, 28 June 1988, both in NPBI/2.

94 Cragg to Sarosy, 28 June 1988, both in NPBI/2.

95 In 1987 it was 0.01 per cent – see Cragg to Kingston, 23 October 1987, NPBIV/1. It hadn't changed by the following year – minutes to Taxol Working Group Meeting of 8 September 1988, 21 September 1988, NPBI/1.

96 This is a point Gordon Cragg emphasized when he discussed the taxol issue with Weyerhaeuser on his site visit in April 1988. See 'Trip report, Oregon and Washington, 17–22 April 1988', in FRD2.

97 Interview with Boettner, 10 November 1997. Boettner retired from Polysciences in 1986 at the age of sixty-eight. Polysciences were particularly under capacity for extraction, their largest vats capable of a maximum volume of 2,000 gallons. This is why they subcontracted the work to Madis Laboratories. Information on Polysciences' inability to expand is from a personal communication with Janice Thompson, 15 July 1998. Cragg had been asking around for companies that had the capacity to handle large-scale isolation of natural products since (at least) late 1986 – see, for example, Douros to Cragg, 3 December 1986, NPBIII.

98 'HAUSER Chemical Research, Inc.: an introduction, 12 May 1986' in NPBIII. Ray Hauser set up an engineering firm in 1961. Dean Stull took it over in 1983, changed its focus to process development and the scale-up of chemical reactions and its name to Hauser Chemical Research.

99 'Visit to Hauser Chemical Research, Inc.', 27 January 1987, NPBIII. The subject of taxol was mentioned in a letter from Dean Stull, Special Projects Manager to Cragg, 27 January 1987, NPBIII.

100 Hauser Chemical Research, 'Taxol', p. 13.

101 'Extraction and purification of 60,000 pounds of *Taxus brevifolia* bark', NPBII.

102 'Extraction and purification of 60,000 pounds of *Taxus brevifolia* bark', NPBII.

103 The isolation and purification process was difficult at the best of times. On several occasions, particularly in March 1988, taxol had to be returned to Polysciences because it contained an unacceptable level of impurities. See Cragg's notes in NPBII.

104 Total processing costs for a pound of bark was estimated at $20.60, of which $3.60 was accounted for by the collection, NPBII.

105 The following is based on Information Specialist SSS to Sarosy, 14 July 1988, NPBI/2.

106 Cragg to Philpot, 23 May 1988, Luscher to Cragg, 19 August 1988, both in NPB(S) and Cragg to Sarosy, 28 June 1988, NPBI/2.

107 Suffness to Douros, 6 July 1988, FRD4.

108 See, for example, Bonnem (Schering) to Wittes, 15 August 1988 and Cragg's notes, all in NPBI/3.

109 Wittes to Bonnem, 15 August 1988, NPBI/3.

110 The following is based on Suffness to Douros, 6 July 1988, FRD4.

111 Pierre Potier of the CNRS in France was also told of Weyerhaeuser's interest in taxol – Cragg to Potier, 9 November 1988, GCB1. Potier wrote to Weyerhaeuser in January 1989 telling the company of his group's work on taxol and its soluble derivatives, and his collaboration with Rhône-Poulenc – Potier to Trotter and Wheeler, 30 January, GCB1.

112 Cragg to Philpot, 12 September 1988, NPB(S).

113 The minutes of the August 1988 meeting are in NPBI/3. The following discussion is based on this document.

114 Charles Philpot, Station Director of the Pacific Northwest Research Station, responded to Gordon Cragg's request for research proposals leading to a greater understanding of *Taxus brevifolia* and alternative methods of supplying taxol that was put at the Portland meeting in April. Philpot sent Cragg a research prospectus drawn up by what was called the 'Pacific Yew Committee', which members included Chuck Bolsinger and Nicholas Wheeler (of Weyerhaeuser), under the chair of Don Minore, Plant Ecologist with the Pacific Northwest Research Station of the Forest Service in Corvallis, Oregon. The research prospectus listed seven major research projects with a total budget requirement of just short of two million dollars, if all were undertaken. The prospectus was also, at the time of writing (31 May 1988), the most up-to-date and comprehensive compendium of yew information available, exceeding that compiled by Richard Spjut. See 'Pacific Yew (*Taxus Brevifolia* Nutt. – A Research Prospectus' in NPB(S)).

115 Suffness to Douros, 6 July 1988, FRD4.

116 Denis et al., 'A highly efficient', published on 17 August 1988, and Colin et al., 'Preparation'.

117 Matthew Suffness and Pierre Potier had been on first-name terms since at least 1981 – Potier to Suffness, 7 July 1981, GCB1. The NCI certainly knew about the French work – see Greene to Suffness, 7 September 1988 and 3 November 1988 and Suffness to Greene, 14 September 1988 – in GCB1. Curiously, on 9 November 1988, Gordon Cragg wrote to Potier, 'your process for producing taxol has certainly generated a lot of interest amongst NCI staff and at Weyerhaeuser' – in GCB1.

118 Blume, 'Investigators', p. 1122.

119 Interview with Wender, 8 April 1996.

120 However, a memo from Matthew Suffness dated 31 August 1989 reports that 'a proposal was written for an RFA (Request for Applications), but in view of the already on-going work in several prominent labs and the low probability of producing a commercially viable synthesis, this RFA did not go forward.' – GCB2.

121 Interview with Kingston, 29 March 1996.

122 Swindell, 'Taxane diterpene'.

123 Zurer, 'Chemists', p. 22.

124 Interview with Holton, 22 May 1998.

125 'Putting the side chain on at 13' refers to the carbon 13 position mentioned in Chapter 3. A 'protection scheme' is a way of making sure that a reaction takes place at the desired site and not elsewhere, by temporarily blocking other possible reactive sites.

126 Eisenberg, 'Public research'.

127 Stereoisomers of a molecule have the same formula and functional groups but differ in the arrangement of the groups in space.

128 Potier's group studied the order of reactivity of the different OH groups. Guéritte-Voegelein et al., 'Chemical studies'.

129 Holton, R., *European Patent Application* 400971 (1990); 'Method for preparation of taxol using an oxazinone'. US Patent 5,015,744 (1991).

130 Reviewed by Nicolaou et al., 'Chemistry and biology'.

131 Holton, R., *European Patent Application* 428,376 (1991); 'Method for preparation of taxol using a β-lactam'. US Patent 5,175,315 (1992).

132 The details are contained in a memo from Suffness, 29 July 1988, NPBI/2.

133 No decision was made at the time. Indeed, the company did not come to a decision as to what part it should play in the development of taxol until 1990, by which time Bristol-Myers Squibb had been selected as the research and development partner of the NCI – this aspect of taxol's development is discussed later in this and in the following chapter. Because of the delay in coming to a decision, Weyerhaeuser lost the initiative in being a leader in the field. Interview with Nick Wheeler, 14 June 1999.

134 Christen's research on tissue culture was brought to the attention of the Taxol Working Group meeting of 23 June 1988. She was subsequently admitted to a subgroup called the 'Friends of taxol'. See NPBI/2.

135 According to Nick Wheeler, the plant geneticist most closely associated with taxol at Weyerhaeuser, the company debated to what extent it should get involved in the business of taxol and to what extent this would fit in with the company's core activities. Going into extraction and purification of taxol was considered an option but was apparently dismissed in the summer of 1988 in favour of the more limited role of providing biomass.

136 Suffness to Douros, 6 July 1988, FRD4.

137 Vida to Suffness, 8 July 1988, NPBIV/1.

138 Suffness to distribution, 12 May 1988, NPBIV/1.

139 See the minutes, dated 21 September 1988, in NPBI/1.

140 Bristol-Myers was involved in discussions to license this compound, isolated from *Begula neritina*, an aquatic invertebrate animal, with Arizona State University and the NCI. See Suffness to distribution, 12 May 1988, NPBIV/1. Gordon Pettit, of Arizona State University, has been deeply involved in the development of this compound – interview with Pettit, 22 October 1997. See also Persinos, 'Bryostatin 1'.

141 The memo, from Gisele Sarosy, dated 12 September 1988, is in NPBI/3.
142 Any new pharmaceutical can be given status as an orphan product if it is useful for rare conditions, defined as affecting a population not exceeding 200,000 people. Designation as an orphan product is made under the Orphan Drug Act of 1983 that provides marketing exclusivity, tax incentives and other financial incentives to the product's manufacturer. A fuller discussion of the orphan drug designation with respect to taxol appears in Chapter 5. Taxol would have qualified as an orphan product because ovarian cancer with 20,000 cases annually in the United States was considered a rare disease under the terms of the Act.
143 The following discussion is based on the minutes of the meeting of 7 December 1988, written up on 9 January 1989, and in GCB2.
144 The CRADA is the subject of Chapter 5. A good discussion of this act appears in Eisenberg, 'Public research'.
145 Courses at the NIH were offered 'to sensitize and educate' staff to the 'opportunities, responsibilities and potential rewards' of the CRADA – Philip Chen (Chair, Patent Policy Board) to NIH Staff, 3 May 1988, NPBIII.
146 Shoemaker to distribution, 17 January 1989, NPBI/3.
147 Dale Shoemaker, personal communication, 13 July 1998.
148 The solicitation date was 19 January 1989. The following is based on information from contract for collection in NPBIV/2.
149 Robert Warner bid $2.75 per pound for his 1984 contract.
150 Advanced Molecular Technologies, 'Executive Summary', 1989, DST. See also Hays, 'Advanced Molecular Technologies'.
151 Nalder, 'Trials of taxol', *Seattle Times*, 15 December 1991.
152 Suffness to Destito, 15 November 1988, DST.
153 Haverfield to Destito, 19 December 1988, DST.
154 Suffness to Destito, 11 October 1988, DST. Suffness's search for other employment at this time has been confirmed by Gordon Cragg, personal communication, 14 July 1998.
155 Personal communication, Gordon Cragg, 14 July 1998.
156 Personal communication, Janice Thompson, 15 July 1998.
157 Connolly to Downes, 28 February 1990, CON.
158 Destito to Vishnuvajjala, 15 November 1989, NPBIII.
159 Destito to Downes, 16 February 1989, NDPIII.
160 Open letter to the Northwest Timber Industry, 1 June 1989, DST.
161 The following is based on Destito to Vishnuvajjala, 15 November 1989, NPB/III.
162 Memo, Jackson to file, 1 September 1989, NPB/III.
163 According to Dale Shoemaker, the relatively long span of time between his draft (January 1989) and the Federal Register announcement was accounted for by bureaucratic red tape as the document wound its way, slowly, through the offices of the NIH – Dale Shoemaker, personal communication, 15 July 1998.
164 *Federal Register*, 1 August 1989.
165 The best data available at that time showed that taxol was indeed most active in ovarian cancer. Aside from ovarian cancer, the only clinical trials of taxol were on melanoma and renal cancer. The melanoma trials were proving disappointing, in contrast with some of the earlier pronouncements, in the press and elsewhere. One trial at the MD Anderson Cancer Center showed an overall response rate of less than eight per cent and

another but much smaller trial showed no response. The best results came from the Eastern Cooperative Oncology Group where the response rate was about fifteen per cent. The renal cancer trial at the Albert Einstein College of Medicine showed no response. The only other ovarian cancer trial, also at Albert Einstein, and still accruing patients, was showing a response rate of about twelve per cent. Taken altogether, the clinical trial data were, at this point at least, at best mixed. See Annual Report to the Food and Drug Administration, Taxol, February 1989, p. 25.

166 McGuire et al., 'Taxol'.
167 News release, The Johns Hopkins Medical Institutions, 'Hopkins uses new drug extracted from tree bark for ovarian cancer', 15 August 1989, NCI/4.
168 Silent because ovarian cancer typically produces symptoms only when it is in an advanced stage.
169 The Task Group met in 1985. It was an idea that surfaced during a series of discussions among Franklin and his colleagues at the Forest Service in the Pacific Northwest – Jerry Franklin, personal communication, 17 July 1998.
170 Old-Growth Definition Task Group, 'Interim definitions'.
171 The definition rested on four stand characteristics and minimum standards for each. For example, a Douglas-fir stand would classify as old-growth if (i) there were two or more species of live trees with a wide range of age and size – any of western hemlock, western redcedar, bigleaf maple, more than twelve per acre and exceeding sixteen feet in diameter: the Douglas fir should exceed thirty-two feet in diameter or be over 200 years old. (ii) A deep-layered canopy. (iii) Conifer standing dead trees, exceeding twenty feet in diameter and fifteen feet in height. And (iv) down logs, more than fifteen tons per acre, exceeding twenty-four feet in diameter and fifty feet in length. Old-Growth Definition Task Group, 'Interim definitions', p. 4.
172 See Ervin, *Fragile Majesty*, p. 15 and Norse, *Ancient Forests*, pp. 56–61.
173 Flournoy, 'Beyond the "spotted owl problem"', p. 288. A Management Indicator Species is an organism that is identified as representing the health of the entire biotic community under discussion – monitoring its biological course is a proxy to monitoring the entire ecosystem. The literature on the spotted owl and old-growth issues is enormous. A good place to begin is with the following: Yaffee, *The Wisdom of the Spotted Owl*; Flournoy, 'Beyond the "spotted owl problem"'; Wilcove, 'Turning conservation goals'; Levi and Kocher, 'The spotted owl'; Lange, 'The logic'; Strong, 'Special feature – spotted owl'; Proctor, 'Whose nature?'; and Proctor, 'The owl'.
174 Dietrich, *The Final Forest*, p. 54.
175 Flournoy, 'Beyond the "spotted owl problem"', p. 294 and Yaffee, *The Wisdom of the Spotted Owl*, pp. 108–109.
176 Flournoy, 'Beyond the "spotted owl problem"', p. 294.
177 Flournoy, 'Beyond the "spotted owl problem"', p. 295 and Yaffee, *The Wisdom of the Spotted Owl*, p. 116.
178 Flournoy, 'Beyond the "spotted owl problem"', p. 276.
179 See Flournoy, 'Beyond the "spotted owl problem"', pp. 285–289 and Yaffee, *The Wisdom of the Spotted Owl*, p. 114.
180 In the Pacific Northwest region of the National Forests, the amount of timber sold in 1988 was seven per cent below the level of 1987 but in 1989 it was forty-seven per cent below the same level – see Farnham and Mohai, 'National forest timber', p. 269.

Part III

Controversies

5

The Politics of Exclusivity and the Business of Taxol

If, by 1989, the American public was being excited by the images of an anti-cancer drug hiding in the bark of a virtually unknown tree growing in the Pacific Northwest, during the next few years they would be subjected to a barrage of stories that would lead them into laboratories in universities, companies and Federal agencies; into the boardrooms of major pharmaceutical companies and a host of start-up biotechnology companies; into the offices of the country's leading Federal agencies; into the old-growth forests of Oregon and Washington; into cancer clinics throughout the country; and into hearings on Capitol Hill.

It became increasingly difficult to follow the traces of taxol as it wound its way simultaneously through these sites. Fortunately, the public was given a moment to reflect on the events and to see taxol in the bigger picture, when some of the major players associated with taxol were asked to appear at three separate Congressional hearings. The first was held on 29 July 1991 and was prompted by a set of exclusive agreements drawn up between the pharmaceutical company Bristol-Myers Squibb and the NIH, the USDA and the Department of the Interior. The hearings focused on whether such agreements were in the public's best interest. The second hearing occurred on 4 March 1992. Its subject was the Pacific Yew Act of 1991, an extraordinary piece of legislation, perhaps the only one of its kind in concentrating on a plant. The final hearing was on 25 January 1993, the issue being the pricing of drugs co-developed by Federal laboratories and private companies, especially taxol.

Whose Molecule? Whose Drug?

The *Federal Register* notice for a CRADA partner had appeared on 1 August 1989.[1] It was a very straightforward notice and, in most respects, reflected precisely what the Taxol Working Group wanted. The only major difference between the document as it appeared in draft form in January 1989 and its final form on 1 August was that the clause 'The United States Government will receive a reasonable share of income once the drug is marketed for general use' was deleted.[2] It called specifically for a pharmaceutical company to pursue the clinical development of taxol. Over the previous years, the NCI had been in touch, in one way or another with a number of individuals and organizations who had shown an interest in taxol, either directly in a taxol-related activity, or indirectly by inquiring into the molecule and the NCI's news about its progress. Included were most of America's large and long-established pharmaceutical companies, such as Eli Lilly, Lederle, Merck Sharpe and Dohme, Sterling, Schering, DuPont and Bristol-Myers, some smaller biotechnology companies, Weyerhaeuser, several Federal agencies and a few others. These twenty-three interested parties were each sent a copy of the *Federal Register* notice; a further twenty-two individuals and organizations made inquiries about the taxol CRADA before the deadline for proposals set for 15 September 1989.[3]

By the deadline, only four companies had submitted proposals. They were: Bristol-Myers (the company merged with the pharmaceutical company Squibb in October 1989 to become Bristol-Myers Squibb), Rhône-Poulenc, Unimed and Xechem.[4] Time was of the essence for the NCI. The Regulatory Affairs Branch of the Division of Cancer Treatment decided to rate the proposals on pre-clinical and clinical grounds using a panel of experts from within the NCI. This group of individuals, constituted as the 'Taxol CRADA Review Committee' met for the first time on 10 October 1989 to begin the selection process.[5] At this meeting, the Committee decided that the most promising proposals came from Bristol-Myers Squibb and Rhône-Poulenc. Both these companies were informed that each was in the running by the 23 and 27 October, respectively, and asked to provide answers to a few specific questions.[6] Letters to Xechem and Unimed were sent on 1 November informing both that they were unsuccessful in their bid for the taxol CRADA.[7]

Bristol-Myers Squibb and Rhône-Poulenc were given until 17 November to respond to the supplementary questions. On 29 November, Dale Shoemaker of the Regulatory Affairs Branch sent the final proposals to all the members of the Taxol CRADA Review Committee. There appears to have been a clear preference for Bristol-Myers Squibb as the CRADA partner even before the final proposals were received. In the memo covering this final stage in the selection procedure, Shoemaker asked his colleagues on the Committee to 'review the proposals and let me know if you still feel Bristol-Myers should be selected for the Taxol CRADA'.[8] Within a few days the Committee concurred and the decision was taken that Bristol-Myers Squibb should be selected for the taxol CRADA.[9] By the second week of December, every individual and organization who had shown interest in the CRADA, although not enough to submit a proposal, was informed that Bristol-Myers Squibb had been selected as the CRADA partner.[10]

The small number of applicants for the taxol CRADA requires some comment. Before that, however, it might help to look more closely at the selection procedure. What transpired in the meetings of the taxol CRADA Review Committee and the reasons why Bristol-Myers Squibb emerged as the successful contender remains hidden from public view. Nevertheless, there are some issues that are not as clear-cut as they are often presented.

The CRADA notice was explicit about the criteria the NCI would adopt in choosing a pharmaceutical company as its partner.[11] As one might expect from a pharmaceutical company, the NCI required experience in preclinical and clinical drug development and experience in handling and interpreting data from a compound selected as an IND and from clinical trials. This was standard. The other criteria were not standard but specific to the taxol case. In particular, the NCI wanted to have a pharmaceutical company partner that had experience in the development of natural products for clinical use and would be willing to share in the costs of collecting bark, extracting, purifying and formulating taxol.[12] The NCI was satisfied with the natural products experience of both Bristol-Myers and Rhône-Poulenc but not with that of Unimed and Xechem who were both criticized particularly on this point.[13]

The first Congressional hearing to enquire into the development of taxol was held on 29 July 1991 before the House Small Business Subcommittee on Regulation, Business Opportunities and Energy, chaired by Congressman Ron Wyden, Democrat of Oregon. It focused directly on the procedure by which Bristol-Myers Squibb had been chosen as the taxol CRADA partner.[14] In the run-up to the hearing, Wyden's staff were directed to find out more about the 'development, implementation and likely result of a series of agreements involving the development and commercialization of taxol'.[15] One of their concerns was the small number of companies that had applied for the taxol CRADA. Although they did not draw any firm conclusions, Wyden's staff reported back, on the basis of interviews with pharmaceutical company executives, that firms had backed off from applying because there was a feeling in the community that Bristol-Myers enjoyed 'overall competitive advantages', although these were not spelled out.

Wyden's staff were clearly concerned about the nature of the competitive process, trying to get to the bottom of why so few companies made a bid for the taxol CRADA and why it was Bristol-Myers Squibb that was successful. One of the events they referred back to Wyden was the case of Robert Wittes. Between 1983 and 1988, Wittes held the position of Associate Director of the Cancer Therapy Evaluation Program, Division of Cancer Treatment, NCI.[16] Though he was not directly involved in the taxol programme, because of his senior position, he was made aware, through copies of taxol meeting agendas, of the nature of the compound's progress through the NCI machinery.[17] In November 1988 Wittes left the NCI to become Senior Vice President for Cancer Research at Bristol-Myers. In August 1990, he returned to the NCI as Chief of the Medicine Branch of the Clinical Oncology Program.[18]

Wyden's staff raised the issue of Wittes's 'revolving door' experiences and questioned whether the move to Bristol-Myers gave any advantage to the company in preparing its proposal.[19] However, Wyden never referred to the Wittes story in his hearing and never questioned anyone about it, publicly at least.

The story, however, leaked out of Congress. In August 1991, the publication *The Cancer Letter*, in a critical piece on Wyden's handling of the hearing, referred explicitly to the Wittes affair as a case of 'stretching or mangling the facts, or disregarding them completely, in attempting to fire up an issue that might look good on television'.[20] The Wittes affair, the article argued, was entirely misrepresented and amounted to an affront to all the parties involved: Wittes's move from the NCI to Bristol-Myers and back to the NCI had nothing to do with the CRADA.

The matter didn't end there, however. Less than a year later, the journal *Multinational Monitor*, a Washington-based publication focusing on the politics of multinational business, returned to the case of Robert Wittes and what it called the 'Great Taxol Giveaway'.[21] Daniel Newman, the author of the article, was unswerving in his condemnation of the CRADA as a vehicle for the privatization of public property, linking Wittes to the give-away.[22] Wittes refused to be drawn into the controversy and refused to answer any of Newman's questions concerning his position at Bristol-Myers Squibb and his role in the CRADA.

This time Wyden picked up the story. He wrote to Bernadine Healy the Director of the NIH in July 1992, asking her to put an end to speculations and innuendoes concerning Wittes and the taxol CRADA by setting the record straight. Her response to him detailed Wittes's movements within the NCI prior to taking up the position at Bristol-Myers Squibb and his subsequent return to the NCI nearly two years later.[23] Healy's position about Wittes was clear and unequivocal: he had nothing to do with the CRADA and Bristol-Myers Squibb's success at getting it, neither at the NCI nor at the company. She ended her letter by recounting that the Special Counsel for Ethics had reviewed the matter and concluded that nothing was amiss. This was the last that was heard on the matter and Wittes himself has never spoken about the issues publicly.

We do not have enough evidence on this episode to make a judgement. The point of recounting it is simply to show that the taxol CRADA was controversial not simply because of the politics of the legislation – the Federal Technology Transfer Act of 1986 – that paved the way for its operation, but specifically because concern was expressed that the competition might have been unfair. The frequent references to the CRADA being awarded 'following a full, and I stress open competition'; and Bristol-Myers Squibb being successful 'on the basis of the merit of their proposal' and 'their extensive experience in the cancer drug field, and their proven ability to bring drugs to marketing status' simply served to stir the interest and raise specific questions about how the competition actually proceeded.[24]

Perhaps one should not be surprised by the suspicions raised by the success of Bristol-Myers Squibb. What these suspicions reflect are, in the wider sense, not so much the possibilities of wrong-doing or undue influence as we've already seen, but, rather, the nature of the public/private organization of cancer research and the specific case of taxol.

Cancer is the West's second major disease but oncology is of minor interest to pharmaceutical companies: anti-cancer drugs in 1990 accounted for less than three per cent of the world's drug market.[25] Most pharmaceutical companies have no product line in oncology. Bristol-Myers Squibb, as it is now, produces most of them. Bristol-Myers, as it was then, had a special relationship with the NCI because of the high profile of oncology agents in their portfolio. It was, for example, the first pharmaceutical company in the United States to be awarded an agreement by which it would market anti-cancer drugs developed and tested by the NCI. This was in 1972.[26] In the year before the taxol CRADA was announced, Bristol-Myers was arranging a licence with Arizona State University to develop and market bryostatins and discussing proposals for the long-term supply and development of these compounds with the NCI.[27] As for personnel, it was not unusual for senior NCI people to end up working for Bristol-Myers Squibb. Robert Wittes was just the latest in a line of transfers. John Douros who was Chief of the Natural Products Branch was another, as was Stephen Carter who had been Deputy Director of the Division of Cancer Treatment between 1967 and 1975 and subsequently employed by Bristol-Myers from 1981 until 1995.[28]

When Bruce Chabner, Director of the Division of Cancer Treatment of the NCI, appeared before the 4 March 1992 hearing on the Pacific Yew Act, he mentioned that at the time of the CRADA competition, taxol was 'of minor interest to drug companies'.[29] There were, he also stated, 'formidable problems in producing the drug'.[30] While we have no definitive explanation of why so few pharmaceutical firms entered the competition, it is highly likely, nevertheless, that the perception of taxol as a difficult drug was real enough. Certainly, this appears to be the case with Upjohn which, after showing initial interest in the project, declined to submit a proposal for reasons we discuss later in this chapter.

What we also do not know is how much pharmaceutical companies knew about taxol although it must have been considerable. By mid-1989, there was certainly quite a lot of technical literature about the molecule, biological, chemical and clinical. On this score, knowledge of its existence and progress would have been widely available. In addition, as the last chapter showed, several pharmaceutical companies, Bristol-Myers, Rhône-Poulenc and Unimed among them, had already expressed an interest in the NCI's experiences with the molecule before the CRADA was announced.

That the NCI was actively seeking a way out of taxol has also been discussed in a previous chapter. Senior people at the Natural Products Branch were, as we have seen, envisioning some kind of alliance between Weyerhaeuser and a pharmaceutical company, Bristol-Myers in particular. These discussions were proceeding well before the NCI settled on the CRADA as the mechanism for the transfer of taxol. As Matthew Suffness said to members of the taxol working party in May 1988: 'They (Bristol-Myers) were . . . interested in the recent trip by Drs. Suffness and Cragg to Weyerhaeuser Co., and the possibility of a sole source supply agreement which could be as good as a patent or license in terms of exclusivity. If a marriage can be arranged between Weyerhaeuser and Bristol, or another large pharmaceutical company, the long term supply situation on taxol could be resolved.'[31] Weyerhaeuser, we know, was looking at the possibilities of a pharmaceutical partner in mid-1988.[32] It should therefore not be assumed, as it was in the various Congressional hearings, in the testimonies presented and in the media reports, that 1 August 1989 was the first time that anyone outside the NCI heard of the agency's intention of seeking a CRADA partner to bring taxol to the market.

Long before the *Federal Register* CRADA notice, complicated moves were already well underway involving various kinds of alliances and joint ventures to bring taxol to the market. Even before he placed his bid for the 1989 yew bark collection, John Destito had included taxol as one of the natural products his company, Advanced Molecular Technologies, would seek to develop as part of their portfolio of compounds. In seeking scientists to join his team, Destito was circulating the company's Executive Summary in November and December 1988, which included taxol in the list of interesting compounds.[33] Early in December 1988, Destito and his company executives paid a visit to Weyerhaeuser where they discussed their possible respective roles in a taxol programme with a pharmaceutical company.[34] By the beginning of January 1989, Destito informed both Nick Wheeler and Judd Haverfield, the two Weyerhaeuser scientists most closely involved in the discussions with the NCI about taxol, that 'as you are aware by now, the National Cancer Institute has prepared a draft for the purpose of placing the entire Taxol Program up for bid on the commercial market, perhaps as early as February'.[35] He also let them know that he had been advised by 'sources within the National Cancer Institute to make immediate contact with both Bristol-Myers Company and Eli Lilly & Co. in regards to our interest and impending capabilities regarding taxol'.[36] At this point, Destito was discussing his company's role in a taxol programme in terms of extraction and purification and not the collection of yew bark.[37] By the end of February 1989, having put in his bid for the collection of bark and confident of its acceptance by the NCI, Destito informed Haverfield of the company's new activities.[38] Weyerhaeuser was already talking to Bristol-Myers and Eli Lilly.[39]

By April 1989, Destito had involved Toray Industries, a Japanese chemical company, primarily producing artificial fibres, but for the past twenty-five years involved in pharmaceuticals and medical devices, in a proposed alliance with Weyerhaeuser and Advanced Molecular Technologies in a taxol programme.[40] Destito sensed that an American company should be included in the proposed alliance and that company he felt should be Sterling Drug Co. He also seemed to know that Bristol-Myers was aware of the NCI's intentions and, as he put it, 'seems to be sandbagging, with a desire to keep the program to themselves'.[41]

It is not clear what happened to the plan to involve Sterling Drug but by the beginning of July, Destito was contacting executives at Merck, Sharp and Dohme and at Dupont to interest them in a plan to co-develop taxol with Advanced Molecular Technologies, Weyerhaeuser and Toray Industries, in which the American pharmaceutical company would be the bidder for the NCI taxol programme.[42] Dupont, in particular, was interested and a meeting was arranged in Wilmington, Delaware, on 28 July 1989 to discuss the proposed worldwide alliance.

In any event, Dupont decided not to participate in the proposed alliance and did not submit a CRADA application. Toray, at that point, pulled its interest, deciding to await the outcome of the competition to see with whom they would be speaking about the development of taxol in Japan and Asia.[43] Destito had hinted to his opposite number at Toray that Bristol-Myers would be the likely winner.[44]

Destito planned that both Toray Industries and the American pharmaceutical partner would provide equity in Advanced Molecular Technologies to finance the taxol extraction and purification programme as well as long-term plans to develop and manufacture new products from plant and marine organisms.[45] Any company intent on submitting a CRADA proposal needed to contact Destito as he was the NCI's official yew bark collector: the CRADA notice expressly required the successful applicant to provide the necessary funds and resources to complete the 60,000 pound bark collection. One of the companies to get in touch with Destito was Upjohn. Destito's lead contact in the company was Pat McGovern, Associate Director of Cancer Research. Destito placed his proposed alliance in front of McGovern including a proposal for Upjohn to take a forty-five per cent stake in Advanced Molecular Technologies ($13.5 million).[46] He reiterated that Advanced Molecular Technologies and Weyerhaeuser needed an American pharmaceutical company in the alliance and that Bristol-Myers was the company to beat.[47] A meeting of the interested parties was scheduled for 31 August 1989, leaving two weeks before the submission deadline.

It is not clear whether this meeting took place, but in any event, Upjohn pulled out of the plan and did not submit a CRADA application on the grounds that the company 'eventually decided to decline this opportunity because of higher priority projects competing for our limited corporate research funds and *our uncertainty that development of a commercially practical process for bulk taxol production was feasible* (our italics)'.[48] With Upjohn gone Destito turned to the Director of Research at Rhône-Poulenc attempting, once again, to forge an alliance and informing him that Advanced Molecular Technologies had been collecting *Taxus brevifolia* needles in addition to bark.[49] But nothing came of this venture either. Destito's corporate initiatives had failed so far.

As discussed earlier, only four companies submitted proposals. What each wanted from Destito varied widely. Bristol-Myers simply wanted him to work with the company and supply them with the rest of the bark under contract to the NCI. It was Bristol-Myers's intention that Hauser Chemical Research would supply it in the future once Destito's contract with the NCI expired.[50] From Unimed Destito could expect their support for the present collection but the future was less clear: the company had already been in touch with Patrick Connolly about that.[51] Rhône-Poulenc had little interest in bark in general and Destito's contract in particular because, as we have seen, they intended to make taxol semi-synthetically from needles.

Xechem, the final applicant, however, presented a more complicated case. Together with a number of other organizations, the company had worked out an alliance to cover all aspects of the requirements of the taxol CRADA. The venture included: Advanced Molecular Technologies for the collection of bark; Polysciences for extraction, isolation and purification of taxol; the College of Pharmacy of the University of Illinois in Chicago for formulation; the Research Institute of Pharmaceutical Sciences of the University of Mississippi for the development of new sources of raw materials in addition to the semi-synthetic approach to taxol manufacture; Weyerhaeuser for stock plants and genetic improvement of the species; and, finally, Xechem itself for the pharmaceutical development.[52] Such a network of small and large companies was certainly in the spirit of the Federal Technology Transfer Act that sought to encourage small firms to participate.[53]

Destito's association with Xechem was probably his best hope of becoming an integral part of a corporate joint venture with, possibly, long-term existence, rather than as an adjunct expedient in the short-term only. Xechem was, however, unsuccessful. Destito and Advanced Molecular Technologies were cast adrift. Weyerhaeuser, by contrast, for so long part of the solution package to taxol's supply problem, and, therefore, more central to the plans of any of the bidders, was in a much stronger position. Destito's lack of success on the corporate front was matched by his lack of success in the forest as Chapter 6 shows.

Both Bristol-Myers and Rhône-Poulenc proceeded through the first stage of the competition, leaving Xechem and Unimed out of the field. The contending companies were asked to verify or expand upon certain claims made in their respective submissions. Bristol-Myers and Rhône-Poulenc were both asked to clarify their statements about the supply of taxol. The Review Committee remarked that Bristol-Myers's estimates of the yield of taxol from bark was off by a factor of two to five.[54] The Natural Products Branch, with years of experience behind it, was working with a figure of one kilogram of taxol from 30,000 pounds of bark, yet Bristol-Myers reported that it expected to get one kilogram of taxol from 10,000 pounds of bark. As evidence of this, the company produced a letter from Hauser Chemical Research, in which Dean Stull, the Chief Executive Officer, wrote that his company was 'projecting a yield of one (1) kilogram per 10,000 pounds of bark'.[55] Whether the Review Committee accepted Bristol-Myers's claim is uncertain, but there is little doubt that the claim was unfounded. Such yields had never been achieved in practice.[56] Still, Bristol-Myers assured the NCI that even if they were overestimating the amount of bulk taxol that could be made, this would not affect the development effort.[57]

Bristol-Myers were also asked to expand on their plans for the long-term supply of taxol and specifically on the chemical conversion of related materials to taxol. In their reply, the company stated that semi-synthesis was the key approach to resolve the long-term supplies of taxol. To this effect, they were negotiating with Robert Holton of Florida State University to license his patented technology for the conversion of baccatin to taxol.[58] Holton had filed his patent in June 1989 and, on the strength of this, he had written to many companies that he thought would be filing a CRADA application, between June and September of that year, to try to interest them in his approach to the supply problem.[59]

Rhône-Poulenc, for their part, were asked to elaborate on their semi-synthetic approach to taxol production and to address the issue of their presence in the United States.[60] They responded by saying that the conversion of 10-DAB into taxol took four steps with an overall yield of fifty-two per cent – they referred the committee to the key article published by Andrew Greene and his colleagues in 1988. In the short-term, Rhône-Poulenc would continue to collaborate with the contacts involved in bark collection but, at the same time, they would be asking for the collections to expand into needle harvesting. In the long-term, however, the company envisioned setting up their own needle collection and drying facilities in the United States as they had already done in Europe.[61] In their original submission, Rhône-Poulenc had made it clear that they would be using *Taxus brevifolia* needles to make taxol: according to their research, the 10-DAB content of *Taxus brevifolia* needles was similar to that of *Taxus baccata* needles with which the company had already worked.[62] Though at the time of submission the company did not have manufacturing facilities in the United States, it was their firm intention to establish these and to develop and supply taxol in the United States for the United States market.[63]

Among other questions, both companies were asked under what circumstances they could envision turning the CRADA project (all the data and the drug) back to the NCI. The answers were very interesting. Bristol-Myers Squibb responded that there were only two conditions under which they would abandon the project. The first had to do with supplies and the issue of access to them. This is how it was stated. 'If further political agitation by environmental groups over the forests in the Pacific Northwest restrict access to the Western Yew before alternative sources can be identified and exploited, we might have to reevaluate the viability of the project.'[64] The only other condition, and highly unlikely according to the company, was if FDA approval was not possible. Rhône-Poulenc also put forth two conditions, although these were wholly unlike those of Bristol-Myers Squibb. The first was if a serious industrial, toxicological or clinical event occurred that would preclude any further development work on taxol; and the second was if a 'taxol-analog or derivative with improved solubility has demonstrated superior clinical activity and could be developed in the same time frame as taxol'.[65]

Shortly after receiving the answers to the supplementary questions, the Review Committee, as we have seen, decided to award the CRADA to Bristol-Myers. Negotiations over the CRADA agreement took most of the next year: the document was undergoing the approval process in the NCI during the month of November.[66] On 19 and 23 January 1991, the CRADA was signed by the NCI and Bristol-Myers Squibb respectively.[67]

The molecule had finally arrived at a pharmaceutical company, twenty-five years after its isolation in Monroe Wall's laboratory in North Carolina. At the same time, it was in the final stage of leaving the NCI and public ownership to become private property. But while the paperwork was being finalized, taxol, the molecule, also became taxol the compound with orphan drug status for use in ovarian cancer on 15 October 1990.[68] Under the rules of the designation, if and when taxol was approved for use against ovarian cancer, Bristol-Myers Squibb could look forward to seven years market exclusivity and tax credits.

The process leading to the filing of a New Drug Application (NDA), as was required by the CRADA, was swift, reflecting, in part, the substantial clinical progress of taxol before the CRADA and, in part, the freeing-up of supplies of raw materials since the CRADA.[69] Eighteen months after the CRADA was signed, on 22 July 1992, Bristol-Myers Squibb filed an NDA for the use of taxol in the treatment of refractory ovarian cancer. On the same day, the company gave up the compound's orphan drug status.[70] The approval process was also fast. Just five months passed between the NDA submission and FDA approval on 29 December 1992. With the orphan drug status removed and no patent on the compound, Bristol-Myers Squibb was granted five years exclusive marketing rights to its drug under the terms of the Waxman-Hatch Act.[71]

Whose Trees?

By the time the taxol CRADA was signed, the NIH had already entered into 120 similar agreements since the programme began in 1987.[72] Of these, only fifteen were established with the Division of Cancer Treatment of the NCI. Many of America's best known pharmaceutical and biotechnology companies had a CRADA with one or more institutes of the NIH. Included were companies such as American Cyanamid, Abbott Labs, Dupont, Sterling Drug, Lilly, Upjohn, Cetus Corporation and Genentech. None of the NIH CRADAs, however, had yet resulted in a marketed product.[73]

Under the CRADA, the NCI and Bristol-Myers Squibb would collaborate on ongoing and future clinical studies to obtain FDA approval for the marketing of taxol, and the NCI would make available exclusively to Bristol-Myers Squibb the data and the results of all taxol studies. As to government-funded taxol data in the hands of extramural investigators, the NCI would urge them to cooperate exclusively with Bristol-Myers Squibb.

Transferring data from the public to the private sector did not, of course, address the critical problem of the supply of taxol which then depended solely on *Taxus brevifolia* bark. Discussions among the various agencies involved, namely the Department of Health and Human Services (the parent agency of the NIH), the USDA and the Department of the Interior, resulted in a Memorandum of Understanding, signed by the respective Secretaries of the three Departments in June 1991.[74] The Memorandum laid out a framework within which these agencies could work together to ensure a supply of *Taxus brevifolia* bark large enough to satisfy the expected demand for taxol in this and future years. The framework hinged on the critical passage of the NIH CRADA with Bristol-Myers Squibb wherein the company was required to secure adequate supplies of taxol for continued development. The objectives of the agreement also delineated an exclusive access to Federal *Taxus brevifolia* bark to the current CRADA partner (Bristol-Myers Squibb) and the company manufacturing taxol in bulk for human use (Hauser Chemical Research). A small rider was added that 'limited amounts of raw material' could be made available to other entities, although no details were entered as to amounts and the procedures necessary to obtain them.

Though the Memorandum of Understanding was an interagency agreement, by using the NIH CRADA as a referent, it paved the way for agreements between Bristol-Myers Squibb, the USDA and the Department of the Interior to provide exclusive access to Federal *Taxus brevifolia*. The mechanism, in the shape of two further CRADAs, was readily at hand and these agreements were duly signed by the respective agencies in mid-June 1991.[75]

The CRADAs with the USDA and the Department of the Interior were virtually the same and designed to run for a five-year period with the possibility of one-year renewals. The key point of the agreements was that they gave Bristol-Myers Squibb and/or their appointed agents right of first refusal to Federal *Taxus brevifolia* in accordance with an Annual Pacific Yew Program, the first of which was to begin in fiscal year 1991. For the purposes of the CRADA, Pacific yew was defined as all portions of *Taxus brevifolia* including bark, needles and twigs.

The right of first refusal ensured Bristol-Myers Squibb exclusive access to *Taxus brevifolia* apart from a limited amount that would be made available to other parties.[76] The amount set aside for others was incorporated in the Annual Pacific Yew Program and negotiated between the respective agency and Bristol-Myers Squibb. In the fiscal year of 1991, for example, the Annual Pacific Yew Program Plan of the Forest Service stipulated that the limit for the transfer of Pacific yew to parties other than Bristol-Myers Squibb was 50,000 pounds of bark and 100,000 pounds of needles or other foliage.[77] In the following year the bark limit remained the same but no limit was set for needles.[78] If, for any reason, Bristol-Myers Squibb declined the offer of the Pacific yew sale then both agencies were free, in principle, to make the sales to any interested party.

Bristol-Myers Squibb, for their part, agreed to provide funds to the Forest Service and the Bureau of Land Management to increase knowledge of *Taxus brevifolia* and its management. The most important part of this programme was the undertaking of a comprehensive inventory to determine the quantity and quality of *Taxus brevifolia* on public lands.

All of the CRADAs with Bristol-Myers Squibb worked, in practice, to give the company exclusive access to the source of the raw material and to all of the data that would be needed to file for the clinical approval of taxol. But the issue of how publicly owned *Taxus brevifolia* should be administered was not left to the CRADAs alone.[79] In November 1991, five months after the CRADAS were signed, a bill appeared in the House of Representatives that was aimed squarely at *Taxus brevifolia* and its management as a public resource. The details of the bill and its subsequent passage into legislation in the following year need not detain us here (it is treated fully in Chapter 6). One section of what became the Act, however, needs to be mentioned. Section 5 authorized the Secretary of Agriculture and the Secretary of the Interior through the Forest Service and the Bureau of Land Management, respectively, to negotiate Pacific yew sales only with those parties manufacturing taxol in the United States who complied with the appropriate regulations of the FDA.[80] This effectively meant that the right of first refusal had become transformed into an exclusive agreement. *Taxus brevifolia* belonging to the Bureau of Land Management and the Forest Service was unavailable to anyone other than Bristol-Myers Squibb or for purposes other than medicine until 1998.[81]

Whose Name?

On 20 December 1990, when the CRADA between the NCI and Bristol-Myers Squibb was all but signed, the company applied to the Patent and Trademark Office of the Department of Commerce to trademark the name 'taxol'.[82] The submission was successful and the name was registered on 26 May 1992. Thereafter, all references to taxol would be required to carry the registered sign, hence taxol became Taxol®. The generic name of 'paclitaxel' was approved at the same time.

Monroe Wall had named the bioactive compound from the bark of *Taxus brevifolia* taxol in 1967. Between the time of the first publication in which the word 'taxol' was mentioned – 1969 – and the date of the registration of Taxol®, the medical database MEDLINE had indexed more than 600 articles using the name taxol to refer to the compound isolated from *Taxus brevifolia* and available as a research tool and as an agent in clinical testing, solely from the NCI.[83] Adding in the large but unknown number of articles in other scientific journals not indexed by MEDLINE, together with the countless newspaper and magazine articles, radio and television programmes from which Americans learned about the remarkable molecule, the name taxol was not just in the public domain but belonged to it.

Bristol-Myers Squibb's actions did not go unnoticed, but the extent of public criticism was much less and its tone more muted than one might expect, given the public persona of taxol. The journal *Nature* was one of the few organizations to criticize Bristol-Myers Squibb's registration of taxol as a trademark. One editorial in 1995 urged the company to relinquish the protection granted by the trademark on the grounds that the name 'taxol' had been used by the research community for at least two decades.[84] On the whole, *Nature* found the company's actions to be shameful. The journal concluded that the examiners in the Patent and Trademark Office in Washington must have been asleep when they approved the application.

Bristol-Myers Squibb's lawyers responded to the charge by repeating that trademarks are subject to review by responsible authorities and generic names are sanctioned by the top health authorities in the world, such as the World Health Organization. As to the charge that the name 'taxol' had been used in the literature 'as a trivial name', this, according to the company, had 'no bearing on whether Taxol is a recognized trademark among oncologists'.[85] Changing the name, they concluded would be a mistake, cause confusion and possibly endanger the health of cancer patients.

Nature and *Chemical and Engineering News* were both chastized by Bristol-Myers Squibb lawyers because they had referred in several articles to 'taxol' as the substance derived from the Pacific yew. The lawyers made it clear to them that the name 'taxol' 'should only be used to refer to the anti-cancer preparation sold by Bristol-Myers Squibb Co.'.[86] *Chemical and Engineering News*, for one, capitulated and publicly announced that it would heretofore use the name 'paclitaxel' to refer to the molecule. On the other hand, Gary Strobel, a microbiologist from Montana State University who discovered that taxol was being made by a fungus growing on *Taxus brevifolia*, publicly refused to accede to Bristol-Myers Squibb's demands and said he would no longer be publishing articles on taxol in the United States.[87]

Publications are one thing. But the real issue about trademarks concerns commerce. Trademarks are words, names or symbols used by a manufacturer to identify its goods and distinguish them from those manufactured by others. They are used to protect the firm's goodwill.[88] Bristol-Myers Squibb, in one instance at least, was able to defend their trademark vigorously on the grounds of the confusion engendered by the use of the name 'taxol' for an anti-cancer preparation of another company. The case was brought by Bristol-Myers Squibb in 1994 against Corporation Biolyse Pharmacopée Internationale, a small pharmaceutical company based in Port Daniel, Quebec and begun by Claude Mercure, a biologist, who sought to make taxol from the needles and branch tips of the fast-growing *Taxus canadensis*.[89]

Bristol-Myers Squibb had applied on 1 February 1991 to register the trademark Taxol in Canada. On 29 December 1992, the Canadian Health Protection Board granted approval for Bristol-Myers Squibb to market Taxol for treatment against ovarian cancer; they began selling it in Canada on 21 January 1993. In their case against Biolyse, Bristol-Myers Squibb alleged that the Quebec company was using the names 'taxol' and 'paclitaxel' interchangeably throughout their protocols; and that they had referred to their preparation as taxol, inferring, in accordance with the trademark registration, that Biolyse's product was the Bristol-Myers Squibb product called Taxol, and misleading the medical profession by passing off their products as those of Bristol-Myers Squibb.[90] Bristol-Myers Squibb, it was stated, had invested 'over $350 million dollars U.S. in the research and development of TAXOL (paclitaxel) since 1991 and that the goodwill associated with the trademark Taxol was vital to the continued business success of the company'.[91] Biolyse rejected Bristol-Myers Squibb's claims about misleading the medical profession and doing anything that would cause damage to Bristol-Myers Squibb.[92] They maintained that Bristol-Myers Squibb had no valid right to the trademark Taxol as it had been used for many years by the medical profession; that it was, indeed, the generic name used to refer to the anti-cancer preparation; and that the company could not, therefore, claim authorship or exclusivity in its use.[93] Consequently, there could be no case for damages as Bristol-Myers Squibb's goodwill was not connected to the trademark Taxol.

Biolyse's arguments did not, however, find favour. On 15 December 1995, the Federal Court judged that the Taxol trademark was 'a valid and subsisting trademark owned by Bristol-Myers Squibb' and that

Biolyse should refrain from using the word taxol in reference to their own products.

This was an important victory for Bristol-Myers Squibb. Their trademark was upheld by a court of law. By June 1994, Taxol had been trademarked in more than fifty countries world-wide. There could be no doubt now that taxol had become private property in substance and in name.

But the question still remains as to how the Patent and Trademark Office could have made their decision to accept the name 'taxol' as a trademark. The same question was asked in the *Nature* editorial and by two patent lawyers in London who were interested in the issue.[94]

Alternatives and Complements: The Business of Taxol

The NCI held two workshops on taxol and *Taxus*, the first in Bethesda, Maryland in June 1990 and the second in Alexandria, Virginia in September 1992. Just under 200 participants attended the first workshop and double that number were at the second. One of the objectives of the workshop was to bring together as many people as possible who were interested in the development of taxol and its source, *Taxus*. Among those attending were a large number of individuals who were particularly interested in developing both alternative sources of *Taxus* biomass and alternative non-biomass routes to the production of taxol. Some were attached to university departments and research institutes while others were employed by private business.

The reason why there was such a great interest in alternatives to the bark of *Taxus brevifolia* as the raw material for the production of taxol was simply that, whatever the state of the population of trees in the Pacific Northwest, it was a finite resource. Regardless of how quickly it was depleted, as long as it was the only source, someday there would be no more wild *Taxus brevifolia*.

We have seen, in previous chapters, that since the late 1960s, it had been clear that *Taxus brevifolia* bark could only be a short-term resource. Still, in 1990, exactly the same was being said.[95] Needles, it was also recognized, were an obvious longer term solution as they were a renewable resource. The problem was that the taxol content in needles was more variable than in the bark and, even though this by itself was not a good reason for abandoning the resource, it was dismissed in favour of bark. There was, however, a big difference between the 1960s and the 1990s in dismissing needles as a source of taxol.

For one thing, the forest had become politicized. While concepts such as renewability and sustainability were rarely mentioned in the 1960s, by the early 1990s they had become household terms. Secondly, the science of detecting minute quantities of compounds in plant material had advanced considerably. Using a variety of newer analytical techniques, particularly high performance liquid chromatography, scientists in the early 1990s re-examined the taxol content of different parts of a number of *Taxus* species, including *brevifolia*. One of the first large-scale studies of the taxol content by tree part and species was conducted at the Frederick Cancer Research Facility and the Natural Products Branch of the NCI and published in 1990. Finding little difference between the taxol content of needles of several species and the bark of *Taxus brevifolia*, the authors concluded that '*Taxus* needles could provide a renewable source of taxol'.[96] They urged more research on harvesting conditions, drying procedures and extraction methods to optimize yields.

There then followed a number of other studies, all of which differed in certain essentials – such as how, when and from where the parts of the tree were harvested – but the results confirmed earlier observations that the variation in taxol content in the needles was large and, indeed, larger than in the bark.[97] Most studies also concluded that the average taxol content in needles was less than that in bark, although the difference between the two varied considerably from a factor of 10 in one study to a factor of 1.7 in another.[98] Even less difference was observed between the taxol content of needles in other *Taxus* species when compared with *Taxus brevifolia* bark: in the case of the wild *Taxus canadensis*, and the cultivated varieties *Taxus cuspidata* cv. Capitata and *Taxus* × *media* cv. Hicksii, the difference was either non-existent or insignificant.[99] If these results were a surprise to some in the community, they were not news to some others, such as Robert Perdue, who had observed the same thing in the late 1960s and strongly urged a programme of cultivating *Taxus* species expressly for their taxol content.[100]

The old argument that needles could not be considered seriously as an alternative source was no longer acceptable. Even though the taxol content in needles was lower than in bark, there was three times the weight of needles as bark on an average *Taxus brevifolia* and they were renewable.[101] But even better yields could be expected from harvesting the needles from cultivated species. At the same time, during the early 1990s, innovative extraction procedures were able to raise the taxol yield from needles to the extent that they became increasingly an economical, as well as an environmentally-friendly, source.[102] At the Second Workshop on Taxol and *Taxus*, five posters were devoted exclusively to the analysis of taxol content in the needles of several species.

The issue about needles and other natural alternatives to wild *Taxus brevifolia* surfaced at the USDA in 1990. On 7 November, the Department invited representatives of the NCI, the Forest Service, the FDA,

Zelenka Nurseries (Muskegon, Michigan), the Secrest Arboretum at Ohio State University, the University of Mississippi and Bristol-Myers Squibb to a meeting.[103] The point of the meeting was for the USDA to lead a multi-institution project to solve the taxol supply problem through agricultural means. The key partner in this enterprise would be the University of Mississippi which was doing the most work in the United States investigating the possibilities of using cultivated varieties of *Taxus* for taxol production. Edward Croom and James McChesney, both of the Research Institute of Pharmaceutical Sciences of the University had already contacted the NCI earlier that year outlining the work they were doing.[104] They also indicated that they were busy negotiating an agreement with Bristol-Myers Squibb to establish a major research facility to look into producing taxol from the needles of cultivated *Taxus* species from nurseries.

The USDA was extremely interested in moving ahead with the needle project. They were aware, at the end of February, that the University of Mississippi and Bristol-Myers Squibb had not yet reached agreement because of disagreements over who controlled the results of their proposed joint research.[105] So vital was the need to develop adequate supplies of taxol from alternative sources, that Paul O'Connell, Deputy Administrator of the USDA, felt that no time should be wasted waiting for the University of Mississippi and Bristol-Myers Squibb to sort out their differences.[106] The agency, together with the University and the NCI, he argued, should move quickly to collect trimmings from the nurseries and produce taxol. At the same time, someone should begin to work with the FDA to prepare the ground for approving taxol from this new source.

An Interagency Agreement was drawn up by which the USDA, the lead agency, would co-ordinate the collection and drying of *Taxus* biomass to be delivered to the NCI, all stages to be performed according to the University of Mississippi's proprietary specifications. The target plant, a single cultivar, *Taxus* × *media* ca. Hicksii, was growing in the Zelenka Nurseries which would collect and dry – with the help of experts from Ohio State University – the late Spring trimmings.[107] Bristol-Myers Squibb agreed to fund the purification part of the project.[108] The original plan, however, did not go ahead as scheduled for Spring 1991 because of various misunderstandings about what the proposal actually entailed.[109] Instead, a revised and less ambitious project was accepted providing for the extraction of taxol from 100,000 pounds fresh weight, or 35,000 pounds dry weight of needles and small twigs from *Taxus* × *media*; it got off the ground in September 1991.[110]

By the end of December of the following year, 1992, Ken Snader of the NCI's Natural Products Branch, was able to report that the project was a success. Just under 40,000 pounds of dry biomass had been collected with an average content of 0.0164 per cent, or 50 per cent more than the working yield of 0.01 per cent for *Taxus brevifolia* bark.[111] This exercise showed that the laboratory results achieved at the University of Mississippi which gave significant taxol yields from the needles of *Taxus × media*, together with the specific harvesting and drying procedures that they had developed, could be scaled-up to commercial levels without much loss on the laboratory values.

One of the interesting developments to occur during the time of the interagency agreement and largely contingent upon it was the establishment of an Alliance for the Production of Taxol, an organization to bring *Taxus* growers in the United States together, to make them aware of the taxol programme and to enlist their help in making trimmings from cultivated stock available for sale. The first meeting of the Alliance was held on 22 March 1991, hosted by the Secrest Arboretum of the Ohio State University.[112] Many nurseries attended the meeting and gave their support to the Alliance. The responsibilities of the individual nurseries included providing the Alliance with a detailed inventory of their *Taxus* holdings. The number of plants growing in the nurseries surveyed totalled more than 30 million from which it was estimated that enough taxol could be produced to treat between 3,000 and 4,000 ovarian cancer patients annually – maybe thirty per cent of all patients who could receive taxol.[113]

As a complement to *Taxus brevifolia* bark, needles from nursery cultivars were, therefore, an excellent source for the production of taxol. But if taxol was shown to be effective in more common cancers, such as breast cancer, then the nursery sources would not be able to meet the anticipated demand.[114] The NCI's strategy at this point, in 1991 and 1992, was to explore as many different avenues as possible to solve the long-term supply problems, initiated by itself or with the co-operation of Bristol-Myers Squibb.

Chief among these alternatives to *Taxus brevifolia* bark was the possibility of using *Taxus* growing in Canada, Russia, India and China; extracting taxol from the heartwood of *Taxus brevifolia*; and a number of grants to support research into semi-synthesis, synthesis, biosynthesis, cell and tissue culture and plant genetics and propagation.[115]

Under the terms of the CRADA, any information coming from the NCI itself or via the NCI from other parties would be made available to Bristol-Myers Squibb. But there was another source of information concerning alternative solutions to the long-term taxol supply problem that came from elsewhere, from the private sector. Taxol caught the eye of several firms who thought they had a solution within their grasp.

Their solution, and one which would appeal most to any pharmaceutical company, was to end the reliance altogether on harvesting raw
materials from both wild and cultivated plants whether they were
intended for the direct extraction of taxol or for the extraction of a
precursor to be made into taxol semi-synthetically. The most fruitful
approach that had already produced results in agriculture, was to make
taxol using plant cell and tissue cultures.[116] By 1991, several groups in
North America were working in this research area, prominent among
them being the Agricultural Research Service in New Orleans that
had taken out a patent on their method in May;[117] a biotechnology unit
at the University of Toronto, headed by Frank DiCosmo;[118] and a group
at Cornell University headed by Michael Shuler.[119]

The cell and tissue culture approach certainly interested biotechnology companies. One of them, Phyton Catalytic, based in Ithaca,
New York, was formed in 1990 and entered into a CRADA with the
USDA in January 1991.[120] By this route, Phyton gained access to
the patent filed by Alice Christen, Donna Gibson and John Bland of the
Agricultural Research Service. Taxol was Phyton's first research and
development interest. The company also received funding from Bristol-
Myers Squibb. Its direct competitor, also a biotechnology company,
based in San Carlos, California, and called ESCAgenetics, had achieved
commercial success in producing vanilla through cell culture techniques.[121] In 1991, just after the granting of the cell culture patent to the
USDA, ESCAgenetics announced that it, too, had produced taxol from
cell tissue culture.[122] Both ESCAgenetics and Phyton Catalytic received
considerable funding from the NCI.[123] In attempting to woo Bristol-
Myers, ESCAgenetics lost out to Phyton Catalytic.[124]

Another group, based at Montana State University, in their search for
an alternative source, however, focused not on cell culture but on the
discovery that a fungus, *Taxomyces andreanae*, growing on *Taxus
brevifolia*, also produced taxol.[125] Further work not only confirmed this
result but also showed that other fungal endophytes associated with
other species of *Taxus* produced taxol as did some fungi associated with
a different plant genus.[126] The group recognized the possibilities and
advantages of using microbial fermentation to produce taxol. Rights for
the technique to produce taxol from fungal endophytes were licensed at
various times from 1993 to Cytoclonal Pharmaceutics, a Dallas-based
biotechnology firm.[127]

The Race to Synthesize Taxol

'Devising a total synthesis of the anti-cancer drug taxol has engaged the
attention of chemists for more than 20 years. But their ingenuity – and

perseverance – has been rewarded.' Thus the journal *Nature* on 17 February 1994 announced the first published total synthesis of taxol by K.C. Nicolaou and his group at the Scripps Research Institute in California.[128] Within a week, Bob Holton and his group at Florida State University also published a total synthesis of taxol.[129] The journal *Chemistry and Industry* described the two events as a 'photo-finish in the race to artificial taxol'.[130]

The various approaches to developing methods of obtaining taxol that we have so far discussed all depended on harnessing biological processes. These included extraction from bark or renewable parts of various *Taxus* species, extraction from the *Taxomyces* fungus, extraction from *Taxus* cell cultures; and semi-synthesis from taxanes related structurally to taxol, extracted from renewable parts of various *Taxus* species and from *Taxus* species that can be cultivated. In contrast to all these, total synthesis uses chemical processes to make taxol from inexpensive starting materials – including naturally-occurring ones – and has nothing to do with yew trees at all.

It was automatic for chemists to try and make taxol by total synthesis as soon as its structure was known.[131] Total synthesis harnesses the specific skills of organic chemists, and represents a major challenge to their chemical ingenuity: 'conquering a molecular Mount Everest'.[132] Tackling the problems of synthesis also generates chemical knowledge about structure, reactions, properties, mechanisms of action, relationships between molecular structure and biological action, and new approaches to synthesis. Moreover, during the process of exploring the synthetic alternatives, analogues are likely to be produced that are potentially simpler and medicinally more effective, or have improved properties (more soluble, or less toxic for instance). Some chemists are also attracted by the aesthetic as well as scientific appeal of complex molecules: the way in which the building blocks of taxol's architecture, for example, are represented by 112 atoms arranged in space.[133]

As we have seen, several groups of chemists began work on taxol in the early 1980s, including Charles Swindell at Bryn Mawr College, Bob Holton at Virginia Polytechnic Institute (later at Florida State University), David Kingston at Virginia Polytechnic Institute, Paul Wender at Stanford University, and Pierre Potier at the Institut de Chimie des Substances Naturelles. All but Potier were primarily interested in total synthesis. Chemists were therefore working on the total synthesis of taxol long before the supply problem had been defined and, with the exception of Potier's group, generally before the work began on semi-synthesis. The earlier work was not aiming at a practical, commercializable route, but was an exercise in developing chemical knowledge. According to Paul Wender, 'we defined the problem initially as ... requiring the development of a new synthetic methodology ... It was a fundamental problem (and) if we were successful ... we would put back into the synthetic chemist's box of tools some significant new tools that will be useful for problems that ... show up in the future.'[134]

Once the clinical trials of taxol revealed the seriousness of the supply problem, the largely academic approach to total synthesis in the United States gave way to a more practical concern. As Paul Wender noted: '(in about 1988) there was a change in the definition of the problem, that led to a change in our approach. We added on this additional component which was designed to yield a result in short order ... All of a sudden you had a fairly rare material but a great deal of potential utility.'[135] Holton agreed that in 1988, 'the need to do something of some practical significance, the opportunity to do something that was really needed and happened to be right on my doorstep' caused him to turn his attention towards a commercially practical route to taxol.[136] From the point of view of the supply problem, if total synthesis were to provide a solution it would have had to be a 'practical' synthesis: that is, one which could be scaled-up from laboratory to industrial preparation, and one which was comparable in cost with existing processes, or cheaper. The cost of the synthetic route would depend not just on the cost of the raw materials, but also on the number of chemical steps needed to get from them to taxol, the yield in which each intermediate product was generated, and the efficiency with which the intermediates and taxol itself could be separated from by-products, and its isomers[137] and enantiomers.[138] The challenge was enormous. Total synthesis of molecules more complicated than taxol had been achieved, but not normally in a practical process for commercialization or bulk production.

Instead of continuing to focus primarily on total synthesis, Bob Holton in 1988 turned his attention, for the time being, to semi-synthesis from 10-DAB as a more practical route than total synthesis for producing taxol. In making this decision, he was particularly encouraged by the results obtained by the groups led by Pierre Potier and Andrew Greene, respectively, in France, and which were published in this same year.[139] Paul Wender, on the other hand, worked on the design of a practical total synthesis that would take few steps, and would start from cheap raw materials.

Holton was unusual in pursuing semi-synthesis. Apart from the French groups, most chemists focused on total synthesis. By the autumn of 1993, shortly before the first publication of successful totally synthetic routes, more than fifty research groups world-wide had published articles on the subject.[140] By this time, Holton too, had his mind once again on the problems of total synthesis, having successfully produced taxol semi-synthetically.

There were, in theory, many different ways to approach the synthesis. The key problem was to reproduce the structure of the ring skeleton, especially the unusual eight-membered ring, and its orientation in space at the various centres of asymmetry; and to construct and attach the side chain and the many functional groups, given that some of the attachments to the molecular framework hindered the sites at which further reactions would have to take place. Constructing and attaching the side chain was, perhaps, the least of the problems because, as we have discussed in Chapter 4, the parallel research on semi-synthesis had by then already found suitable methods for doing this.

The major task, therefore, was to make the three connecting rings of the core skeleton. Two broad approaches to this were possible. One was to construct several subunits and then put them together (the convergent approach); the other was to build the whole molecule up in step by step additions (the linear approach). In taking account of the stereo-chemistry of natural products, a further two approaches were possible.[141] One was to select the correct mirror image, or enantiomer, early on with chemicals of the desired configuration, and maintain their orientation at each subsequent step of the synthesis. The other was to work with a mixture of enantiomers and to select the desired configuration towards the end of the synthesis, a technique known as resolution.

The Holton group chose a linear approach. Holton first reported the synthesis of the tricyclic taxane ring system in 1984,[142] then taxusin in 1988[143] (the first synthesis of a naturally occurring compound that contains the entire taxane ring system, but not the side chain), and finally taxol itself in 1994. Initially, Holton's starting point for making taxusin was patchino, a chemical sold in bulk by International Flavor and Fragrances Inc. At that stage Holton saw the attachment of the side chain at C-13 as presenting a real obstacle,[144] although the groups of Greene in Grenoble and Potier at Gif-sur-Yvette had just published their method for doing this.[145] Bob Holton's method for the total synthesis[146] used some forty steps and arrived at taxol via 10-DAB this time from readily-available camphor, with an overall yield of four to five per cent of the starting materials. The Nicolaou group, by contrast, chose a convergent synthesis, followed by resolution of the enantiomeric forms. Their method[147] comprised a twenty-eight step process in which two of the rings were prepared and joined in such a way that the third eight-membered ring was constructed between them. This resulted in a 0.05 per cent overall yield of taxol.[148] Nicolaou's group submitted their synthesis for publication a month later than Holton, but it appeared a week earlier. Holton had been working on taxol for more than ten years by this time,[149] and had first published on taxol in 1984, but Nicolaou was a relative newcomer, having started on the problem of taxol synthesis only in 1992.[150] Indeed, Nicolaou reported some difficulty in being accepted into the 'taxol community', noting that his first and second project proposals for total synthesis of taxol were turned down by the NCI, his first communication on the project was rejected by the prestigious chemical journal *Angewandte Chemie*, and he was unable to obtain taxol for research.[151]

Another major player in the total synthesis stakes was Paul Wender and a team of twenty-one funded by the National Science Foundation, NCI and Bristol-Myers Squibb. They made taxol from the starting material pinene slightly later in 1994,[152] although they published their planned synthetic approach some two years earlier.[153] Pinene is itself a natural product obtained from pine trees, but as a major component of turpentine and other solvents is both abundant and inexpensive, as well as being a relatively simple molecule. 'One could not ignore the additional aesthetic attractiveness of using the abundant constituent of one tree to produce the trace component of another,' reported Wender's group.[154] Like Nicolaou's group, they used a convergent approach, but isolated the desired stereoisomer early on. Their strategic design approach was also similar to that of the Nicolaou group, which was to work backwards from the ring system, calculating which bonds, when broken, would generate similar sized fragments that, in total synthesis, could be made independently and then joined together.[155] Several fragments were six-membered rings, which led the team to search for commercially available six-membered rings with the desirable stereochemistry, and α-pinene proved to be a suitable candidate, even though 'its relationship to taxol ... is not immediately obvious'.[156] They were able to assemble the taxane ring system in as few as five steps from commercially available α-pinene, although the whole process from pinene to taxol is said to have taken thirty-eight steps.[157]

What is interesting about the attempts to synthesize taxol is the gulf that seemed to separate the chemists and journalists, on the one hand, and the NCI (and probably other bodies as well), on the other hand, on the value of this approach. In the scientific press, total synthesis, from the late 1980s, was persistently discussed in the context of the supply problem.[158] In 1988, for example, *Chemical and Engineering News* reported Holton's preparation of taxusin, one of the intermediates in his total synthesis, in the context of the shortage of supplies of taxol for clinical trials and NCI's consequent support for projects for the synthesis of taxol.[159] Several years later, in 1992, *New Scientist*'s report of the American Chemical Society April meeting suggested that 'commercial quantities of taxol ... may soon be manufactured from readily available raw materials', referring to Wender's and Holton's ongoing work on total synthesis.[160]

The political climate surrounding taxol and *Taxus brevifolia* in the early 1990s certainly helped bolster the link between total synthesis and the supply problem that chemists articulated. In 1992, for example, Wender's group reported their proposed pinene path as a practical, commercializable synthesis: 'our approach to this problem was guided by the goal of producing a practical synthesis of taxol'.[161] The successful synthesis was described as 'an exceptionally concise route to a wide range of analogs of taxol as needed for mode of action studies and a potentially practical synthesis of taxol itself'.[162]

Despite these optimistic statements from chemists and the press, from the NCI's perspective, total synthesis was not seen as a serious commercial route. Bruce Chabner of the NCI was quoted by *Chemical and Engineering News* in the same year as saying 'NCI and Bristol-Myers Squibb are working with the biomedical and agricultural research communities to develop alternative methods... These include total [synthesis]...'.[163] But Chabner went on to say that 'the ultimate source is going to be semi-synthesis from a precursor'. Once total synthesis had been achieved in 1994, the NCI appears to have been little impressed by what others saw as an amazing achievement. In response to Holton's total synthesis, Sam Broder of the NCI was quoted by *Chemistry and Industry* as saying that the 'achievement may enable researchers to devise more effective, less toxic drugs and could thus have a significant effect on cancer treatment'.[164] He was not quoted as saying anything about total synthesis being a goal for industrial production. Matthew Suffness shared Chabner's lukewarm reception of total synthesis as a practical route. He thought that the number of steps in the synthesis would need to be fewer than twenty-five before the process could be said to be practical – all of the total syntheses to date exceeded this number of steps.[165] Susan Horwitz, while greeting Nicolaou's total synthesis as a 'scientific land mark and an intellectual achievement', went on to say that 'it is not clear whether their accomplishment will make large quantities of the drug available to treat patients, or result in a decrease in its cost, but it will allow the preparation of new compounds that otherwise would be unavailable for testing and for studies on mechanism of action'.[166]

Was there a race? Paul Wender thought not: 'most of us are driven by... helping people rather than competing against one another...' The *Los Angeles Times* presented it as a competition '...I am offended by that... I'm not going to be giving you a soap opera for science... It's really stupid if scientists let competition get in the way of scientific progress.'[167] Nicolaou took the opposite position: as he put it, 'there was a competition even if we don't want to admit it'.[168] Whether it was a race or not, casting the several attempts to synthesize taxol in these terms may have made good media copy but as a practical approach to taxol production, the verdict was less than optimistic. *Chemical and Engineering News* stated quite decisively that neither of the two syntheses would be of practical use for commercial production of taxol, although they reported that Holton and Nicolaou had both filed patents.[169] And that seemed to be about right. None of the four successful total syntheses reported by 1996 [Nicolaou's (1994), Holton's (1994), Wender's (1995) and Danishefsky's (1996)][170] have been applied to the production of taxol.[171]

The total synthesis still had a practical as well as a theoretical use, however. Creating analogues of known molecules is, as we have seen, a major goal of total synthesis. The gains from discovering analogues that might be more active, or less toxic, or more soluble or otherwise improved in properties were potentially enormous. As Nicolaou, Guy and Potier have remarked: 'By constructing taxol with simple building blocks, we would be able to modify the compound's structure at any position, thereby creating a variety of taxol derivatives.'[172] '... Many researchers, including the three of us, are pursuing the challenges of developing an entire family of taxol-like compounds – known as taxoids – that may eventually be easier to manufacture and that may also afford more and better therapeutic options than the parent molecule taxol.'[173] Indeed, as it turned out Potier and his group were eminently successful. The analogue they discovered was named taxotere. It was commercialized by Rhône-Poulenc, and approved by the FDA for use in advanced breast cancer in 1995. Early results showed it to be more active and more soluble than taxol.[174]

Notes

1 *Federal Register* vol. 54, no. 146, 1 August 1989, pp. 31734–31735. The CRADA mechanism for the transfer of technology from the public to the private sector, as it applies in the health field, has been subject to little critical comment. For the background, see Eisenberg, 'Public research' and Berman, 'Technology transfer'. For pharmaceuticals and especially the issue of pricing, see Brody, 'Public goods and fair prices' and Marks, 'NIH CRADA'.
2 Shoemaker to Suffness, 17 January 1989, NPBI/1. In the notice and in the CRADA agreement, no money was to change hands. The successful company would need to provide funds but only for development purposes. The financial issues of the CRADA would be the subject of a Congressional hearing on 25 January 1993.
3 Subcommittee on Regulation, Business Opportunities, and Energy, *Hearing: Exclusive Agreements*, pp. 401–408.
4 Bristol-Myers was a large health-care company based in the United States. Rhône-Poulenc was a multidivisional chemical company, based in France, but with international manufacturing and marketing activities. Xechem was a

wholly owned subsidiary of Lyphomed, Inc. Though Lyphomed received the Federal Register notice, it was Xechem that submitted the proposal. In September of 1989, Lyphomed was bought by the Fujisawa, one of Japan's largest pharmaceutical companies. Lyphomed had gone through a rough patch in recent years because of quality control problems but was beginning to turn around thanks to the FDA approval in June 1989 of aerolized pentamidine, used to treat AIDS-related pneumonia – see *Chemical Marketing Reporter*, vol. 236, no. 11, 1989, p. 41 and *Chemical Marketing Reporter*, vol. 235, no. 25, 1989, p. 9. Lyphomed was a small company. Unimed was even smaller, specializing in licensing promising compounds from university laboratories and research institutes. It described itself as a company specializing in cancer chemotherapy compounds and agents used in the care of cancer patients. Its main success before 1989 was the drug Marinol used to lessen the effects of nausea in cancer patients undergoing chemotherapy. Its active ingredient was a synthetic version of THC (tetrahydrocannabinol), the active ingredient of marijuana. In 1989, Unimed received approval from the FDA to begin clinical trials on a nitrogen mustard compound, G-6-M, licensed from Georgetown University. See Unimed, Annual Report, 1988 and 'Marijuana derivative to get FDA okay', *Chemical Marketing Reporter*, vol. 229, no. 14, 1986, p. 5.

5 Shoemaker to Members, Taxol CRADA Review Committee, 2 October 1989, NPBI.

6 Shoemaker to DeFuria (Bristol-Myers Squibb), 23 October 1989 and Shoemaker to Gural (Rhône-Poulenc), 27 October 1989, NPBII.

7 Shoemaker to Pandey (Xechem), 1 November 1989 and Shoemaker to Plasse (Unimed), 1 November 1989, NPBII.

8 Shoemaker to Members, Taxol CRADA Review Committee, 29 November 1989, NPBII.

9 Gordon Cragg, Chief of the Natural Products Branch and one of the four preclinical reviewers, for example, had cast his vote for Bristol-Myers Squibb by 1 December 1989 – Cragg to Shoemaker, 1 December 1989, NPBII.

10 See, for example, Shoemaker to Luce (Adria Laboratories), 11 December 1989 in Subcommittee on Regulation, Business Opportunities, and Energy, *Hearing: Exclusive Agreements*, p. 399.

11 These are to be found in *Federal Register*, vol. 54, no. 146, 1 August 1989, pp. 31734–31735.

12 This may have been somewhat of a tall order as most large pharmaceutical companies had limited experience in natural non-microbial products at this time. Plants, in particular, hardly mattered in most research programs. See O'Neill and Lewis, 'The renaissance of plant research'. Recent research has provided a good quantitative measure of the importance of natural products in pharmaceutical development. Of 520 new approved drugs in the United States between 1983 and 1994, six per cent were derived from unmodified natural products and a further twenty-four per cent were derived from a natural product source (semi-synthetically): in the field of oncology, the corresponding figures were better at seventeen per cent and twenty-nine per cent, respectively of the eighty-seven approved anti-cancer drugs. Unmodified plant-derived anti-cancer drugs accounted for only five per cent and semi-synthetic plant-derived anti-cancer drugs only three per cent of the total. The data come from Cragg, Newman and Snader, 'Natural products', pp. 52–54.

13 Shoemaker to Pandey (Xechem), 1 November 1989, Shoemaker to Plasse (Unimed), 1 November 1989, Shoemaker to DeFuria (Bristol-Myers), 23 October 1989 and Shoemaker to Gural (Rhône-Poulenc), 27 October 1989, NPBII.

14 The hearing was critical of the whole CRADA process, implicitly and explicitly. Others were not so critical of the CRADA, however. Praise for the CRADA and Bristol-Myers Squibb came, for example, in 'Bristol-Myers Squibb's taxol gamble – the Schwartz commentary', *Scrip*, no. 1715, 6 May 1992, p. 17 and Donehower, 'The clinical development'.

15 Subcommittee Staff to Wyden, 22 July 1991, SCH.

16 Wittes's biographical information is from his 'Curriculum vitae', NCI Archives, DC012499.

17 He had also held discussions with the pharmaceutical company Schering-Plough in 1988 about their possible involvement in the taxol programme, as discussed in Chapter 4.

18 *The Cancer Letter*, vol. 16, no. 23, 8 June 1990, p. 1.

19 Subcommittee Staff to Wyden, 22 July 1991, in Subcommittee on Regulation, Business Opportunities, and Energy, *Hearing: Exclusive Agreements*, p. 240.

20 *The Cancer Letter*, vol. 17, no. 32, 9 August 1991, p. 2.

21 Newman, 'The great'.

22 Newman, 'The great', p. 19.

23 Healy to Wyden, *The Cancer Letter*, vol. 18, no. 35, 11 September 1992, p. 4.

24 'Testimony of Bruce Chabner, Director, Division of Cancer Treatment, National Cancer Institute', Subcommittee on Regulation, Business Opportunities, and Energy, *Hearing: Exclusive Agreements*, p. 19. Eric Nalder, a reporter on the *Seattle Times*, who was following the story about taxol and *Taxus brevifolia*, became interested in the CRADA competition to the extent of requesting all documents dealing with it, including the role of Robert Wittes, from the NCI.

25 Calculated from *Scrip Yearbook, 1991*, p. 61 and *Scrip Yearbook, 1992*, p. 73. By contrast, cardiovascular drugs, the principal product of the pharmaceutical industry, accounted for seventeen per cent of worldwide sales.

26 'HEW News Release: National Institutes of Health, National Cancer Institute, 20 December 1982', NCI Archives AR-7212-008808.

27 Suffness to Distribution, 12 May 1988, NPBIV.

28 Interestingly, Stephen Carter was Bruce Chabner's opposite number at Bristol-Myers Squibb for the CRADA. The CRADA agreement contained a clause which authorized Carter and Chabner to decide on an issue in the event that the Joint Steering Committee which oversaw the CRADA could not come to an agreement – see 'CRADA for the clinical development of taxol', NPBIII.

29 Subcommittee on Fisheries, etc., *Hearing: Pacific Yew Act*, p. 31.

30 Subcommittee on Fisheries, etc., *Hearing: Pacific Yew Act*, p. 31.

31 Suffness to Distribution, 12 May 1988, NPBIV.

32 Suffness to Douros, 6 July 1988, FRD4.

33 Advanced Molecular Technologies, 'Executive Summary', attached to letter to Ken Snader, 30 December 1988, DST.

34 Haverfield to Destito, 19 December 1988, DST.

35 Destito to Haverfield, 9 January 1989, DST.

36 Destito to Haverfield, 9 January 1989, DST.

37 Weyerhaeuser, while not being keen on collecting bark from wild *Taxus brevifolia*, nevertheless felt it had the connections to undertake collections and would help Advanced Molecular Technologies do this, if they wished. Haverfield to Destito, 19 December 1988, DST.
38 Destito to Haverfield, 28 February 1989, DST.
39 Destito to Haverfield, 28 February 1989, DST.
40 Soule (Vice President, Research and Engineering, Weyerhaeuser) to Destito, 28 April 1989. In this alliance, Toray was responsible for pharmaceutical development, Weyerhaeuser for selection, cultivation and improvement of plants and Advanced Molecular Technologies for the collection of the bark and for the extraction and purification of taxol.
41 Destito to Haverfield, 2 May 1989, DST.
42 Destito to Oliff (Merck, Sharp and Dohme), 3 July 1989 and Destito to Dexter (Dupont), 3 July 1989. Both letters had attached to them the 'Taxol Co-Development Working Plan'.
43 Imanishi (Toray Industries) to Destito, 18 August 1989, DST.
44 Destito to Imanishi, 10 August 1989, cited in Imanishi to Destito, 18 August 1989, DST.
45 Alan Jones, a biochemist working for Advanced Molecular Technologies, had prepared suggestions on how to improve the procedure of purifying taxol from bark the process time of which, he maintained, he could cut by fifty per cent – see Jones, 'Taxol Preparation Report', 17 July 1989, DST.
46 Destito to McGovern, 21 August 1989. The equity investment Destito proposed was on the same basis as any pharmaceutical company in the co-development plan, that is for long-term expansion and not, as he emphasized, the 60,000 bark collection.
47 Destito to McGovern, 19 August 1989, DST.
48 McGovern to Destito, 23 October 1990, DST.
49 Destito to Fabre, 8 September 1989 and 13 September 1989, DST.
50 Destito to Bristol-Myers Company, 7 September 1989, DST. See also Ziemer (Bristol-Myers) to Destito, 5 September 1989, from which it is clear that Bristol-Myers was shying away from any medium- to long-term commitment to Destito.
51 Destito to Plasse (Unimed) and Plasse to Connolly, 25 August 1989, CON.
52 'Organizational Chart' attached to Pandey (Xechem) to Destito, 1 September 1989, DST.
53 Eisenberg, 'Public research'. 15 USC Section 3710a explicitly encourages CRADAs with small businesses.
54 Shoemaker to DeFuria, 17 November 1989, NPBII.
55 Stull to Fiorenza (Bristol-Myers), 7 November 1989, FRD3.
56 In a memo on 7 May 1990 (six months after the Review Committee's supplementary questions to Bristol-Myers) to the Acting Associate Director of the Developmental Therapeutics Program of the Division of Cancer Treatment, Gordon Cragg and Ken Snader of the Natural Products Branch voiced their scepticism at Hauser's claim that '750 gm can be isolated from 10,000 pounds; this far exceeds their present performance for NCI (approximately 500 gms/10,000 lbs), and they still have to achieve GMP status'. The figure of 750 grams/10,000 pounds of bark was in a presentation Bristol-Myers Squibb gave to the NCI in April or May 1990. Documents in FRD4. In October 1990, Hauser was managing 550 grams of taxol from 10,000 pounds of bark – Canetta (Bristol-Myers Squibb) to Members, Taxol Update

Meeting, 29 October 1990, NPBII. The report on manufacturing at Hauser was presented by Ken Snader of the Natural Products Branch of the NCI. At the hearing on the exclusive agreements between Bristol-Myers Squibb and Federal agencies in July 1991, Dean Stull, when asked how much Pacific yew bark was required to make one kilogram of taxol testified 'We require less than the published data, which is about 30,000 pounds per kilo, and it is proprietary, but it is *approaching* (our italics) two-thirds or so of that or less.' – see Subcommittee on Regulation, Business Opportunities, and Energy, *Hearing: Exclusive Agreements*, p. 63.

57 DeFuria to Shoemaker, 17 November 1989, NPBIII.

58 DeFuria to Shoemaker, 17 November 1989, 'Taxol CRADA Proposal – October 23rd – Questions and Answers', p. 3, NPBIII.

59 Interview with Robert Holton, 22 May 1998.

60 Shoemaker to Gural, 27 October 1989, NPBIII.

61 Gural to Shoemaker, 20 November 1989, NPBIII.

62 Gural to Shoemaker, 15 September 1989, 'CRADA submission', p. 3, NPBIII.

63 Gural to Shoemaker, 15 September 1989, 'CRADA submission', p. 24 and Gural to Shoemaker, 20 November 1989, p. 7, NPBIII. By March 1990, Rhône-Poulenc had purchased controlling interest in the pharmaceutical company, Rorer, based in Pennsylvania, and established the headquarters of their pharmaceutical subsidiary, Rhône-Poulenc Rorer in that state.

64 DeFuria to Shoemaker, 17 November 1989, 'Taxol CRADA Proposal – October 23rd – Questions and Answers', p. 4, NPBIII.

65 Gural to Shoemaker, 20 November 1989, pp. 5–6, NPBIII. This was a veiled reference to the company's own taxol analogue, taxotere, on which it had been working for several years. It entered Phase I trials in Europe in 1990.

66 'Taxol Status Report, 27 November 1990', NPBII.

67 Relationships between the NCI and Rhône-Poulenc did not end with the decision to invite Bristol-Myers Squibb as the CRADA partner. In July 1990, representatives of the NCI met with their opposite number from Rhône-Poulenc in Paris to discuss possibilities of the two organizations collaborating in the development and testing of the company's own anti-cancer compound taxotere – see Chabner 'For the Record', 20 July 1990, FRD2. A CRADA for taxotere was signed later that year. Under the agreement, the NCI would conduct clinical trials in the United States and make the results available exclusively to Rhône-Poulenc Rorer. Taxotere was produced by a semi-synthetic process from the precursor 10-DAB, derived from the needles of the European yew *Taxus baccata*. For an overview of taxotere's clinical performance, see Pazdur et al., 'The taxoids' and Holmes et al., 'Current status'.

68 An excellent overview of the Orphan Drug Act and orphan drug designation is given in Haffner, 'Orphan products'. See also Asbury, 'Evolution and current status' and Shulman et al., 'Implementation'. The rules governing the designation of orphan disease were discussed in Chapter 4.

69 More details on the solution to the taxol supply problem can be found later in this chapter and in Chapter 6.

70 Bristol-Myers Squibb stated that it had relinquished orphan drug status for taxol because the company believed 'the potential use of Taxol for ovarian cancer and other tumor types would place it outside the spirit and intent of the Orphan Drug Act' – see Subcommittee on Regulation, Business Opportunities, and Technology, *Hearing: Pricing of Drugs*, p. 119. The company was

heavily criticized at the Congressional hearing on exclusive agreements on 29 July 1991, both by Rep Ron Wyden and other Congressmen for seeking orphan drug status for taxol. Wyden, in particular, was concerned about why Bristol-Myers Squibb was granted the status before the CRADA was signed or, as he put it, why the company had such favourable treatment. See Subcommittee on Regulation, Business Opportunities, and Energy, *Hearing: Exclusive Agreements*, p. 91 and passim.

71 The Waxman–Hatch Act was passed in 1984 and sought to protect pharmaceutical products that otherwise had no protection such as a patent. A good overview of the Act can be found in Grabowski and Vernon, 'Longer patents'.

72 The data can be found in Subcommittee on Regulation, Business Opportunities, and Energy, *Hearing: Exclusive Agreements*, pp. 436–481.

73 Subcommittee on Regulation, Business Opportunities, and Energy, *Hearing: Exclusive Agreements*, p. 422.

74 A copy of the Memorandum can be found in Subcommittee on Regulation, Business Opportunities, and Energy, *Hearing: Exclusive Agreements*, pp. 279–281.

75 Copies of the agreements are to be found in Subcommittee on Regulation, Business Opportunities, and Energy, *Hearing: Exclusive Agreements*, pp. 271–278 for the Forest Service and pp. 328–336 for the Bureau of Land Management.

76 Congressman Ron Wyden, Chair of the Congressional hearing on exclusive agreements with Bristol-Myers Squibb pressed the representatives of the Federal agencies and the company to explain the circumstances under which other parties would be allowed to collect *Taxus brevifolia* biomass, especially needles, from public lands. Wyden referred to a memo from Bob Leonard, a timber manager for the Forest Service, dated 12 June 1991, that referred to the substantial collection of needles by Hauser Chemical Research, something that surprised Leonard since Hauser's extraction and the whole taxol development programme to date was based on bark. Wyden suggested that this was done to keep others from getting at the needles, thereby making a nonsense of the access provisions in the agreements. See the questions and testimony in Subcommittee on Regulation, Business Opportunities, and Energy, *Hearing: Exclusive Agreements*, pp. 43, 44, 59–60.

77 Subcommittee on Regulation, Business Opportunities, and Energy, *Hearing: Exclusive Agreements*, p. 313.

78 United States Department of Agriculture, Forest Service, *Pacific Yew: Final EIS*, Appendix E. The Annual Pacific Yew Program of the Bureau of Land Management prescribed a limit of 5,000 pounds of bark and no limit on needles: see United States Department of Agriculture, Forest Service, *Pacific Yew: Final EIS*, Appendix E.

79 For a good discussion of Pacific yew management issues, see Wolf and Wortman, 'Pacific yew'.

80 A copy of the Pacific Yew Act of 1992 can be found in Department of Agriculture, Forest Service, *Pacific Yew: Final EIS*, Appendix N. Section 5 is on pp. 3–4.

81 This was date on which the Act effectively expired. See Chapter 6 for further details.

82 We discuss the trademarking issue from a more anthropological perspective in Goodman and Walsh, 'Attaching to things'.

83 The first time that the name taxol appeared in published form was in Perdue and Hartwell, 'The search for plant sources', p. 47.

84 'Names for hi-jacking', *Nature*, vol. 373, 2 February 1995, p. 370.

85 Stephen Chesnoff, 'The use of Taxol as a trademark', *Nature*, vol. 374, 16 March 1995, p. 208.

86 The quote is from the editorial by Madeleine Jacobs, 'What's in a name?', *Chemical and Engineering News*, 21 October 1996, p. 5.

87 See 'Taxol: yew-dunnit', *The Economist*, 2 November 1996, pp. 126–127.

88 A good overview of trademark law in the United States can be found in Carter, 'The trouble with trademark' and Cohen, 'Trademark strategy'. The economic argument for trademarks can be found in Landes and Posner, 'Trademark law'.

89 Gilles Gagné, 'Biolyse pourrait s'emparer du marché de Taxol grâce à l'if du Canada', *Le Soleil (Québec)*, 13 November 1993. The case was reported in the pharmaceutical media – see 'Bristol-Myers Squibb in Canadian legal row over Taxol', *Scrip*, no. 2044, 21 July 1995, p. 13.

90 Affidavit of Christine Poon, President of Bristol-Myers Squibb Canada Inc., Bristol-Myers Squibb (plaintiff) and Corporation Biolyse Pharmacopée Internationale (defendant), Federal Court of Canada, Trial Division, T-946–94, 29 June 1995.

91 Affidavit of Christine Poon, President of Bristol-Myers Squibb Canada Inc., Bristol-Myers Squibb (plaintiff) and Corporation Biolyse Pharmacopée Internationale (defendant), Federal Court of Canada, Trial Division, T-946–94, 29 June 1995, p. 10.

92 This, and the following responses, from Biolyse are in Statement of Defence, Bristol-Myers Squibb (plaintiff) and Corporation Biolyse Pharmacopée Internationale (defendant), Federal Court of Canada, Trial Division, T-946–94, 30 September 1994.

93 Biolyse had opposed Bristol-Myers Squibb's application to register the Taxol trademark in a supposition dated 8 November 1993, but to no avail.

94 White and Cohen, 'Trademarks'.

95 See, for example, Ken Snader, 'Speaker Abstract', Workshop on taxol and *Taxus*: current and future perspectives, Bethesda, 26 June 1990.

96 Witherup et al., '*Taxus* spp. needles', p. 1253.

97 A comparative table showing taxol content by tree part and species derived from studies up to 1994 can be found in Croom, '*Taxus* for taxol', pp. 52–53.

98 The study showing that taxol content in bark was ten times that in needles was Vidensek et al., 'Taxol content', p. 1609; the study showing a factor of 1.7 was Witherup et al., '*Taxus* spp. needles', pp. 1250, 1252. Yet another study concluded that the difference between needles and leaves was a factor of 3.8 – see Kelsey and Vance, 'Taxol', p. 913.

99 Witherup et al., '*Taxus* spp. needles', p. 1252.

100 See Chapter 3 for a discussion of this point. It was also made strongly in Persinos, 'The Pacific yew and cancer', p. 337.

101 See Croom, '*Taxus* for taxol', p. 59.

102 See Snader, 'Detection and isolation'.

103 Suffness and Snader to Distribution List, 13 November 1990, NPBII.

104 McChesney to Suffness, 3 July 1990, NPBI/1.

105 O'Connell (USDA) to Hess (USDA), 28 February 1991, FRD1. Croom and McChesney had earlier expressed disappointment with the slow pace of

Bristol-Myers Squibb's negotiations and doubted the company's sincerity in the project – see Suffness to Files, 3 July 1990, NPBI/1.

106 See O'Connell (USDA) to Hess (USDA), 28 February 1991, FRD1.

107 See Schepartz to Chabner, 9 April 1991, NPBII and 'Interagency Agreement YO1-CM10173-30: Statement of Work', NPBI/1.

108 Schepartz to DeFuria, 12 April 1991 and DeFuria to Schepartz, 24 April 1991, FRD2.

109 Saul Schepartz outlined the problems in his memo to Michael Grever, Acting Associate Director, Developmental Therapeutics Program, 5 June 1991, NPBII.

110 Snader to Schepartz, 18 July 1991 and Minutes, Source Evaluation Group for YO1-CM-10173-30, 22 August 1991, both in NPBII.

111 Snader to Lewin (Contracting Officer, NCI), 15 December 1992, NPBII.

112 Ken Cochran (Secrest Arboretum) to *Taxus* grower, 24 May 1991, NPBII.

113 Hansen et al., '*Taxus* populations'. There were approximately 20,000 new cases of ovarian cancer at this time, of which 60 per cent or 12,000 were in the advanced stage – see Eriksson and Walczak, 'Ovarian cancer', p. 214. See also Averette, Janicek and Menck, 'The national'.

114 By March 1991, for example, the MD Anderson Cancer Center Phase II trial on metastatic breast cancer was showing a fifty-six per cent response rate: recall that the ovarian response rate was thirty per cent. See 'Annual Report to the Food and Drug Administration, Taxol', March 1991, pp. 18–19.

115 These are detailed in 'Taxol Status Report' for 27 November 1990; 8 January 1991; 28 August 1991; 23 January 1992; and 4 August 1992 – all in NPBII.

116 An overview of this technique, its achievements and its problems can be found in Gibson et al., 'Potential of plant cell culture'. See also Gibson et al., 'Initiation'.

117 A.A. Christen, D.M. Gibson and J. Bland, 'Production of taxol or taxol-like compounds in cell culture', US Patent 5,019,504, 28 May 1991. The patent was filed on 23 March 1989.

118 See Fett-Neto et al., 'Cell culture of *Taxus*'. DiCosmo had begun his work on producing anti-cancer compounds using cell culture with *Catharanthus roseus* (vinca alkaloids) – interview with DiCosmo, 24 October 1995.

119 Shuler had been in the business of making plant compounds using cell culture for a long time – see Shuler, 'Production of secondary metabolites'. Shuler's survey of the possibilities of biochemical engineering for the production of taxol can be found in Shuler, 'Bioreactor engineering'.

120 See Subcommittee on Regulation, Business Opportunities, and Energy, *Hearing: Exclusive Agreements*, p. 42.

121 Interview with Walter Goldstein, 12 April 1997.

122 Press release, ESCAgenetics, 25 June 1991.

123 Press release, ESCAgenetics, 26 March 1992 and Erickson, 'Secret Garden', p. 121. The NCI grant was to a consortium including Cornell, Colorado State University, the Agricultural Research Service and Hauser Chemical Research plus Phyton Catalytic.

124 Aside from supplying the National Cancer Institute with small samples of cell-cultured taxol, ESCAgenetics never reached commercial potential. Its financial situation continued to worsen in 1993 and 1994 and, in 1995, it filed for bankruptcy. By contrast, Phyton went from strength to strength. It began to collaborate with Bristol-Myers Squibb for plant cell fermentation technology in 1993. In 1995, Phyton licensed its proprietary technology to

Bristol-Myers Squibb and in 1998, the two companies signed an agreement to commercialize the technology. Bristol-Myers Squibb has reportedly invested more than twenty-five million dollars in the project since 1993 – see 'Paclitaxel production, marketing heats up', *Chemical and Engineering News*, vol. 76, 1998, pp. 11–12.

125 Stierle, Strobel and Stierle, 'Taxol and taxane'.

126 See, Strobel et al., 'Taxol from fungal endophytes'; Strobel et al., 'Taxol from *Pestalotiopsis microspora*'; and Li et al., 'Endophytic taxol-producing fungi'. For an overview of research in this field, see Stierle et al., 'The search for a taxol-producing organism'.

127 'Alternate routes to taxol make headway', *Chemical Marketing Reporter*, 1993, vol. 244, no. 6, p. 5 and 'Taxol: yew-dunnit', *The Economist*, 2 November 1996, pp. 126–127. Cytoclonal signed a license and research agreement with Bristol-Myers Squibb on two microbial technologies in 1998 – Press Release, Cytoclonal Pharmaceutics, 16 June 1998.

128 This quote appears on p. 593, introducing Horwitz 'How to make taxol from scratch'. Nicolaou et al., 'Total synthesis of taxol'.

129 Holton et al., 'First total synthesis of taxol 1' and Holton et al., 'First total synthesis of taxol 2'.

130 Anon, 'Photo-finish', p. 125.

131 Susan Horwitz, for one, says that a complete synthesis of taxol has been a goal for chemists ever since its structure was published in 1971, Horwitz 'How to make taxol from scratch'.

132 Nicolaou, Guy and Potier, 'Taxoids', p. 86.

133 For example, Nicolaou, Guy and Potier make this point in 'Taxoids'.

134 Interview with Wender, 8 April 1996.

135 Interview with Wender, 8 April 1996.

136 Interview with Holton, 22 May 1998.

137 Molecules with the same formula (number and type of atoms), but a different structure, or arrangement of atoms in space.

138 These are isomers with the same formula, the same functional groups but are mirror images of each other.

139 Interview with Holton, 22 May 1998.

140 Wender, Natchus and Shuker, 'Toward the total synthesis'.

141 Stereochemistry is the branch of organic chemistry which deals with structure in three dimensions.

142 Holton, 'Synthesis of the taxane ring-system'.

143 Holton et al., 'A synthesis of taxusin'.

144 Zurer, 'Chemists', p. 23.

145 Denis et al., 'A highly efficient'.

146 Holton et al., 'First total synthesis of taxol 1' and Holton et al., 'First total synthesis of taxol 2'.

147 Nicolaou et al., 'Total synthesis'.

148 Flam, 'Race to synthesize taxol' quotes Nicolaou as saying that he and Holton calculated their yields in different ways, but that in fact they were similar.

149 Anon, 'Photo-finish'.

150 Nicolaou, Guy and Potier, 'Taxoids'.

151 Nicolaou and Guy, 'The conquest of taxol'. Indeed, Nicolaou says just after they had published their synthesis in early 1994, they received a fax from Matthew Suffness offering them their first NCI grant – interview with

Nicolaou, 5 April 1996. The Nicolaou group was financed by the NIH, Merck, Schering Plough, Pfizer, Glaxo, and Rhône-Poulenc Rorer.

152 Wender et al., 'The pinene path', p. 339 was received by the editors of the book in August 1994, shortly after the American Chemical Society symposium at which the work was presented.
153 Wender and Mucciaro, 'A new and practical approach'.
154 Wender et al., 'The pinene path', p. 331.
155 Nicolaou et al., 'Total synthesis of taxol', p. 630. See also Wender et al., 'Toward the total synthesis', table 1, pp. 133–134.
156 Wender et al., 'The pinene path', p. 331.
157 Interview with Wender, 8 April 1996.
158 For example, Joel, 'Taxol and taxotere'.
159 Zurer, 'Chemists'. See also Holton, 'A synthesis of taxusin'.
160 Shannon, 'Chemists', p. 19.
161 Wender and Mucciaro, 'A new and practical approach', p. 5878.
162 Wender et al., 'The pinene path', p. 331.
163 Borman, 'Anti-cancer drug', p. 4.
164 Anon, 'Photo-finish'.
165 Flam, 'Race to synthesize taxol'.
166 Horwitz, 'How to make taxol from scratch', p. 593.
167 Interview with Wender, 8 April 1996.
168 Interview with Nicolaou, 5 April 1996.
169 Borman, 'Total synthesis of anti-cancer agent', p. 32.
170 Danishefsky et al., 'Total synthesis'.
171 Interview with Wender, 8 April 1996.
172 Nicolaou, Guy and Potier, 'Taxoids', p. 87.
173 Nicolaou, Guy and Potier, 'Taxoids', p. 84.
174 Joel, 'Taxol and taxotere'.

6

The Political Life (and Death) of
Taxus brevifolia

In 1991, and then again in 1993, as we have seen, taxol became a hot political issue in the United States as the participants in its biography were questioned and cross-examined in two congressional hearings. The issue that taxol raised for the politics of the nation was whether the arrangements between the public and the private sector were in the public's best interest, either in the matter of exclusivity or of pricing. Of course, taxol is not unique in this debate; but taxol lent itself to a thorough exploration of the issues and sub-issues because it had spent so long in the public domain. And, of course, taxol was controversial. Despite the intensive questioning and the long parade of witnesses, testimonials and other types of documentation, the Congressional hearings seemed to take the whole process for granted. The issue for them was not: did it have to turn out this way? But rather: as we have this system, is this the best way of managing it?

   In this the concluding chapter, we wish to pursue the theme of contingency by shifting the focus back on to the source of taxol, *Taxus brevifolia*. The tree, too, became a political phenomenon in the early 1990s and it, too, was subjected to its own Congressional hearing. Seeing the possibility of a confrontation between 'environmentalists' and 'cancer patients', the American media, especially but not exclusively in the Pacific Northwest, followed the trials and tribulations of *Taxus brevifolia* as its identity was changed from a 'trash' tree to the most valuable species in the forest. Though newspapers, in particular, tried to characterize the debate in strictly polarized terms, it was, as is true of most debates on such difficult subjects, much more complicated than that.[1] In their attempt to simplify matters, the newspapers obscured the quite important point that *Taxus brevifolia* had many voices speaking for it, with their own agendas, not always in unison but not always in confrontation either. This chapter will let these voices speak for themselves.

The voices speaking on behalf of *Taxus brevifolia* were heard loudly in 1990, 1991 and 1992. The tree sustained a substantial interest in the Pacific Northwest and elsewhere in the country. It became an important symbol for the fate of the American temperate rainforest in particular and the planet's ecosystem in general. *Taxus brevifolia* took its place next to the northern spotted owl as an icon of resistance to what many believed was the imminent disappearance of an entire ecology. But it played yet another, and perhaps more important part. *Taxus brevifolia* reminded people that they knew next to nothing about the forests, about how they worked and, particularly, what hidden human benefits there were waiting to be discovered. In short, *Taxus brevifolia* gave a concrete meaning to the word 'biodiversity'.[2]

Yet, as the saying goes, here today, gone tomorrow. No sooner had the tree hit the headlines and appeared on prime-time television than it disappeared from the public conscience. At the beginning of 1993, Bristol-Myers Squibb announced that it was effectively pulling out of the Pacific Northwest ancient forests and sourcing its raw materials as far away from this political hot-spot as it could get. Almost overnight the networks built around the voices of *Taxus brevifolia* began to disintegrate as the voices themselves stilled. With one action, Bristol-Myers Squibb cut all the networks that had sustained *Taxus brevifolia* as a political actor. A few die-hards continued to speak out against the destruction of the tree, taking, now, a more global than local perspective, but the days of *Taxus brevifolia*'s fame were over.

The theme of contingency is implicit throughout. This chapter explores the transformation of a plant species from being waste to being precious and back again. The energy and money that accompanied this transformation and went into the actions and reactions of all those who participated in the drama is incalculable. But it was not inevitable. For one thing, taxol threw the spotlight on *Taxus brevifolia* not because of some 'natural' or 'inevitable' connection, but because the decisions taken by key actors along the historical path from the 1960s led to this outcome. It could have been quite different. Had, for example, decisions been taken in the late 1960s and 1970s to seek cultivars as the raw material for taxol production, then, with the possible exception of one or two individuals, no newspapers would have been carrying stories about *Taxus brevifolia*, no Congressional hearing would have been held, and no special yew conferences organized and attended. Or, had the NCI followed the path pursued in the 1980s by natural product chemists in France on semi-synthesis, there would have been no NCI-sponsored workshop on taxol and *Taxus* and no creation of the Native Yew Conservation Council, the tree's most public voice.

Politicizing Old-Growth Forests

In the reawakening of an environmental consciousness focused on the destruction of the world's rainforests, the growing hole in the ozone layer, industrial pollution and waste, to name but a few issues, nature has come to be viewed by many as fragile and in need of protection.[3] Plants and animals and biospheres such as rainforests receive special attention because they are perceived to be in an endangered state. Beginning in the late 1980s and continuing during the 1990s, an avalanche of material, both scholarly and popular, has been produced alerting the world to the unique majesty, on the one hand, and the near extinction, on the other hand, of the rainforest.[4] But it was not always so. As Catherine Caufield noted in her book on the South American rainforest: 'When I was researching and writing this book in the early nineteen-eighties, I dreaded being asked what I was working on, because experience had taught me that the answer, "tropical rainforests," could kill a conversation stone-dead as people struggled to think of something to say on such an obscure subject . . . In recent years, however, people have discovered that tropical rainforests *are* interesting and important and that their extinction is a tragedy.'[5] While the subject of tropical rainforests continued to receive the greatest attention, that of temperate rainforests especially of the Pacific Northwest, also came under the spotlight as commentators reminded their American readers that they didn't need to look further than their own backyards to see the destruction and its tragedy. By the late 1980s and early 1990s, Pacific Northwest forests were hot material, both in the sense of their media exposure and their political currency.[6]

What made the Pacific Northwest rainforest a particularly potent subject was the realization that the destruction of that ecosystem had been progressing since the European settlement of the region in the late-nineteenth century and at an alarming rate since World War II. Americans, in other words, were paying for their increasing material comforts by destroying their own environment. By the time the public was alerted to the situation, most of the rainforest was gone. In the late 1980s, various estimates were made about what was left and, although these varied, the picture they painted was much the same.[7] Very little was left; between eighty-two per cent and eighty-seven per cent of old-growth in the Pacific Northwest had been destroyed, leaving about 2.5 million acres, of which only five per cent was reserved in national parks and wilderness areas.[8]

Listing the spotted owl as a threatened species in June 1990 was, as we have learned, the closest that anyone came to protecting the old-growth ecosystem as a whole. Even though the original listing did not designate critical habitat for the owl, political and legal pressure on the Fish and Wildlife Service forced a change. On 6 May 1991, in direct response to Judge Thomas Zilly's order to the agency to do what it was legislated to do, the Fish and Wildlife Service designated 11.6 million acres as critical habitat; 6.5 million acres of this was under Forest Service control, 1.4 million acres under the Bureau of Land Management and 3 million acres in private hands.[9] Through a long series of bitter disputes, in the legislature, in the courts and in the localities of Oregon and Washington, the Fish and Wildlife Service critical habitat designation came under fire, particularly from logging companies who managed to have their 3 million acres restored.[10] By April 1993, the controversy had reached such a high pitch that President Clinton called a Forest Summit in Portland where so-called Option 9 was offered as the best strategy – designating 7.4 million acres or thirty per cent of federal lands as 'late-successional reserves' in the range of the spotted owl, which was predominantly a protected area, although it allowed some silviculture.[11] The amount of timber sold and cut in the Pacific Northwest collapsed, while prices rose. Although, for example, annual sales of 5 million board feet had been common through the 1960s, 1970s and most of the 1980s, this figure was more than halved in 1991 and fell to just over 400,000 board feet in 1995, a level of sales not seen in the region's timber industry since 1941.[12]

It is important to understand that the spotted owl was a surrogate, an indicator of and a perfect vehicle for the much broader issue of the old-growth ecosystem. Though it was threatened (or even endangered) according to the definitions of the Endangered Species Act, it was not a creature that elicited the kind of anthropomorphisms lavished on some species. Much as it was admired (or loved) by some such as Eric Forsman who devoted a considerable part of his career to studying its behaviour, it was hated and vilified by others for whom it was a symbol of interference with and destruction of their economic livelihood.[13]

As far as the Pacific Northwest was concerned, therefore, the wider debate from the early 1980s was the fate of the forest. This continued to be the case right through the debate over the management of the spotted owl.[14] And so it was for *Taxus brevifolia*.

Taxus brevifolia Redefined

In March 1992, a hearing was held before three subcommittees of Congress. The purpose of the meeting was to discuss a bill HR 3836, to become the Pacific Yew Act, a piece of legislation requiring the appropriate Federal agencies to improve their management of the Pacific yew in order to ensure continuing supplies of taxol. Two of the witnesses called were Zola Horovitz, Vice-President for Business Development and Planning at Bristol-Myers Squibb and Dr Bruce Chabner, Chief of the Division of Cancer Treatment of the NCI. Robert Smith, a Representative from Oregon, asked Horovitz how long he had known that *Taxus brevifolia* 'might possibly have ingredients to treat cancer'.[15] Horovitz did not answer; instead he passed the question on to Chabner. Here is the exchange between Chabner and Smith.

> *Chabner*: The active principal (sic) was isolated about 15–20 years ago but it had no demonstrated activity against cancer until about 1988 . . . When we discovered that it had significant clinical activity, then we faced the problem of scaling it up and finding a commercial partner to market it because the Cancer Institute doesn't market drugs. That is what happened in the period between 1988 and 1990.
>
> *Smith*: So when did the Federal agencies, as far as you know, know that the yew tree was going to be a valuable resource?
>
> *Chabner*: None of us knew that the yew would be a *valuable tree* (our italics) until late 1988 perhaps 1989 . . . they became aware of the clinical activity at the same time we did. It was in late 1980's.

Later in the hearing, it was the turn of Jim Jontz, Democrat Representative from Indiana and a member of the Committee on Agriculture, to question Bruce Chabner.[16]

> *Jontz*: OK. Dr. Chabner, again, I want to follow up on my colleague from Oregon, Mr. Smith. As I understand what you told him, it was late 1988 or early 1989 when you made your substantive conversations with the Forest Service came about (sic)?
>
> *Chabner*: No, I said that was the time at which we realized that the drug had activity in ovarian cancer. We had been dealing with people from Agriculture and the Forest Service about obtaining small amounts. Actually, we were doing this through a contractor.
>
> *Jontz*: For how long?
>
> *Chabner*: Well, it began in the early 1980's.
>
> *Jontz*: So really the Forest Service should have had reason for 10 years to know that there was something important?
>
> *Chabner*: No, I wouldn't say they knew something was important.
>
> *Jontz*: Well, why would you be dealing with them if it weren't important?
>
> *Chabner*: Well, we didn't know it was important.
>
> *Jontz*: When did you determine it was important?
>
> *Chabner*: In late 1988 or early in 1989.

The exchange is important in that Chabner related taxol to *Taxus brevifolia* historically at the moment when the compound was reported as being active in patients with ovarian cancer. That is, the value of the one determined the value of the other at a particular point in time. There is, however, much at stake in this testimony. For one thing, Chabner was careful to say that taxol had 'no demonstrated activity' against cancer until 1988. As we have seen, taxol would not have been in the clinical stage to yield the 1988 results (whatever they may have been) had the compound not shown significant activity in the experimental stages until that point; that is, against malignant cells, mouse tumours and human xenografts covering a period between 1966 and 1982. Taxol had, therefore, been showing activity for a much longer time. The anomaly between Chabner's statement and the record turns on the word 'cancer'. In the NCI, the word 'cancer' was reserved exclusively for the disease state in humans, emerging as a word only with Phase II trials that did not begin until 1985. By referring to taxol's activity against cancer, Chabner was able to deflect attention away from all those years when the portfolio of taxol's activity was becoming increasingly rich in information.[17] At the same time, and speaking on behalf of the Forest Service and the Bureau of Land Management, Chabner dextrously deflected attention from their practices and, effectively, severely shortened the span of time over which *Taxus brevifolia* could have been viewed as an important species.[18]

As we have seen, the Forest Service, or at least some of its regional foresters, knew well before 1988 of the growing interest in taxol by the NCI and of the interest shown in *Taxus brevifolia* both by them and by the USDA, when it was part of the interagency programme. Yet there is no doubt that both the Forest Service and the Bureau of Land Management treated *Taxus brevifolia* as a species without value.

How can we make sense of this? The answer lies in the practices of both agencies. If we think about *Taxus brevifolia* not as an actor but as an actor–network in the old-growth Pacific Northwest, then we can begin to understand how its identity was made and changed.[19] The key point is the one that Michel Callon has elucidated on many occasions: the identities, shapes, forms of actors, be they human or non-human, are a product of the relations established within a network.[20] One can, therefore, only understand identity as a product of the network not as something that is determined at a point in time or in space. It is something that is performed as a network effect.[21] This is as true of humans as it is of forests and the species within them.[22] Before the 1960s, *Taxus brevifolia* was an actor–network consisting of the Forest Service, the Bureau of Land Management, logging companies, loggers, fencepost makers, firewood gatherers, Douglas fir, and slash piles.

The relations within this network were built around Douglas fir.[23] The practice that delivered Douglas fir from the old-growth forest was clear cutting. All other vegetation, including *Taxus brevifolia*, was destroyed in the process and hauled to slash piles to be burned.[24] The fact that *Taxus brevifolia* was not taken in pre-logging operations and was destroyed in the clear-cutting operation was the result of the relations within the network and determined, therefore, the identity of *Taxus brevifolia* as a 'trash' tree, whatever competing identities existed for it outside this network.[25] The appearance of the NCI and taxol as actors in this network in the late 1960s and continuing right through until the late 1980s did little to alter the identity of *Taxus brevifolia* as a species without value because the relations and practices in the forest remained unchanged. The bark harvests in the 1970s and 1980s were, in practice, equivalent to the salvage of other parts of *Taxus brevifolia* as firewood and fenceposts. The knowledge that *Taxus brevifolia* was valuable as a source of a medicinal compound was inherently unstable in this network because the stability of the network rested entirely in the relations around Douglas fir.

At the very end of the 1980s and for the early years of the 1990s, the actor network that was *Taxus brevifolia* became increasingly complex as many more actors appeared on the scene. These included the spotted owl, the Environmental Defense Fund, the Oregon Natural Resources Council, Bristol-Myers Squibb, Hauser Chemical Research, the Native Yew Conservation Council, biodiversity, various testaments and Congress.[26] These actors attempted to destabilize the network whose practices were focused on Douglas fir and to place *Taxus brevifolia* in a venerable role within a new set of practices. In this, as we will see, they were successful, although it was a process whose outcome, the changed identity of *Taxus brevifolia* as an important and valuable species, did not become stable before 1992 or 1993, not until the forestry agencies altered their practices.

The Breast Cancer Clinical Trial

In December 1992, slightly more than thirty years after USDA botanists sampled *Taxus brevifolia* in the Gifford Pinchot National Forest in Washington State, taxol received FDA approval for use in refractory ovarian cancer. The approval was momentous in several senses: it gave women suffering from ovarian cancer who had not responded to the standard available therapy another chance at treatment; and it was the first compound discovered in the NCI–USDA plant screening programme to get FDA approval.

Clinical trials of taxol, as we have seen, were severely limited during the late 1980s because of the shortage of the compound. Though a broad programme of trials was envisioned and planned, most trials remained on hold during these years. Taxol was only tested for activity against ovarian and renal cancer and melanoma. The results for ovarian cancer were, it will be recalled, considered excellent; the melanoma trials were somewhat disappointing while those for renal cancer showed no activity.

In 1985, one of the Phase II trials that was planned was in breast cancer. Recall that taxol had shown significant activity against an experimental breast cancer model, the human MX-1 mammary tumour xenograft. Because of the shortage of taxol, this trial, approved to be undertaken at the MD Anderson Cancer Center at the University of Texas in Houston, did not, in fact, get underway until January 1990. By September, the trial had enrolled enough patients to derive meaningful results and was closed to further patients.[27]

In this same year, 1990, the NCI also gave the green light for a large number of other backlogged trials to begin to run. These included colon cancer, gastric cancer, head and neck cancer, prostate cancer, cervical cancer and small-cell and non-small-cell lung cancer. Also included was a large-scale Phase III trial on ovarian cancer, conducted by Dr William McGuire. The supply of taxol for these crucial clinical trials was just about all that the NCI had on hand. Yet another supply crisis was in the offing.[28]

The breast cancer trial at the MD Anderson Cancer Center began to yield results by October of 1990. Officials at the NCI learned of the unconfirmed results very quickly and, by November of that year, these began to be distributed to other interested parties within the NCI. The November Taxol Status Report cheerfully stated that nine of twenty-five patients with advanced and refractory breast cancer had responded. This represented a response rate of thirty-six per cent, a figure larger than that of the, by now, famous ovarian cancer trial at Johns Hopkins.[29] By the time that the next Taxol Status Report was written at the beginning of January 1991, the response rate had risen to forty-eight per cent and, when in March, the final, confirmed results were in, the response rate was now fifty-six per cent.[30] Frankie Ann Holmes, the oncologist in charge of the clinical trial, presented her findings at the annual meeting of the American Society of Clinical Oncologists in Spring and then published them later the same year.[31] The results were outstanding and they were confirmed in 1992 by a trial at the Memorial Sloan–Kettering on both pretreated and untreated breast cancer patients.[32]

What Gordon Cragg, the Chief of the Natural Products Branch, feared would happen now happened. Taxol was found to be active in a cancer affecting a larger population than ovarian cancer. Cragg had done his calculations in 1988 on the basis of the ovarian cancer and melanoma results and estimated an annual consumption of two grams of taxol for each cancer patient: for ovarian cancer, for example, with an annual affected population of 20,000 women, the consumption would be a maximum of forty kilograms.[33] For breast cancer, with an affected population reaching 200,000 in the United States alone, annual consumption of taxol could be as high as 400 kilograms, assuming that the drug became front-line therapy.

This impasse lay in the future. For the present, the problem lay in meeting the requirements of the large number of clinical trials it was necessary to complete before an NDA could be sent to the FDA. And that in turn depended on what had by now become a perennial problem but with a new twist – the forest and its chief inhabitant, *Taxus brevifolia*.

The Political Economy of Bark

As we have seen in earlier chapters, developments and events from 1962 onwards conspired to equate taxol with the bark of *Taxus brevifolia*. This was not inevitable. Many attempts to steer away from this course were made throughout the period and, as far as the record allows us to gauge, bark stripped from living trees was widely seen as a short- to medium-term solution to the supply of taxol. Yet, despite these efforts, bark as source became locked-in and the politics of taxol became inexorably linked to the political economy of bark. The effect of this was far-reaching.

Focusing on bark had three main effects. First of all, alternative solutions to making taxol receded both in memory and in reality. This was especially true of those alternatives, put forth at various times since 1962, that required investment and a long gestation time – solutions such as using yew cultivars or other parts of the tree. Secondly, collecting bark meant killing the tree and, as the demand for bark grew, the mortality of *Taxus brevifolia* also grew. Not that this would go unnoticed because, as we have also seen, there was in the early 1980s a small but growing concern for the fate of the yew in the Pacific Northwest. Finally, and perhaps most importantly, the bark lock-in in terms of supply for taxol, also locked in the approval procedure. The taxol used in clinical trials was made exclusively from the bark of *Taxus brevifolia*, and, therefore, any approval for the clinical use of taxol would be made on the strict understanding and requirement that commercial supplies, too, would be made from bark using an industrial method approved in the NDA – what is called Good Manufacturing Practice (GMP). Taxol made in any other way would need to go through a new round of clinical trials and a new process of approval at the FDA.

John Destito held the NCI contract for supplying 60,000 pounds of bark which he was awarded in April 1989. As we have seen, his contract got off to a bad start because of delays in awarding it to him even though he was the lowest bidder. The delay cost Destito the best season for stripping the bark and by September he had only managed to secure 8,000 pounds. A return to the forest was scheduled for the following spring. Destito's problems in the forest and with the NCI were just beginning. His contract with the NCI was short and not entirely successful but it came at a time of immense change in the whole taxol project. Peering into Destito's experience gives us a rare glimpse into the kind of turmoil that, to a greater or lesser extent, informed the development of taxol over the next few years.

Recall that Destito had experienced several delays in being awarded the contract to collect 60,000 pounds of bark. As he explained to Dr Rao Vishnuvajjala, the Project Officer at the NCI, a series of hold-ups with both Forest Service and Bureau of Land Management officials resulted in the first deliveries of yew bark arriving by mid-August.[34] By November, Advanced Molecular Technologies had about 500 pounds of bark ready for processing, instead of the 30,000 pounds called for.[35]

Destito now entered a bureaucratic maze. In order to speed up the operations, he decided to collect as many yew logs as he could during the autumn season, when it was impossible to peel the bark from the trees, stockpile them and then peel them by first steaming the cut log to a temperature of 40°C.[36] The contract stipulated the hand-peeling of yew bark without mechanical aids because this was the established practice and the taxol content using such a technique well-known. Ken Snader, a chemist at the Natural Products Branch, was confronted with this problem during his site visit to Advanced Molecular Technologies in the early part of November. Because of the urgency of the problem, Gordon Cragg moved very quickly to analyse the taxol content of bark using the steam technique.[37] By 21 November, an analysis of the taxol content in this bark had been made and declared to be acceptable.[38]

The site visit to Advanced Molecular Technologies in early November included Snader and Richard Spjut, the USDA plant collector in the 1970s who had compiled the first report on *Taxus brevifolia* for prospective bark collectors. The site visit, to judge from both Destito's reaction to it and the report on it from Wayne Jackson, the Co-Project Officer of the Pharmaceutical Resources Branch of the NCI, was anything but smooth. For one thing, there was the misunderstanding about how much bark was on hand – 8,000 pounds as Jackson believed on the basis of an earlier conversation with Destito; there was disquiet on the part of the NCI that Destito had referred to the agency in an advertisement without prior approval; and finally, and perhaps most importantly, there was apparently an accusation that Destito was withholding yew bark for personal profit.[39]

Notwithstanding these issues, the NCI visitors were impressed with the facilities and with the new technique for peeling bark. Though 'under normal circumstances it would be recommended that the contract be terminated for default' they recommended that the contract be extended to 31 December in the hope that between 8,000 and 10,000 pounds of bark would be made available. Defaulting on this delivery would spell the end of Destito's contract.[40]

Destito was on the defensive as he tried to regain the NCI's confidence in him as a contractor. He put his side of the events to the NCI and assured them of his commitment to honour his contract.[41] He also responded to the accusation about collecting bark for himself. In his defence, he stated that alongside the bark he was also collecting needles and stems as part of 'clean-up operations'. The bark was exclusively for the NCI but because, as he said, the NCI was uninterested in the other material, he was making the needles and stems available to Calbiochem, a natural products company and supplier of research grade biochemicals in southern California, from which they were hoping to extract and purify the taxol content. Destito had received permission from the Forest Service to collect all of these parts of *Taxus brevifolia*.[42]

This seemed to satisfy the NCI and with no further problems, Destito pushed ahead with his plans to get between 8,000 and 10,000 pounds of dried bark by the end of the year.[43] When the due date of 31 December came around, however, Destito could only muster up just under 5,000 pounds of bark; he was certain that he could supply a further 5,000 pounds by the end of January 1990. He pleaded for an extension to the contract until this date.[44] By the end of January, and after assurances, documentation and photographs supporting his claim to be able to deliver 10,000 pounds of bark, Destito was able to wrest a new delivery contract out of the NCI, one that would both relieve pressure on winter operations and provide an incentive to return to standard practices in the spring. He was given until 7 March 1990 to deliver the 10,000 pounds: if successful, the contract would be extended to 7 June 1990 and, if he could provide 30,000 pounds by 7 May 1990, then there would be an automatic extension until 7 November 1990.[45] A return inspection of Advanced Molecular Technologies' facilities was scheduled for 17 March 1990. These were probably more generous terms than he could have imagined. But new trouble in the form of an old adversary was brewing.

Late in February 1990, Patrick Connolly complained again to the contracting officer at the NIH that they should have listened to his earlier protest which, he argued, had been borne out by the inability of Advanced Molecular Technologies to deliver on time.[46] He maintained that only he could deliver the amount required (and more) and that the NCI's contract with Destito should not be extended and instead should be given to him. In his bid for the NIH's heart and mind, Connolly presented himself as being extremely sensitive to the new contexts for bark collections. He suspected, for example, that the CRADA with Bristol-Myers Squibb would mean that future collections would be made by them or by a company selected by them. In addition, he felt that future collections, besides being of much greater volume than they had previously been, would need to be mindful of concerns about the destruction of *Taxus brevifolia* and its impact on the gene pool, as well as the particular role of the Forest Service and the CRADA partner.

Destito had, in fact, warned the NIH of this protest at the end of December 1989, as he suspected that his ex-plant production manager had taken up with Connolly.[47] As far as one can tell, the protest did not affect Destito's contract, although several of Connolly's arguments and predictions did come true. Back at Advanced Molecular Technologies' facilities, things were going much better. By mid-March, Destito informed Wayne Jackson that 10,000 pounds of bark were ready for shipping in time for his inspection visit scheduled for 17 March.[48] By the beginning of April, the shipment had been received by Hauser Chemical Research, the NCI's contractor for extraction and purification of taxol.[49]

All, finally, seemed to be going well for Destito. He had managed to provide the NCI with bark and his explanation for the delay was beginning to be seen in a more sympathetic light. Then, at the beginning of April, a new problem emerged. Dean Stull, Chief Executive Officer of Hauser Chemical Research, informed NCI's Gordon Cragg of a substantial number of *Taxus brevifolia* that were going to be destroyed in a clear-cutting operation.[50] Cragg acted swiftly to save the situation by issuing a general letter so that Forest Service officials would co-operate with Hauser to save the bark from the trees before clear cutting.[51] This important letter informed the officials that Hauser was 'currently working under contract with the National Cancer Institute in the isolation and purification of the anti-cancer drug, taxol' and that they should allow Hauser to collect the bark because the company 'has identified areas where large numbers of this tree might be destroyed in clearcutting operations'.[52] Cragg noted that the programme could not afford to waste any *Taxus* bark and appeared thankful that 'Bristol

[Bristol-Myers Squibb] has agreed to finance an HCR [Hauser Chemical Research] collection to save the bark'.[53]

What happened next can only be described as bizarre yet it reflected the messiness of this scientific programme. Early in April, Neil Jans, Business Development Manager at Hauser, wrote to Destito declaring that 'we [Hauser] have gotten formal approval from Bristol and NCI to immediately begin procuring additional Yew bark'.[54] As proof of this, Jans referred to and attached Cragg's 4 April memo to forestry officials. The key word in Jans's letter was 'additional', which one might be forgiven for thinking referred to the bark in the clear-cutting areas that, as Hauser had alerted Cragg, were scheduled for destruction: hence, the attached memo from Cragg. Yet the rest of the letter used the word 'additional' to refer not to the one-off collection sanctioned by Cragg but to bark collections over and above those performed by Advanced Molecular Technologies. Jans asked Destito whether and to what extent he would be willing to supply Hauser with *Taxus brevifolia* needles and limbs.[55]

Jans's letter was somewhat confusing. Destito was outraged by, as he put it in a letter at the end of April, 'Hauser's sudden authorization to collect *Taxus* bark for the NCI and Bristol-Myers'.[56] As far as he was concerned, and he had not been informed otherwise, he was the sole contractor for the NCI. Forest Service and Bureau of Land Management officials, he remarked, were confused about who was authorized to collect yew bark. He implored the NCI immediately to 'notify Hauser Chemical Research, Inc. to stop its activities in regards to *Taxus* bark and needle collections until AMT [Advanced Molecular Technologies] completes its current contract and Bristol-Myers receives the opportunity to thoroughly review AMT's future collection proposal accompanied with a site visit'.[57]

It is unclear how Destito's demands were received at the NCI but we can be sure that they did not much matter at this point. Destito was correct that he was the NCI's official contractor for *Taxus brevifolia* bark, but was incorrect in thinking that his pleas for the intervention of the NCI in Hauser's collection would be heard. The reason was quite simple. During the month of April and possibly before that date, Hauser and Bristol-Myers Squibb were discussing a partnership agreement whereby Hauser would act as the supplier of *Taxus brevifolia* bark as well as purified taxol once operations under the CRADA began. These discussions were part of the overall negotiations that were taking place at the time between the NCI and Bristol-Myers Squibb with respect to the CRADA. By the end of April or early May, the discussions between Hauser and Bristol-Myers Squibb reached a satisfactory conclusion and Hauser emerged as the official collector for Bristol-Myers Squibb.[58]

The CRADA negotiations between the NCI and Bristol-Myers Squibb dragged on for most of the rest of the year, but this had no impact on the separate agreement between Hauser and Bristol-Myers Squibb.

During this same month of April, Hauser was carrying on its own discussions and negotiations with Patrick Connolly and Floyd Ehrheart, another bark collector, for them to do the collecting on behalf of Hauser. Neil Jans offered Connolly a contract on 23 April 1990, for one season only, to collect bark from trees in clear-cutting areas.[59] Jans provided Connolly with two documents to help him in discussions with forestry officials: a letter from himself identifying Connolly as working under contract for Hauser; and the 4 April open memo from Cragg authorizing Hauser to collect from specifically identified clear-cutting areas. Hauser would purchase 50,000 pounds of bark and limbs from Connolly at a price of $3.50 per pound.[60]

By early May, therefore, both the Forest Service and the Bureau of Land Management were made aware that Patrick Connolly would be collecting in the northern part of Oregon and that Floyd Ehrheart would be doing the same in the southern parts of the state.[61] Hauser stressed to all parties that the collection would be made in an environmentally-friendly way, from clear-cut areas only and that the whole tree would be taken, harvesting the bark and the limbs. The delivery of 50,000 pounds of material was scheduled for 1 June 1990.[62]

The CRADA negotiations involving Hauser, Bristol-Myers Squibb, the NCI, Patrick Connolly and Floyd Ehrheart did not directly affect Destito's collection because the latter was contracted to the NCI alone. Whatever was going on elsewhere, Destito was still under contract to provide the NCI with its supply of bark. Destito promised to have ready for inspection and shipping 20,000–25,000 pounds of bark by 7 June 1990.[63] On the basis of this, Destito's contract was extended to 7 June but he was told that the Pharmaceutical Resources Branch of the NCI would not grant another extension.[64] In the event, the inspection didn't take place until 14 June and, rather than the 20,000–25,000 pounds promised, only 3,671 pounds were on hand to be inspected and shipped to Hauser for extraction and purification.[65]

Inspecting the shipment was Richard Spjut who had done the same in the autumn of the previous year. Spjut was, in fact, part of a Taxus Survey Trip, covering the period 11–15 June 1990 and headed by Gordon Cragg and Ken Snader. There were four main objectives to the trip: to identify areas in Idaho and British Columbia where clear-cutting operations were underway in areas where *Taxus brevifolia* was growing; to enlist the help of forestry officials in those areas to regulate timber harvesting; to estimate the potential for harvesting both bark and needles from these areas; and, finally, 'to introduce representatives

from Bristol-Myers/Squibb [sic] (BMS) and their procurement contractor, Hauser Chemical Research (HCR), to the forestry officials as the
only collaborators of the National Cancer Institute (NCI) in the yew
bark collection project'.[66] Salvatore Forenza and James Matson represented Bristol-Myers Squibb and Neil Jans represented Hauser
Chemical Research. The group visited various forests and people in
Idaho, Montana and British Columbia, but they also paid a visit to
Weyerhaeuser where they were told of the company's research on the
taxol content of various parts of *Taxus brevifolia* and *Taxus* cultivars.[67]

Before they left for British Columbia, Cragg, Snader and Spjut were
scheduled to inspect Destito's impending shipment of bark. In the
event, Spjut went on his own because Destito had, by then, threatened
legal action against the NCI; Cragg and Snader thought it inappropriate
to accompany Spjut. Destito's lawyers had written to both the Acting
Director and the Director of the NCI outlining their client's charge that
'certain representatives of the NCI have been acting improperly in
concert with Hauser Chemical Research, Inc. to prevent AMT from
being able to continue to perform the contract and to cause irreparable
damage to the contractual rights and business prospects of AMT'.[68] The
actions that Advanced Molecular Technologies wished of the NCI
included letters of retraction on the 4 April memo, a cessation of
acceptances of deliveries from Hauser, its collectors or any other party
that had not been successful in a bid award from the NCI and a
reinstatement and amendment to the company's contract with the
NCI to 7 November 1990.[69] Having not heard anything in reply,
Destito's lawyers advised the NCI, on 14 June, the day of the inspection, that they were putting the matter into the hands of their litigation
attorneys and were bringing the matter to the attention of certain
Congressional authorities in order to begin an investigation into the
NCI's activities.[70]

To the surprise of Cragg and Snader, Destito turned up at their
meeting with representatives of the British Columbia Ministry of
Forestry and the Council of Forest Industries of British Columbia in
Vancouver, the day after the inspection. Destito spoke at the meeting,
outlining his bark collecting experiences and his ideas on collecting in
British Columbia.[71] At the end of the meeting, Destito remained in
discussion with Neil Jans of Hauser and John Mann, a consultant to the
British Columbia Forestry Industry, about the possibility of collections
in Canada.

On 26 June 1990, the NCI held its first workshop on taxol and *Taxus* in
Bethesda. Nearly everyone connected with both the molecule and the
tree was present. Destito was there, too, and held discussions with both
Neil Jans of Hauser and James Matson of Bristol-Myers Squibb who had

been in the group travelling together in the Taxus Survey Trip earlier
that month. Several important events occurred. First Destito told both
Cragg and Snader that he would not be pursuing his legal actions.[72]
Secondly, Destito agreed to work with Hauser and Bristol-Myers, to join
their collection team and 'maximize our efforts for the good of the Taxol
Development Program'.[73] More than 24,000 pounds of *Taxus* material
was ready for shipment, Destito told Jans early in July, and they would
have it once he received a contract from Hauser. Destito attached his
own 'Taxus collection proposal' detailing long-term supply arrangements and prices.

At this point, Destito also confirmed to Jans that his legal action
against the NCI and, by implication Hauser and Bristol-Myers Squibb,
had come to an end. A letter to this effect was sent by Destito's lawyers
to the NCI on 11 July and the matter effectively closed.[74] Jans sent Destito
a draft agreement in July but nothing came of it, certainly not by the end
of the summer.[75] By then, however, Destito's mind was caught up in
boardroom politics, involving a take-over of his company by a Seattle-
based investment group and the redeployment of Advanced Molecular
Technologies' staff and assets to the former's offices. Acrimony, alle-
gations, counter-allegations and interventions by the state of Washington's Security Division finally led to the entire collapse of Advanced
Molecular Technologies. It was wound up in December 1990.[76]

What would have happened to Advanced Molecular Technologies as
part of the Hauser-led collection team is anyone's guess. Though he did
not strictly adhere to the timetable laid down by the NCI for the 1989
contract, undoubtedly Destito had produced the connections necessary
for collecting bark. He also significantly changed the NCI practices to
allow for the mechanical debarking of *Taxus brevifolia* out of season, a
change that would become crucial in future collections.

The spotlight turned away from Destito and on to Hauser, their
subcontractors Connolly and Ehrheart, and the forest. Hauser's goal for
bark collection during 1990 was 100,000 pounds.[77] Despite the fact that
they employed someone like Connolly with experience of collecting
bark in Oregon, the amount of material shipped to Hauser's plant in
Boulder fell short of this amount. By the end of the season, just over
86,000 pounds of bark had been collected. Once again, the unpredictability of the forest had intruded. The Forest Service had closed much of
the forest because of the fear of forest fires. Weather that was drier than
expected not only increased the risk of fire but it also resulted in the
bark tightening earlier than usual, slowing down the process of stripping and reducing the quantity of bark taken.[78]

To make up the shortfall, Hauser planned on a winter collection
whereby *Taxus brevifolia* would be cut down and then the logs

transported to a mill where they would be debarked mechanically.[79] Connolly estimated total equipment costs at $175,000 but was confident that he would recover these expenses given the amount of bark he expected to handle:[80] he had made a verbal agreement with Hauser to supply them with 200,000 pounds of bark by March of the following year.[81] Connolly purchased some of the machinery immediately, investing more than $40,000 in special equipment, particularly a debarker and drying equipment.[82] Despite Connolly's excitement and optimism in the deal with Hauser, there were already some signs of a souring of the relationship. It began with a decision by Hauser not to purchase limbs and needles from Connolly and Ehrheart.[83] This had two main effects. It increased costs by more than fifty per cent and decreased the income earned by the pickers themselves, as they were no longer paid for the limbs and needles.[84] Ehrheart asked for a hike in the price Hauser paid for bark to reflect the changed circumstances: Jans answered that he thought Ehrheart had been making a good enough margin.[85] Connolly also remarked that several of his pickers had left him once they stopped taking limbs and needles.[86]

A more serious problem began to emerge sometime in September when Connolly learned of several of Hauser's logging deals and their interest in increasing the number of bark suppliers. Connolly was steadfastly against this, arguing, as he had done on an earlier occasion when awarded the NCI bark contract in 1987, that Hauser was better off with one contractor only.[87] Oregon alone, Connolly maintained, could supply 1.5 million pounds of bark: there was simply no reason for Hauser to look elsewhere in the forests of California, Washington and Idaho. Besides which, costs at his plant would continue to fall as he reached full potential.[88]

By mid-October, the relationship between Hauser and Connolly was in tatters. Connolly accused Jans of not supplying yew logs to him from Hauser's buyers. Without this supply, the plant was idle. Connolly's suggestion that he purchase logs on his account was turned down by Jans. A stand-off ensued. Jans broke the silence by offering to buy Connolly's company at a price of $80,000. After some negotiations that did not go Connolly's way, and after turning to Bristol-Myers Squibb for help in finding an outlet for the bark he could supply to no avail, he and Jans agreed on a buy-out price of $76,000 on 26 October 1990.[89]

By buying Connolly's plant and changing its name in November to Hauser Northwest, Inc., the company centralized its operations in Cottage Grove from where it organized the collections and processed the bark before it was shipped to the chemical plant in Boulder. The big players were now in charge. Connolly was out of the yew business as Destito before him. The only survivor was Floyd Ehrheart who continued to work with Hauser for the next few years, collecting bark on private land.[90]

The Politics of Identity

The demand for *Taxus brevifolia* bark was still primarily determined by clinical trials that were expanding not only into disease sites not tested with taxol before, but moving into the third and virtually final stage, Phase III. These are the largest tests, in terms of the patients that are enrolled, and are used to test the activity of the new drug compared with the standard therapy on a disease site that has already shown good activity in Phase II.[91]

The amount consumed in a clinical trial was substantial but now that the real possibility existed for preparing an NDA for regular clinical use of taxol in refractory ovarian cancer and, in time, metastatic breast cancer, the issue of the supply of bark and, consequently, taxol, took on a new dimension.[92] Hauser and Bristol-Myers Squibb now planned for the largest single collection to date. For 1991 they planned to collect 750,000 pounds of *Taxus brevifolia* bark, four times more than had been collected altogether since 1962. In terms of *Taxus brevifolia* mortality, the amount would translate into the removal of up to 100,000 trees.[93]

The Environmental Defense Fund and the Voice of the Threatened Species

By the time of that announcement, as we have already seen, substantial concern for the fate of *Taxus brevifolia* had built up, caused by a combination of bark harvests and the more general destruction of old-growth forests. Jerry Rust, the Lane County Commissioner, and his friend and colleague, Hal Hartzell, had by now attempted, by writing their book on *Taxus* and by political persuasion, to raise some kind of public awareness of what was occurring. That, of course, was mainly local awareness. In the middle of 1990, *Taxus brevifolia* found a new voice in the Environmental Defense Fund, a Washington-based activist group seeking legal and economic solutions to environmental problems.

On 17 July 1990, Michael Bean and Bruce Manheim, lawyers with the Environmental Defense Fund, met with Saul Schepartz and Gordon Cragg of the NCI.[94] Bean and Manheim were seeking support from the NCI for their ideas on the preservation of *Taxus brevifolia*. At the time, they were considering either petitioning the Forest Service and the Bureau of Land Management to declare *Taxus brevifolia* a 'sensitive species', requiring the agencies to maintain viable populations within their management practices; or, alternatively, petitioning the Fish and

Wildlife Service to list *Taxus brevifolia* as a 'threatened species'.[95] Schepartz and Cragg were sympathetic with the Environmental Defense Fund's overall concern, but could not lend their support officially because one government agency cannot petition another government agency in the absence of official policy.[96] In the absence of direct support, Schepartz and Cragg offered contact names.

The Environmental Defense Fund had had several noted successes in the past, particularly the campaign against the use of DDT and the campaign to list hunted whales through the Endangered Species Act.[97] This was the first time, however, that they had ventured into the area of attempting to declare a plant as being in a precarious state. Though plants were covered by the Endangered Species Act, listing them was a much more complicated procedure than listing animals. By the early 1980s, for example, ten times as many animals as plants had been listed as either threatened or endangered.[98]

Bean and Manheim had been alerted to the plight of *Taxus brevifolia* by Elliott Norse, a scientist working for the Center for Marine Conservation in Washington, DC. Norse had appeared at a general meeting in Washington in the summer of 1990 where issues about old-growth forests and the recent controversy over the spotted owl were being discussed.[99] At that meeting, also attended by Bean and Manheim, Norse spoke about *Taxus brevifolia*, using it as an example of the potentially enormous and more likely than not unknown human value that lay in protecting nature. Norse had, in fact, made a similar point in his book that had just been published. In it, he outlined for his readers the meaning of *Taxus brevifolia* within the context of the fight over old-growth forests, linking the plight of the yew with that of the ancient forest and the health of humans.[100]

> For people today, the most remarkable thing about Pacific yews
> is their bark. It is unusual to the eye, true enough: dark red or
> purplish, occurring in very thin, long, wavy strips. But it is the
> yew bark's chemical composition that has scientists so excited,
> for it contains a compound – taxol – that could help humankind
> to fight one of our most feared enemies: cancer . . . These very
> shade-tolerant trees grow exceptionally slowly, which limits
> them largely to ancient forest . . . So much ancient forest is now
> gone that it will be difficult to get enough bark for clinical trials . . .
> Between losing their habitat and being stripped of their bark,
> Pacific yews could become the spotted owls of the plant world . . .
> The only way to have enough yews in the years to come is
> to protect our remaining ancient forests and to manage lands
> where logging is allowed with far more care than they are now
> given. We can do this only if Congress, foresters, and citizens

recognize that forest management is more than timber management. Managing for biological diversity is essential to maintain
our options for the future. We will never know how many
potential cures for cancer, heart disease, or AIDS have already
been clearcut to extinction.

To all those concerned about old-growth forests, Norse's reference to
this tree, virtually unknown outside the Pacific Northwest, opened up
an important space in a debate that had become exceedingly polarized.
Shifting the focus from the spotted owl to *Taxus brevifolia* was a way of
complicating the old-growth issue and challenging the alliances that
had been constructed in the spotted owl debate. In particular it allowed
for actors, who in other instances might have been on opposite sides of
an argument, to find a common ground and to align their political
interests with that of *Taxus brevifolia*.

Bean and Manheim recognized the political currency in *Taxus brevifolia*. On 6 August 1990, Bruce Manheim wrote to Cragg and Snader at
the NCI enclosing a draft petition to Manuel Lujan, Secretary of the
Department of the Interior, to list *Taxus brevifolia* as a 'threatened
species'.[101] He explained that the Environmental Defense Fund deliberately chose to petition for the designation 'threatened' because, if
successful, it would make federal agencies, such as the Forest Service
and the Bureau of Land Management, take action not to jeopardize the
tree while allowing for it to be harvested. This was, of course, precisely
how they could protect the habitat for *Taxus brevifolia* – old-growth
forests – while ensuring a supply of bark, in the short to medium term.
It would be very difficult, even for the timber industry, to argue against
the spirit of the petition.

The petition was sent to Secretary Lujan on 19 September 1990. As
co-signers, the Environmental Defense Fund was able to enlist the
support of the following organizations: The Wilderness Society, the
Natural Resources Defense Council, the National Wildlife Federation,
the Center for Marine Preservation, the Oregon Natural Resources
Council, the Defenders of Wildlife, and the Friends of the Ancient
Forest. Both William McGuire, the oncologist in charge of the ovarian
cancer trials at Johns Hopkins and Susan Horwitz, who had discovered
taxol's unusual mechanism of action, also signed. The American Cancer
Society sent a separate letter expressing their support in seeking
threatened status for *Taxus brevifolia*, although they declined to sign the
petition.

Launched with substantial media coverage, the petition is a landmark document in the history of taxol and *Taxus brevifolia*.[102] It based its
case on the argument that logging practices in the past had reduced the
number of *Taxus brevifolia* substantially and that these same practices

were presently further reducing their numbers.[103] By designating *Taxus brevifolia* as a 'threatened species' not only would the tree receive the protection, in the form of management, research and interagency consultations it needed, but, under the Endangered Species Act, bark would still be allowed to be harvested. The petition provided the most up-to-date information on both taxol and *Taxus brevifolia*, culling this from both published and unpublished sources. It was, therefore, an extremely comprehensive compilation of the state of knowledge of *Taxus brevifolia*, bringing Spjut's 1974 account into the early 1990s.

Despite its eloquence and scholarship, the petition failed to move the Fish and Wildlife Service to list *Taxus brevifolia* as threatened. The agency turned down the petition in 9 January 1991.[104] Their key contention was put in the following statement: 'insufficient scientific information exists to determine whether regulatory protection under the Act may be justified'. The detailed response consisted of a refutation of a number of facts that the petition put forth to support its case of which two are particularly important to consider. One of these was the argument the petitioners insisted on, namely that there had been and continued to be a severe reduction in the number of *Taxus brevifolia*, primarily because of the indiscriminate destruction of the yew and its habitat by current logging practices. The Fish and Wildlife Service countered that, according to their data, the tree was not threatened, either in the past or in the present. Though they agreed that there may have been a decrease in the range of *Taxus brevifolia*, particularly in lowland areas because of land clearing, countering this was evidence that, because of a reduction in the frequency of fire, there was a likely increase in the size of populations. In short, they maintained that 'no data exists to show that any historical reduction in yew abundance has occurred'. As to the Environmental Defense Fund's charge that 'although the Pacific yew occurs over a large part of western North America, it is generally rare throughout most of its range', the Fish and Wildlife Service answered that it is 'not rare, but merely often subdominant throughout millions of acres of forest-land habitat'.

At no point in their petition did the Environmental Defense Fund offer an estimate of the size of the population of *Taxus brevifolia* in the Pacific Northwest. Indeed, there had been, to date, no inventory of *Taxus brevifolia* on Forest Service lands where most trees could be found.[105] The petition referred to data assembled by Charles Bolsinger of the Forest Service, but this information related to the age distribution of *Taxus brevifolia* on private as compared with Bureau of Land Management land. Even had there been an estimate of the size of the *Taxus brevifolia* population, this would not have altered the petition's main argument, which was based on the estimation of how quickly they were declining in numbers, an estimation derived from knowledge of how quickly old-growth forests were disappearing.[106]

Surprisingly, given that there was no inventory of *Taxus brevifolia* on Forest Service lands, the Fish and Wildlife Service, nevertheless, reported in their rejection document that the 'Forest Service estimated that 130,000,000 yew trees occur on 1,778,000 acres of National Forest lands in the Washington and Oregon Cascades, and Oregon Coast Range'. As to Bureau of Land Management and private lands, the Fish and Wildlife Service remarked that there, too, one could find *Taxus brevifolia* on 2.5 million acres. This was their justification for not accepting that *Taxus brevifolia* was rare.

The other main argument made by the Fish and Wildlife Service centred on taxol. They were not impressed by the argument that the harvest of bark for the production of taxol posed a significant threat to the species as a whole. They were even less impressed by the argument in the petition that listing *Taxus brevifolia* would have the effect of ensuring a supply of bark to the taxol programme. Their main point and one that required no specific data, was that, in their interpretation, the purpose of the Endangered Species Act is 'not to provide needed supplies of drugs for medical research, but to provide for the conservation of endangered and threatened species and their ecosystems'.

Whatever may be said about the quality of the facts the Fish and Wildlife Service brought to bear on their decision to reject the petition, and whatever may be said about the merits of the case one way or the other, this whole episode pointed up one crucial issue. Despite the decades of interest in taxol and the continuing stripping of bark, almost nothing was known about the tree itself. Ironically, the argument for rejecting the petition, that of insufficient information, was precisely the problem with the rejection case itself.

The Environmental Defense Fund chose not to appeal. Nor did it pursue its other strategy of cajoling the Forest Service to treat *Taxus brevifolia* as a 'sensitive species'. For the time being, an action of this kind, petitioning a government agency at the highest level, had not borne results. The Fish and Wildlife Service would, therefore, not become the voice of the yew.

The Native Yew Conservation Council and the Voice of the Strategic Resource

Because taxol was so long in the making, it had become associated with many people from various different backgrounds and interests.

Table 6.1. *Participants at workshop on Taxol and* Taxus, *June 1990, Bethesda*

A	*Agronomics* Includes people interested in collection, ecology, forestry, conservation, germplasm, cultivation, strain improvement, and tree genetics.
B	*Chemistry* Includes analytical chemistry, isolation, bulk production, total and semi-synthesis, medicinal chemistry, prodrugs, formulation, and process development.
C	*Clinical studies* Includes all clinical aspects.
D	*Biological production* Includes biosynthesis, tissue culture and genetic engineering.
E	*Biological effects* Includes mechanism of action, experimental therapeutics, resistance, and pharmacology.
F	*R&D Support* Includes licensing, venture capital, NCI staff, publicists, regulatory affairs, and miscellaneous.

Moreover, for the same reason, the development of taxol reflected the wide array of changes that had been occurring in science, medicine and technology, not to mention society and politics over the period.

As mentioned in the previous chapter, the first taxol and *Taxus* workshop met in Bethesda on 26 June 1990. The participants, totalling just under 200, reflected the huge number of sites in science, medicine and business into which taxol had become insinuated. At this meeting were individuals who had been crucial in getting taxol to this point, many of whom had never met before. Present among the crowd were Fred Boettner, Charles Bolsinger, Patrick Connolly, Gordon Cragg, Dianne DeFuria, John Destito, Floyd Ehrheart, Frankie Ann Holmes, Susan Horwitz, Wayne Jackson, Neil Jans, David Kingston, William McGuire, Jerry Rust, Ken Snader, Matthew Suffness, Monroe Wall, and Mansukh Wani, all of whom have already appeared in this book. Reflecting the momentous developments in molecular sciences, there were biotechnologists, cell culture experts and biogeneticists amidst the organic chemists and chemical engineers.

Reproduced is Table 6.1 showing the interests of the participants broadly divided into the categories the workshop itself used. Though the list did not make it clear, about one-quarter of the audience came from the corporate sector representing pharmaceutical companies, biotechnology companies, bulk chemical producers, small-scale log-gers and major timber companies. As an object, taxol drew upon many diverse practices. The workshop was there to celebrate this achieve-ment and to announce to the public that trusting the NCI, and therefore the State, to find a cure for cancer, was paying off.

One thing the meeting did not discuss as a problem was the fate of *Taxus brevifolia*. Despite the nearly 200 participants, the tree itself did not figure as an actor. It was not given a space in which to act, even though, on reflection, there would have been no such workshop, no such molecule, had there been no *Taxus brevifolia* and even though some of the participants were explicitly concerned with its fate. The assumption that ran through the workshop was that in the short term and medium term, taxol would continue to be made from the bark of *Taxus brevifolia*. Ken Snader, from the Natural Products Branch of the NCI, made this argument in his contribution but reminded his audience that even though the medium-term plan (three to five years) involved other approaches to supply, namely semi-synthesis of both taxol and other taxane analogues and the cultivation and harvest of other *Taxus* species and cultivars, there were substantial problems with the alternative approaches.[107] He also commented that, according to the good clinical results that had been accumulating, once FDA approval was granted for taxol, the minimum requirement annually would be twenty-four kilograms, equivalent to 720,000 pounds of bark.[108] Charles Bolsinger's contribution, providing valuable information on the distribution, abundance and stand characteristics of *Taxus brevifolia* was also delivered with the assumption that the tree would continue to be harvested.[109] The only speaker to address the issue of a sustainable source of supply was Ed Croom from the University of Mississippi who remarked that 'clinical supplies must be based on a reliable, sustain-able, abundant and economical source'. And that source, he stated, existed in the form of ornamental *Taxus* cultivars.[110]

In bringing together what might be called the 1990 taxol network, the NCI had scored an important success. But not everyone came away from it satisfied. Certainly this was true for those whose concern was for *Taxus brevifolia* and who felt that issues about it were not being addressed. One of those present at the workshop with these concerns foremost in his mind was Jerry Rust. Listening to the presentations left him with questions unanswered. He met informally in Bethesda with a few other participants sympathetic to his concerns who vowed to proffer another voice.[111]

The group sympathetic to the fate of *Taxus brevifolia* was from the Pacific region and returned there to spotlight the tree and to consider their next move. Within a few weeks of the Bethesda workshop, a number of individuals met in Eugene, Oregon to form the Pacific Yew Conservation Group. Assembled together by Jerry Rust, the group's brief was to 'review the status of yew harvesting practices in the Northwest, and to define a conservation plan for this strategic resource in the fight against cancer. Protection and harvesting of the Pacific yew, a small tree native to northern California and other western states, has become a critical issue in forest management'.[112] This call was made more urgent by Samuel Broder, Director of the NCI, who at the workshop had commented on the need for a rapid expansion of the limited supply of taxol.

To ensure a sustainable and renewable supply of taxol, the group discussed a number of policy positions including declaring *Taxus brevifolia* a national strategic resource, demanding an inventory of the tree, adopting specific yew harvesting guidelines guaranteeing in particular, that all plant material containing taxol be used efficiently, and encouraging regeneration. Rather than dwell on the medium- and long-term possibilities, as had been done at the workshop, this group of concerned individuals fundamentally sought to give *Taxus brevifolia* their immediate attention. They agreed to continue discussions at another meeting, held on 12 August 1990, at the University of California, Berkeley.

Jerry Rust was in the chair surrounded by ten other people. The agenda reflected the discussions held in Eugene in July. This time, rather than simply hashing over ideas, they hoped to draft a comprehensive conservation strategy. Their objective was to publicize the status and likely fate of *Taxus brevifolia*, to enter it into the political consciousness and to invite the public and the authorities to participate in this crucial exercise.

A small aside. One of the aims of actor–network theory is to draw attention to the way in which heterogeneous actors with different interests, backgrounds, hopes and aspirations, are enrolled in projects, the outcome of which depends entirely on the actors sticking to the script and leaving their differences aside. One device to aid this process of translation, as it is called, is to fix the actors' gaze on to an 'obligatory point of passage' through which they must all pass in order to satisfy the project's objective.[113]

The group that met in Berkeley was unquestionably heterogeneous. Some of them, indeed, had very little time for each other, positively distrusted and maybe even despised each other. Jerry Rust placed *Taxus brevifolia* as a 'national strategic resource' as the 'obligatory point of passage' of this network, now called the Native Yew Conservation Committee. By forcing the members of this group to focus on *Taxus brevifolia* in the identity he provided for it, he was able to keep an

inherently unstable, even chaotic, network, stable and working, at least
for the time being.

Attending the meeting were Jerry Rust, County Commissioner; John
Destito, one-time official bark collector for the NCI, suspicious of
Hauser's role in undermining his bark collection efforts and now under
the shadow of a hostile take-over bid for his own company; Patrick
Connolly, another one-time official bark collector for the NCI, author of
several petitions to discredit Destito as a collector and currently collecting bark for Hauser; Floyd Ehrheart, also currently collecting bark
for Hauser and critical of them in rescinding the contract to buy *Taxus
brevifolia* limbs and needles; Phil Hassrick, field co-ordinator for
Hauser; Neil Jans, Director of Business Development at Hauser; Brian
Stone, representing the Forest Service from California; Stan Scher, a
silviculturalist with several years research interest in *Taxus brevifolia*;
and Bert Schwarzschild, an environmentalist interested in the conservation and sustainability of *Taxus brevifolia*.[114]

The meeting discussed a number of issues, some contentious and
others not.[115] The objective was to draw up a draft resolution but many
of those around the table had very different ideas on what shape such a
declaration should have. Scher and Schwarzschild veered towards
issues of protecting *Taxus brevifolia* as a resource by adopting prudent
harvesting techniques and further research on the tree itself. Brian
Stone, on the other hand, spoke little of protection or conservation.
Instead, his interest in *Taxus brevifolia* was as a source of revenue to the
Forest Service, looking for the right price and for the right management
policy to ensure a continuing supply of demand. The representatives of
Hauser, Phil Hassrick and Neil Jans, saw things very differently. As for
the Forest Service's financial interests in *Taxus brevifolia*, they felt that,
on the contrary, the agency should see the harvesting of bark as a
humanitarian programme and keep costs at a minimum, even zero. Of
course they were interested in protecting the yew, but, as they saw it,
the real issue was to keep the tree as an American resource, to keep it
locked up between Hauser and Bristol-Myers and as a source of revenue for these companies. Indeed, they went so far as to recommend
that all of the interests around taxol, the present group, the NCI, the
collectors and cancer patients, should be represented by Hauser. Jerry
Rust, as one might expect, was more political, more pragmatic than
most, reflecting his years of experience in Oregon politics. He outlined a
seventeen-point conservation programme and argued strongly for
action in the form of sending the group's resolutions to forestry officials, members of Congress and the press in Oregon.

Though they differed on tactics and overall objectives, the members
of this fledgling Native Yew Conservation Committee saw their

common purpose as the provision of taxol at the same time as the protection of *Taxus brevifolia*. And, they pointed out clearly, protection here meant conserving it as a resource, not, as some people thought, forbidding its exploitation.[116] Despite Hauser's bid to position itself as the 'obligatory point of passage', for the moment, at least, Rust managed to hold *Taxus brevifolia* in this tactical position. During the meeting, and seemingly unnoticed by the other participants, Rust dextrously managed to engineer another 'obligatory point of passage', not a species but a place, the State of Oregon. He would continue in the future to equate *Taxus brevifolia* with the State of Oregon, for his own and for the Committee's best interests. The meeting adjourned and agreed to meet again on 12 October, this time in Medford, in southern Oregon, hosted by Floyd Ehrheart.

If the purpose of the Berkeley meeting was to map out the political terrain, that of the Medford meeting was to put it into practice. Rust's pragmatism ruled. The committee members, now enlarged to include a representative of the Rogue River National Forest, Pat Kenyon from Advanced Molecular Technologies and Hal Hartzell, Jerry Rust's friend and colleague, worked out an agreed resolution and a strategy for publicizing their thoughts.[117] They agreed that the Native Yew Conservation Committee's mission was 'to foster the sustainable harvesting of yew, to assure a continuous source of taxol in the fight against cancer and to guarantee the health of the species for future generations.' To accomplish these goals, the Committee also agreed on an eleven-point programme including the demand for a yew inventory, plans to use the yew resource more effectively, extending beyond taxol, demands to alter current timber practices to be more mindful of the yew and, finally, because 'any waste of this resource is unconscionable', that *Taxus brevifolia* should be declared a national strategic resource 'with appropriate management considerations given to this important species'. A resolution covering the policy recommendations was sent to a number of influential (and sympathetic) members of Congress soliciting legislative assistance; to the Secretaries of Interior and Agriculture, pressing, as a matter of urgency, the need for 'wise stewardship of the yew resource'; and to F. Dale Robertson, Chief of the Forest Service, urging an early meeting.

Also under discussion at this meeting was the Environmental Defense Fund's petition to list *Taxus brevifolia*. Not everyone at the meeting supported the petition or, at least, the manner by which the Environmental Defense Fund and its backers were attempting to protect the tree. Though August and worthy environmental bodies put their signature to the petition, this should not be read as an indication of far-reaching support in this constituency. The Native Plant Society of

Oregon, a group of amateur and professional botanists, for one, certainly did not support the petition and requested the petitioners to withdraw their demands: instead, the society invited concerned parties to join them in drawing up a 'regional interagency management plan'.[118]

The similar timing of the Environmental Defense Fund's petition and the Native Yew Conservation Committee's resolution invites comparison between the two in achieving objectives. The Environmental Defense Fund sought the channels of current legislation and the courts, if necessary, to carve out a protective space for *Taxus brevifolia*, as had already been done for other plants and, more spectacularly, for the spotted owl. Their methods, indeed overarching concerns, lay within the context of forest politics, especially that of ancient or old-growth forests. If *Taxus brevifolia* could be listed, then a critical habitat would need to be designated as for all listed species. And, of course, that critical habitat was the old-growth forest itself. As the drafters of the petition maintained, while the focus was *Taxus brevifolia*, the object was the forest and that 'conflict in the Pacific Northwest was not simply the choice between protecting owls or providing jobs for the loggers, but rather it was the choice of sustaining a diverse forest type that had within it a lot of potentially useful organisms and chemicals of which the yew and taxol were examples ... that the loss of those old-growth forests in the Northwest threatened more than just spotted owls, it threatened other resources, some of which had the potential to be of substantial value to human beings for medical research ...'.[119] The Environmental Defense Fund was not attempting to position *Taxus brevifolia* as an 'obligatory point of passage', but rather to give it a voice in terms of its proposed identity as an threatened species. Once listed, the job of the Environmental Defense Fund would be over, and the wheels of legislation and other actors would begin their work.

The Native Yew Conservation Committee, by contrast, sought to become the voice of *Taxus brevifolia* on a continuing basis by making it not only an 'obligatory point of passage' for its own members but, even more significantly, for the entire taxol programme and its networks. To achieve that required some legislation but mostly a great deal of politicking, lobbying and pressure. Even more, as the official voice of *Taxus brevifolia*, the Native Yew Conservation Committee, would be in a strong position, it hoped, to draft scripts for other actors as the occasion arose. Importantly, the Committee, at this point at least, did not wander into the thicket of old-growth forest politics, opting instead for the less controversial strategy of anchoring *Taxus brevifolia* securely in the taxol story.

Their resolution completed, the Committee agreed to meet shortly, on 30 November, in Olympia, the State capital of Washington, hosted by John Destito and Advanced Molecular Technologies. On the agenda were proposals to formalize the structure of the Native Yew Conservation Committee, as well as further discussions of those issues raised at previous meetings. This meeting was extremely well attended, numbering over thirty individuals, many more than at any of the previous meetings. Moreover, the constituency had broadened significantly, reflecting, as had the NCI-sponsored workshop on taxol in the summer, the varied and numerous sites where taxol was of interest. Dianne DeFuria, representing Bristol-Myers Squibb was invited, although, in the end, she was unable to attend.

The substance of the meeting might best be described as a continuation of past efforts but with an increasing presence. The number of participants had risen as had the mailing list. In one respect, however, there was already some hint of a honing of the demands of the Committee and, significantly, the emergence of a practical definition of a word used in its mission statement – sustainability.

This would become clear at the next meeting, scheduled for 18 January 1991 in Cottage Grove, Oregon. At this point, the Native Yew Conservation Committee went public, in the sense that it presented itself as a public forum for the discussion of *Taxus brevifolia* issues. The Cottage Grove meeting took the form more of a workshop or symposium than of a meeting. Speakers were invited to discuss a number of specific issues focusing on *Taxus brevifolia*. The objective was to air these concerns publicly. The subject of this meeting was foliage as an alternative raw material source.

Two papers, in particular, reflected both changed and broader concerns. One of these, given by Stanley Scher, focused squarely on the question of foliage as an alternative source to bark in the production of taxol. Scher's paper coincided with a number of developments in the analysis of taxol content in various parts of the tree, particularly the needles. These had been tested on several occasions during the 1960s and 1970s but the taxol content, it was then concluded, was both inferior to and more variable than bark.[120] Now, however, and largely in response to the changed politics of taxol and *Taxus brevifolia*, the needles were being revisited using new and, by all accounts, more sensitive assays to detect the presence of taxol. One of these analyses, conducted by scientists at the NCI, showed remarkable results, certainly challenging the received wisdom about the inferiority of needles head on. Published in the autumn of 1990, the researchers showed that in four *Taxus* species (the wild *brevifolia*, *canadensis* and *cuspidata* and the cultivated *media*), the 'dry weight percentage of taxol ... is roughly equivalent to the amount of taxol found in the bark of *T. brevifolia* (0.01% dry wt)'.[121] Scher referred to this study in his presentation.

The other paper, given by Jerry Rust, took a broader approach by looking at the whole of *Taxus brevifolia* as an economic, yet renewable, resource.[122] In it, Rust outlined his vision of sustainable economic development based on *Taxus brevifolia*, involving a multifaceted industry, providing several thousand jobs and a guaranteed supply of taxol. The key to Rust's model was an insistence on using *Taxus brevifolia* on a sustained yield basis ad perpetuum. He foresaw a mini-economy emerging out of, yet sustaining, *Taxus brevifolia*, in the same manner as other forest economies in the Pacific Northwest, particularly those based on the dominant commercial species, such as Douglas fir. Consequently, he envisioned *Taxus*-based job creation, research and development, conservation, extraction and manufacture. In this scheme, taxol, made from both bark and foliage, was only one, albeit the most important, cog in this perpetual economy. As he himself put it, in almost evangelical terms, 'we have an opportunity to create a truly sustainable forest product industry based on the yew species. This could create revenue, jobs and wealth for the Pacific Northwest in perpetuity and supply the needed taxol for cancer research.'[123] He contrasted his broad and sustainable approach to taxol to that of the NCI and, by implication, Bristol-Myers Squibb. They, he pointed out, saw the forest as a short-term expedient. According to their own estimates, they would continue to strip bark from *Taxus brevifolia* for the next five years, after which they would leave the forest as the medium- and long-term programmes – nurseries, semi-synthesis and synthesis, for example – were phased in.[124] Put this way, the NCI and Bristol-Myers Squibb were not true friends of the forest and did not have the welfare of the people of the Pacific Northwest at heart. Only people like himself and, also by implication, the Native Yew Conservation Committee, could engineer divergent interests towards a common and laudable goal.

Rust's paper was an inspired piece of master building. Whatever one may have thought of his arithmetic, or of the specifics of his plan, there is little doubt that his vision of *Taxus brevifolia* as the generator of a new economy, ground it even deeper and wider as an 'obligatory point of passage'. After all, these were hard times for the Pacific Northwest forests.

Rust's vision, however, was just that, a vision. The reality was that of bark and its political economy, and the Native Yew Conservation Committee worked to wean all interested parties from this material in favour of sustainable alternatives. Over the year, following the January 1991 meeting in Cottage Grove, the Native Yew Conservation

Committee became incorporated and changed its title to the Native Yew Conservation Council. Its Officers and Board of Directors continued to reflect that heterogeneous character, obvious from the first. It sponsored at least two more meetings, organized on the symposium model, covering the themes of the manner of extracting taxol and *Taxus* and the pharmaceutical development of taxol and other taxanes. Speaking at these symposia were experts representing taxol and *Taxus* and much in between. In this sense, the Native Yew Conservation Council was the only continuous forum in the United States where all the issues about taxol and *Taxus* could be discussed as they came up. Reflecting this growing interest, the membership of the Native Yew Conservation Council increased enormously, reaching between 500 and 1,000 people by year's end.

Although the Native Yew Conservation Council could rightly proclaim itself as the voice of *Taxus brevifolia*, there was little it did or could do to make policy. It seemed to be responding to events, not making them. This is precisely the tone of the editorial update of events during 1991 in the first issue of 'Taxofile', the newsletter of the Native Yew Conservation Council. As Hal Hartzell, the editor lamented: '1991 was a year in which the embattled yew gained a little respect but lost a lot of ground. Newspapers and magazines across the country, indeed the world, carried major articles on taxol and Pacific yew. Estimates range from 50,000 to as many as 200,000 yew trees destroyed in the combined processes of burning logging slash, and legal and illegal bark harvesting in 1991.'[125] Hartzell was referring to the harvesting of more than 825,000 pounds of bark from Forest Service land.[126] Ironically, and not going unnoticed by Hartzell, it was Hauser Northwest who was responsible for collection, one of whose chief officers, Phil Hassrick, was on the Board of Directors of the Native Yew Conservation Council.[127]

Nevertheless, as with any heterogeneous assemblage, the fact that actors hold conflicting views does not affect the stability of the network so much as the translation processes. For Hauser Northwest did have a big stake in keeping eyes and minds fixed on *Taxus brevifolia* as the source for taxol. Threats to the mission of the Native Yew Conservation Council, at this time at least, came not from within but from without. Specifically, the Council's policy on sustainability and renewability, summed up in the letter from Shimon Schwarzschild, President of the Council, to its members, in 1992: 'NYCC is working to secure a renewable source of taxol ... NYCC advocates sustainable approaches to yew harvesting to prevent further destruction of the depleted native yew resources ... renewable harvesting of yew foliage will assure a continuous supply of taxol for today and tomorrow.'[128]

Yet, while advocating the use of foliage, the evidence about its taxol content was becoming as variable as the content itself. Late in 1990, for example, another group of researchers, at Stanford Research Institute, reported disappointing results on the taxol content of *Taxus brevifolia* needles, showing it to be one-tenth of that of the bark.[129] Ken Snader, chemist at the Natural Products Branch of the NCI, in response to a request for information from the Secretary of the Council, was also less than optimistic about the chances of needles becoming the raw material for making taxol.[130] Recall, too, that in 1990, Hauser had decided to abandon its interest in any part of *Taxus brevifolia*, apart from the bark. The call for foliage was beginning to sound hollow.

In the spring of 1991, Hal Hartzell, published his book on the yew tree adding a biography to its voice.[131] The book was the most up-to-date collection of information about the entire genus and, for the first time, was able to include substantial material on taxol itself. However important and interesting, it could not get around the fact that events were shaped by the big players. Jerry Rust went so far as to try and persuade the editors of *Time* to propose an award similar to that of man-of-the-year, and declare 1991 'The Year of the Yew'.[132] Certainly, judging from the media coverage that *Taxus brevifolia* received that year, 1991 was an unusual year in the extent to which Americans were fed stories about a single tree.

The Oregon Natural Resources Council and the Voice of the Environment

The Oregon Natural Resources Council was another organization that attempted to be a voice for, or, at least, to add its voice to *Taxus brevifolia*. This organization came into being in 1982, although it previously exis-ted under the name of the Oregon Wilderness Coalition. Its two most outspoken and active members were Andy Kerr and James Monteith.[133] Their political battle was fought out over the fate of the old-growth forests of the entire Pacific Northwest, but principally in Oregon. It was Monteith who is credited with coining the expression 'ancient forest'.[134]

The Oregon Natural Resources Council's interest in *Taxus brevifolia* dated back to 1987 when Monteith inquired into the nature of the 60,000 pound collection of that year: he further highlighted the tree in the following year when he proposed to the Bureau of Land Management that they designate a forty-acre site near the town of Saginaw in central Oregon an 'Area of Critical Environmental Concern' because it con-tained a large population of old-growth Pacific yew – he suggested calling the designated site 'Cougar Mountain Ancient Yew Grove'.[135] In his letter to the Bureau, Monteith displayed his knowledge of the tree and of the growing clinical uses of taxol. He took the opportunity to remind the Bureau that modern timber management regarded *Taxus brevifolia* as a weed tree and that unless there was a change in this attitude, current forest practices would certainly eliminate options in the future. In a somewhat veiled allusion to biodiversity, Monteith reiterated a point made by many others: that forest management in the Pacific Northwest was blindly dedicated to a single species – Douglas fir – to the exclusion of all other forest products.

Assuming that Monteith was representing the views of the Oregon Natural Resources Council, and there is no good reason to suppose otherwise, they were arguably, together with Rust and Hartzell, the first group to realize what was going on in the forests and to recommend changes. However, no further action appears to have taken place until the Oregon Natural Resources Council teamed up with the Environmental Defense Fund in presenting the petition to list *Taxus brevifolia* as a threatened species.

Since its establishment, the Oregon Natural Resources Council has worked on changing policy by three main methods: putting pressure on agencies concerned with natural resources to alter their practices; litigating against those agencies that they feel are breaking the law with regards to natural resources; and, finally, lobbying Congress to tighten natural resource laws in those cases where the other methods have not borne fruit.[136]

According to Wendell Wood, who in the early 1990s was the Oregon Natural Resource Council's Conservation Co-ordinator, the group's position on *Taxus brevifolia* was that it was being underutilized as a resource.[137] That is, most of the bark was not being taken for cancer research but was being destroyed indiscriminately in logging operations on private and, especially public lands. The goal of the Oregon Natural Resources Council was to pressure the Forest Service and the Bureau of Land Management to adopt measures to ensure that the bark was not destroyed but made available. This was not going to require any great legislative effort because, they argued, the legislation already existed in the form of the National Forest Management Act, the Federal Land Policy and Management Act and the National Environmental Policy Act.[138]

In the early 1990s, the Oregon Natural Resources Council's major preoccupation was the whole issue of the ancient forest and not any species in particular. Wendell Wood became involved specifically in the issue of *Taxus brevifolia* on behalf of the Council through relations with Jerry Rust. As the Native Yew Conservation Council held meetings and sponsored symposia, Rust and the Oregon Natural Resources Council were raising public consciousness by writing letters, issuing press statements and appealing timber sales on public lands. After the failure of the Environmental Defense Fund to list *Taxus brevifolia*, the Oregon Natural Resources Council stepped up its activity during 1991 using the tactics it had already honed in the larger ancient forest campaign.

Focusing on publicizing needles as the source of the precursor 10-DAB, from which taxol could be made as had already been demonstrated by Pierre Potier and his team in France; and the gross underutilization of bark as a result of the continued destruction of the resource during routine timber sales and consequent clear-cuts, the Oregon Natural Resources Council pressed Forest Service and Bureau of Land Management officials to adopt specific guidelines not to waste *Taxus brevifolia*.[139] In November 1991, for example, the Oregon Natural Resources Council held a well-publicized media conference in Oregon at which Wendell Wood reminded his audience that there was a large gap between what the public believed was occurring with *Taxus brevifolia* and what his group's research revealed.[140] The public, he argued, were under the mistaken impression that *Taxus brevifolia* had made the transition in identity from that of a waste to an extremely valuable product. They should not be complacent, he warned, because the identity of *Taxus brevifolia* was more ambiguous than the public had been led to believe. While in some places and times it was being harvested correctly, at other places and times, it was being wasted at a colossal level. Less than a fortnight later, a similar charge was levelled specifically at Weyerhaeuser.[141]

The underutilization argument was certainly a powerful one, particularly as it tried to break the argument widely promulgated in the media that pitted 'environmentalists' against 'cancer patients'.[142] A prominent article published in the *Wall Street Journal* in 1991 was typical of many that year, in which the argument about underutilization of *Taxus brevifolia* bark because of current timber practices on Federal lands got no mention at all: instead, the reading public was given the following headline: 'Clashing priorities: A new cancer drug may extend lives – At cost of rare trees. That angers conservationists who say taxol extraction endangers the prized yew'.[143] Not only was the argument about underutilization and waste not sticking in the public mind, but, because of its very nature, it was very difficult, if not impossible, to get precise information on how much bark ended up in slash piles. Anecdotal evidence was not sufficient. We will return to this point shortly.

Because of the close association between Jerry Rust and the Oregon Natural Resources Council, the latter was not only kept closely informed of developments in the wider contexts of *Taxus brevifolia*, but could prod and cajole state and Federal agencies in a way that was not available to the Native Yew Conservation Council. Together the two organizations probably did as much as they could to alert the American public to events in the forests of the Pacific Northwest, although not always to their advantage.

The Pacific Yew Act and the Voice of Legislation

In an important respect, however, the voice of *Taxus brevifolia* became truly public when on 20 November 1991, Gerry Studds, Democratic Congressman for Massachusetts introduced legislation (The Pacific Yew Act) into the House of Representatives to 'promote the availability of taxol . . . by requiring the Federal government to vastly improve its management of the Pacific yew tree – the primary source of the drug'.[144] Studds was perfectly placed to introduce a bill that straddled vital environmental and health issues, as he was the Chairman of the House Merchant Marine and Fisheries Subcommittee on Fisheries and Wildlife Conservation and the Environment and had many legislative interests in the field of health. This legislation, co-sponsored by Ron Wyden, Democrat, from Oregon, who also had intimate knowledge of the vast number of issues tied up with taxol, reflected the inertia demonstrated by the Forest Service and the Bureau of Land Management in changing their practices and awakening fully to the central importance of *Taxus brevifolia* in their forests. It also vindicated so many of the arguments made on various occasions by the Native Yew Conservation Council and the Oregon Natural Resources Council and also present in the Environmental Defense Fund's petition of 1990.

The underutilization argument was at the heart of the bill's objective, being to 'direct the Forest Service and the Bureau of Land Management to develop and implement sound management guidelines for the Pacific Yew to provide for the efficient harvest and utilization of yew resources, while also ensuring the continued survival of the species for future use.'[145] Among other policy measures, it provided for an inventory to be made of *Taxus brevifolia* on all Federal lands and for appropriate management guidelines to prevent the wasting of Pacific yew resources.[146]

The bill was referred to the Committees on Agriculture, Interior and Insular Affairs and Merchant Marine and Fisheries. On the 4 March 1992, a hearing was held jointly by all subcommittees of all three committees at which a number of individuals made statements. One of them was Bruce Manheim, Senior Attorney at the Environmental Defense Fund and who, with colleague Michael Bean, had drafted the petition to list *Taxus brevifolia* under the Endangered Species Act.[147] One of the issues Manheim addressed was the underutilization of bark. He had two main points to make. One was that National Forests within the same administrative region were following different practices when it came to *Taxus brevifolia*. Three National Forests – Willamette, Mount Hood and Umpqua – had adopted policies to ensure that bark was harvested from trees before they were burned in slash piles but other National Forests had not followed suit. Secondly, he presented some evidence of the scale of wastage, alleging that officials at the Willamette National Forest conceded that sixty to seventy-five per cent of *Taxus brevifolia* bark was being destroyed during logging operations on other tree species. He also calculated, on the basis of the 1991 bark harvest compared with the timber harvest on both Forest Service and Bureau of Land Management land, that 585,000 pounds of bark, enough to treat 9,750 patients could have been harvested but was, in fact, simply destroyed.[148] Manheim's case was amply supported by the testimony presented the same day by James Duffus III, Director, Natural Resources Management Issues of the General Accounting Office. He reported that during 1991, yew bark was not always collected before commercial timber was harvested (despite instructions to field per-sonnel to do just that); collectable yew bark was being left behind on branches and stems of smaller diameter; and that bark was not being collected from trees scattered over a large area but rather where they were found in close proximity to each other.[149] The General Accounting Office pointed its finger at the Forest Service, the Bureau of Land Management and Hauser Northwest.

The Pacific Yew Act was signed into law on 7 August 1992, after having passed through the House and the Senate in July. But the Act that came into being was not exactly the one that had been originally introduced. While it required a policy on Pacific yew conservation and management; encouraged research on the tree; and stipulated that careful records of sales and other collection data be kept, all worthy and generally well-supported concerns and included in the original, the Act differed from the original in that it contained a 'sunset clause'. Section 8 allowed for the Act to expire when the Secretary of Health and Human Services deemed that 'quantities of taxol sufficient to satisfy medicinal demands are available from sources other than Pacific yew trees harvested on Federal lands'. This clause, however, introduced two problems. One of these was that by using the imprecise word 'sufficient', it gave the Secretary of Health and Human Services substantial power in exercising judgement and terminating the Act.[150] Secondly, by insisting on an expiration or sunset clause, specifically that legislation would only exist while *Taxus brevifolia* on Federal lands continued to be the most important source, the Act did not seek to protect *Taxus brevifolia* and 'the long-term conservation of the species'. A legislative distinction was being drawn between a public and a private *Taxus brevifolia*. Implicit in both the Bill and the Act were instrumental values that identified *Taxus brevifolia* solely as the provider of taxol for human use, and the broader argument that many were trying to make about preserving ecosystems and biodiversity was entirely sidelined.[151]

Apart from waste, the Act addressed another concern of harvesting bark. Section 5 directed the appropriate agencies to 'ensure the development, implementation, and enforcement of processes for the collection and sale of Pacific yew resources that will minimize the illegal harvest and sale of such resources'. This may seem an unusual requirement but, in the circumstances, it was understandable, although, as one commentator maintained, a bit excessive.[152]

Thefts of bark from Federal lands first came to public notice when they were discovered in the Willamette National Forest on 14 May.[153] Whether this was the first theft is impossible to say, but there was a definite upward trend. By the height of the summer, four National Forests in Oregon and one in Washington reported yew thefts. Charges were brought against five men in Eugene in October, accused of stripping about two tons of bark from trees in the Sweet Home Ranger District.[154] A sting operation went into action during the same summer and netted Bill Reisinger, a farmer in Chehalis, Washington, and sole collector for Hauser Northwest in the state: it was said that he grossed $400,000 on illegally poached yew bark.[155]

The Forest Service took action to thwart the thieves. They drafted more agents to check permits in the field and to weigh the bags of bark ensuring that it did not contain more than the allotted amount; posted substantial rewards leading to the arrest of suspected felons; and tightened the permit system.[156] By the summer of the following year, forestry officials were confident that they had beaten the problem: thefts, they maintained, were all but eliminated.[157]

Hauser and the Voice of Business as Usual

In 1990, after becoming Bristol-Myers Squibb's official contractor, Hauser Northwest managed to collect only a fraction of what it intended. Yet, at over 80,000 pounds by the end of the year, it was still the largest collection to date. In 1991, however, this paled into insignificance as the scale of collection reached a level never seen before. More than 850,000 pounds was collected from Federal lands in 1991, a further 225,000 pounds from State lands and 525,000 pounds from private lands, making for a grand total of 1.6 million pounds of bark.[158] The harvest for 1992 was also 1.6 million pounds, but this time it was split almost 50/50 between public and private land.[159] The increasing role of private lands in the supply of *Taxus brevifolia* bark should be noted.

Hauser Northwest was the subsidiary of Hauser Chemical, based in Boulder, Colorado, where the bark eventually ended up to make taxol. According to Hauser, the 1991 collection of bark yielded 130 kilograms of taxol in 1992.[160] This reflected a substantial improvement in the yield of taxol from bark, from 20,000 pounds of bark for one kilogram of taxol in 1988 to a figure of between 16,000 and 13,000 pounds of bark for one kilogram of taxol in 1992.[161] Because the 1992 collection volume was virtually the same as in the previous year, in the absence of hard evidence, we can assume that at least a similar amount of taxol was made by Hauser Chemical Research. Assuming an average yield of 14,500 (mid-way between 16,000 and 13,000) pounds of bark per kilogram of taxol, we can estimate that taxol produced by Hauser from its collections in 1990, 1991 and 1992 amounted to approximately 230 kilograms of taxol.[162] In terms of chemotherapy for cancer patients, each kilogram of taxol was sufficient, in very general terms, to treat 500 individuals; at the rate at which taxol was coming out of Hauser Chemical Research and the supply of bark out of the Pacific Northwest, annual treatment would be available for something like 65,000 patients.[163]

At the time, this level of output was substantial and drew a veil over the supply crisis that had plagued the taxol programme for more than a decade. We will return to this point later in the chapter. Aside from giving a lifeline to women suffering from ovarian cancer – many more clinical trials were started and treatment referral centres were opened at a large number of NCI cancer centres – and to all those cancer sufferers who looked upon taxol with hope, the increasing harvest of *Taxus brevifolia* bark in the Pacific Northwest, according to Hauser Northwest, also brought some relief to an otherwise gloomy economic future for many people previously sustained by logging operations.[164]

Bark harvesting is labour intensive and most of the demand for labour is accounted for by the harvesters themselves – individuals whose job it is to peel the bark. The size of the operation, all other things being equal, is limited by the size of the labour force. Hauser Northwest employed about 1,000 bark harvesters in the Pacific Northwest during the 1991 and 1992 collections, half of them in Oregon alone.[165] The harvesters worked during the peeling season, usually between May and August. An average day's work could bag about 100 pounds of wet bark, representing an income to the harvester of about $125 per day.[166] Considering that employment in the lumber and wood products industry in Washington and Oregon fell by about 12,000 between 1990 and 1994, the increase in the demand for *Taxus brevifolia* bark took some of the sting out of the decline in traditional forms of employment.[167]

Hauser Northwest organized its harvesters in such a way that they delivered their wet bark to a number of collectors responsible for specific geographic areas. The collectors also handled the bureaucratic details of getting the permits from the appropriate agency. Once collected, the bags were shipped to one of several processing centres, located in Washington, Oregon, Idaho and in British Columbia. This was the capital intensive end of the operations, where the wet bark was dried, chipped and re-bagged for shipment to Hauser Chemical Research in Boulder for the extraction and purification of taxol. In these years, it was expected that about forty weeks would elapse between the start of a collection programme (surveying of sites where *Taxus brevifolia* grew and obtaining permits) and the production of one kilogram of taxol.[168] Thus bark collected in one year would not appear as taxol until the following year, at about the same time of the year.

Ironically, the discourse surrounding *Taxus brevifolia*, particularly about the need to protect it from wanton destruction and to curb what some saw as an unreasonably excessive level of wastage, took place within the context of a quite extraordinary level of harvesting. This mismatch, this tension between scarcity and plenty, was not simply abstract but was reflected in much of the public discussions about taxol and *Taxus brevifolia* and would come up time and time again. Aside from manifesting different perspectives, the tension was also a result of the state of science and the quality of the statistics available.

Scarcity, the Supply Issue and Yew Knowledge

In 1993, William Boly, a contributing editor to the magazine *Health*, published a critical essay on taxol, something almost unheard of at the time.[169] Most of the article focused on the contrast between the 'hype' surrounding taxol and the dismal state of cancer in the United States as reflected in unyielding mortality rates. Chemotherapy, long the favoured option in the oncology community, he argued, had a lacklustre career. Few dared to prick taxol's halo.

The article's headline ran: 'Almost everything you've heard about taxol, the wonder drug, is wrong.' Aside from the hype, what also caught Boly's eye was what might be described as the politics of scarcity. He recounts that alongside tales of wonder were narratives of scarcity, drawing on images of lonely yew trees in dark corners of the forest, of cancer researchers desperate for experimental supplies, of cancer patients desperate to get on clinical trials to get access to taxol on compassionate grounds. But, as he points out, scarcity was a myth.

It 'suited a lot of agendas' but it was based not on accumulated knowledge but the lack of it.[170]

Scarcity was certainly a theme that ran through the reports on taxol. But what was it that was scarce? Boly misrepresents the case. As we have seen, no one who spoke for *Taxus brevifolia* ever said it was scarce, just that, under then current forestry practices, its existence was threatened while it was being treated as a useless species. Others chimed in reminding everyone that even when *Taxus brevifolia* was being spared the fate of its past generations, as forestry officials maintained, the bark (and needles) were still being wasted. The figure of 130 million yew trees as reported in the rejection of the Environmental Defense Fund's petition was not taken seriously because those in the know knew that no inventory had been taken. The Native Plant Society of Oregon refused to support the Environmental Defense Fund's petition precisely because its officers believed that the species was abundant, a point made on several occasions, both publicly and privately by Charles Bolsinger at the Forest Service.[171]

What was scarce, in the sense of being in short supply, was taxol, but that bottleneck had been broken by 1991 and 1992. The question that Boly should have been asking was why was it scarce before 1992 and what was so different in 1992 that would lead to the ending of scarcity?

Part of the answer to these questions has already been given in earlier chapters but it would be well to revisit them here. Prior to 1990, no single collection of *Taxus brevifolia* bark exceeded 60,000 pounds. There is nothing magical about the figure. It is simply based on a calculation of what the expected needs for taxol would be at a future time using a conversion formula to get from taxol back to bark. Before 1990, the demand for taxol came from those involved in clinical trials and, as we have seen, partly because of taxol's unique mechanism of action and partly because of the nature of the experimental tumours in which it had demonstrated activity, there was intense interest in the compound. The trouble was that there was more interest in it than supply of it. The supply problem turned on several factors. On the technical side, scaling-up was proving difficult but not impossible. Capacity was also a major problem. As we have seen, during the 1980s, it was believed within the NCI that there were very few companies in the United States capable of extracting and purifying large quantities of natural compounds. Scaling-up required capital investment and given the general lack of interest both in natural product medicines and anti-cancer agents among pharmaceutical manufacturers, there was probably a reluctance to invest. Added to that was the long process time between receiving the bark and formulating taxol ready for human consumption.

It is also important to remember that it took an enormous amount of bark to produce a tiny amount of taxol. During the 1980s, the generally accepted figure was 30,000 pounds of bark for one kilogram of taxol. Bark collections were costly. They also proved difficult. Forests were frequently shut down during part of the summer months and sometimes inaccessible because of late springs. We have provided evidence that costs, both of collecting and processing bark, were cutting into NCI budgets for which there was strong and growing competition from other programmes.

All of these factors, in their time and place, conspired to keep the supplies of taxol at a level below that of demand. But there was another and perhaps even more serious limiting factor: the extremely cautious nature of the procedure at the NCI by which compounds proceeded from experimental product to commercial drug and the assumptions about the kinds of compounds passing through the system.

The Decision Network, the NCI committee that decided which experimental compounds should progress through preclinical studies and then clinical trials, was established at a time when the vast majority of compounds passing through the system were synthetic. Indeed, the Decision Network operated on this assumption because the issue of supply was not built into any stage of the process. Supply was, therefore, seen as automatic. Samuel Broder, the Director of the NCI, said as much when he was quoted in 1991: 'Many times we have assumed in our development program infinite supply'.[172] Natural products, however, cannot be requisitioned at will. Because the Decision Network had not been tested on enough natural products, and because the NCI had cut its links with the botanists at the USDA, taxol's experience was, in many ways, a test case. Or, as Broder put it: 'This is a warning shot across the bow'.[173] This, compounded by the conservative nature of the Decision Network, doomed taxol to a state of crisis.[174]

Boly, as we argue, misrepresented the discourse of scarcity but on one point he was absolutely correct – the embarrassingly low level of knowledge about *Taxus brevifolia*. It is well to remember that what triggered environmental concern for the plight of *Taxus brevifolia* was, first, the call for 60,000 pounds of bark in 1987 and then for 750,000 pounds in 1991. Remember also, that the Fish and Wildlife Service declined the petition to list *Taxus brevifolia* because it was claimed to be abundant, quoting a figure of 130 million trees in support of its argument. Yet, as we know, the Forest Service had not done an inventory of *Taxus brevifolia*. Even Charles Bolsinger was taken aback by what he termed a 'crude approximation', and not knowing its provenance.[175]

The figure of 130 million *Taxus brevifolia* trees was reported several times in the press during 1991, but was supplanted by the figure of twenty-three million trees on Forest Service lands around the middle of the year. This figure, together with a tally of 6.5 million trees on Bureau of Land Management lands, first appeared in the press on 20 June 1991 and was culled from a joint Forest Service and Bureau of Land Management statement, published on 19 June 1991.[176] Shortly thereafter, James Overbay, the Deputy Chief of the Forest Service, restated the twenty-three million figure and it passed into the *Taxus brevifolia* discourse as a scientific fact.[177]

It was, however, only an estimate of the number of *Taxus brevifolia* trees and not an inventory. That had still not been done, despite the overwhelming need for it. Indeed, the mechanisms for undertaking an inventory of *Taxus brevifolia* on all Federal land were not instituted before 19 June 1991, when both the Forest Service and the Bureau of Land Management signed co-operative agreements with Bristol-Myers Squibb to supply the company exclusively with bark. From this point, it took eighteen months before the Forest Service, on 12 December 1992, declared that the results of its first inventory showed that there were approximately forty-one million trees over one inch in diameter.[178] The Bureau of Land Management had conducted its inventory during the summer months, using a different method, on its lands in Oregon and reported that there were over ten million trees growing.[179] A further ten million trees, it was estimated, were growing on private and State lands in Oregon, Washington and northern California.[180]

The slow manner by which a fairly reasonable count of *Taxus brevifolia* was made typified the slow pace of knowledge accumulation in general. At a conference on *Taxus brevifolia* in 1992 held in Corvallis, Oregon, and sponsored by the three leading Federal agencies involved in taxol and *Taxus*, the Forest Service, the Bureau of Land Management and the NCI, Tom Spies, a leading research ecologist with the Forest Service, remarked how little was known about the biology and ecology of the tree while it was being cut down and destroyed in the thousands.[181] The point was underlined and, indeed, made all the more urgent, in the Final Environmental Impact Statement on the Pacific Yew, published in September 1993, which decried the lack of knowledge of the tree's ecological role.[182] As Spies remarked, 'the lack of basic biological information on yew is a reminder that we know very little about the biology and ecology of most of our non-commercial forest plants'.[183]

The lack of knowledge about *Taxus brevifolia* had the effect of adding to its mystery as an understory species living a slow existence in the shadow of the giant species in the ancient forests of the Pacific Northwest. It certainly underpinned much of the media's construction of a battle between the tree and people. It provided for an easy slippage between the scarcity of taxol – that is, its low level of supply before the early 1990s – and the scarcity of *Taxus brevifolia*.

Cutting the Network

The year for *Taxus brevifolia* was 1992 when it had become indisputably a valuable species. It had a molecule, an approved drug, its own Act, its own management plans, a Council, an Environmental Impact Statement, a book and a biography, not to mention media coverage and countless millions in the United States and elsewhere who had heard, read about and were speaking of it.

Appearing again as a witness to a Congressional hearing on 25 January 1993, held by Oregon Democrat Ron Wyden, Chairman of the Committee on Small Business Subcommittee on Regulation, Business Opportunities, and Energy, focusing this time on the issue of the pricing of taxol, Zola Horovitz, the much-questioned Vice-President of Business Development and Planning at Bristol-Myers Squibb, announced that 'we do not plan to harvest pacific yew bark from Federal lands in the 1993 growing season'.[184] The announcement came as a surprise, even as a shock, to nearly everyone.

Horovitz's statement needs careful consideration. He announced that Bristol-Myers Squibb would not be taking bark from *Taxus brevifolia* from Federal lands during 1993. He also stated that Bristol-Myers Squibb would be producing significant amounts of taxol from a semi-synthetic process during 1993 and that the reliance on Pacific yew bark would come to an end in 1995.[185]

Horovitz said nothing about private or, indeed, state lands. The point is an important one because of how the various voices or interests around *Taxus brevifolia* aligned themselves with respect to space.[186] While one could be forgiven for thinking that *Taxus brevifolia* was a single species, this would be too simplistic. Indeed, there was the private *Taxus brevifolia*, the state *Taxus brevifolia* and the Federal *Taxus brevifolia* (split between the Forest Service and the Bureau of Land Management). Strange as it may seem, the voices we have heard speaking on behalf of *Taxus brevifolia*, those of the Native Yew Conservation Council and the Oregon Natural Resources Council, for example, were, in fact, only speaking for the Federal species partly because this was the most numerous and partly because they could realistically only hope to change Federal practices. It becomes far less strange when one remembers that, in the bigger picture, the controversy over *Taxus brevifolia* was a subset of the controversy over public lands.

Not least of those who reeled from the announcement was the team charged with conducting *Taxus brevifolia's* Environmental Impact Statement, which had just published its draft proposal and was preparing for the final version.[187] Reacting to the announcement, Susan Whitney, a member of the Forest Service's organizing team, was reported as saying that the plan, consisting of a proposal to harvest ten per cent of *Taxus brevifolia* over the following five years, was now hypothetical.[188] The anticlimax of the Environmental Impact Statement did not go unnoticed. Many of those who responded to the public invitation to comment early in 1993 questioned the purpose of the exercise given Bristol-Myers Squibb's announcement.[189] The agreements between the Forest Service, the Bureau of Land Management and Bristol-Myers Squibb led to the creation of a bureaucratic machinery that was now unsure of its position. As Susan Whitney put it: 'There's a lot of things we need to do to make this transition. We had geared up to provide the material for Taxol production. Now we see ourselves phasing that out.'[190]

The other casualty was the Native Yew Conservation Council. Though it tried to put a brave face on matters, Bristol-Myers Squibb's announcement undercut the Native Yew Conservation Council's raison d'être. David Pilz, the Council's President at the time, attempted to find a new way for the organization. He suggested that the Council turn its attention to encouraging yew regeneration programmes; to pressing for the use of *Taxus brevifolia* needles as a sustainable resource; to promoting the scientific study of yews; and to extending the practice of sustainable harvests to yews growing in other countries.[191] In this, Pilz was attempting to put *Taxus brevifolia* in a new context, focusing on the species in all of its spaces, public and private, domestic and foreign, and to redirect support for the tree outside the old-growth forest narrative. As he said: 'The tree of death: weapons, poisons, and hunting instruments; The tree of meaning: musical instruments and religious symbolism; The tree of life: indigenous medicines and now taxol. We owe this tree a great deal.'[192] Pilz strongly advocated a regeneration programme to return the population of *Taxus brevifolia* on public lands to their pre-timber harvest numbers.

But the fire was out in the Pacific Northwest. The International Yew Conference, the first of its kind convened by the Council on 12 and 13 March 1993 in Berkeley, California, took a broader political stance than the Council had been used to. They urged President Clinton, who had called for a Forest Summit in Portland on 2 April, 'to consider conservation of old growth forest ecosystems as a primary issue.'[193] Phil Hassrick, Vice-President of Hauser Northwest, a Board member and one of the Council's longest serving members, tendered his resignation on 3 March 1993. The membership list shrank and meetings became a rare event, attended by a mere handful.[194]

Hauser was another fatality. Amid dire predictions of lay-offs, the company's share value collapsed early in February by twenty-nine per cent to fourteen dollars per share.[195] In August of the same year 1993, Bristol-Myers Squibb announced that it would not be renewing the supply contract for taxol and that it would not be needing *Taxus brevifolia* after the expiry of their contract on 15 August 1994: Hauser shares plummeted, losing more than half their value and ending the day at $6.625.[196] Pulling the plug on Hauser was serious for the firm. Late in 1992, at the height of its relationship with Bristol-Myers Squibb, taxol-related business accounted for ninety-five per cent of the company's revenues.[197]

Jerry Rust's vision of a thriving mini-economy based on sustainable yew harvests fell apart immediately. Instead he applauded Bristol-Myers Squibb's decision. 'It's a tremendous victory for industry, science, cancer patients and the environment', he was quoted as saying.[198] As for the Oregon Natural Resources Council, they turned their attention to how other agencies, such as the FDA, were acting in respect of environmental practices and to the protection of other Pacific Northwest species.

Though newspapers routinely reported Bristol-Myers Squibb's announcement as 'out of the woods', in fact, it initiated a process of retreat from and not an abrupt departure from the forests of the Pacific Northwest. In the first place, Bristol-Myers Squibb and Hauser were required by the Pacific Yew Act to 'prevent the wasting of Pacific yew trees while successful and affordable alternative methods were developed.'[199] In other words, on those sites on Federal lands that had already been sold for timber and were destined for clear cutting, the companies involved were obliged to salvage the yew bark.[200] A representative of the Bureau of Land Management was quoted as saying that Hauser was expected to harvest almost one million pounds of green bark from Federal sites during 1993.[201] According to the Bureau of Land Management's own figures, the 1993 fiscal year harvest netted more than 100,000 pounds of green bark and the 1994 fiscal year harvest just over 86,000 pounds of green bark.[202] The Forest Service reported a harvest of 674,000 pounds of green bark in the 1993 fiscal year (October 1992–September 1993).[203] Hauser increased its relationships with private landowners and, in its own statements, reported that it was shifting the balance of its supply as much over to private sources as possible.[204] According to Hauser, they collected 1.5 million pounds of dry bark during 1993 from all sources.[205]

Bristol-Myers Squibb's decision, therefore, needs to be seen as one of phasing-out one process in favour of another. Without doubt, considering the level of bark harvests in 1991, 1992 and 1993, there was a substantial stockpile of taxol and more to come as the production process turned bark into compound.[206] In addition, the company had already agreed to purchase Bob Holton's semi-synthetic process. Holton's process used the taxol precursor, 10-DAB, extracted from the needles of *Taxus baccata* growing in the Himalayas and in Europe, and supplied to Bristol-Myers Squibb by Indena, a Milan-based bulk natural products supplier – early results of the semi-synthetic process were very encouraging.[207] Other explanations that peppered the media especially included the rising costs of bark collection attributed to environmental constraints and the growing success of Weyerhaeuser's plantation programme.[208]

Whatever the reason for their withdrawal, Bristol-Myers Squibb did shift towards the semi-synthetic process rapidly. On 23 December 1993, they filed a Supplemental New Drug Application with the FDA for the process. It was granted approval in the United States on 19 October 1994.[209]

The manufacture of taxol by a semi-synthetic process using renewable biomass from outside the United States had considerable impact on the political climate. For one, it finally broke the bark lock-in that had, for so long, driven taxol development. Bristol-Myers Squibb was no longer dependent on a finite and politically charged resource and free from the environmental politics of the Pacific Northwest. For another, Bristol-Myers Squibb could now take over the manufacturing of taxol directly. The company decided to locate its taxol manufacturing in its plant in Ireland. Except in its final form as a commercial product, taxol had now lost its American identity.[210]

With taxol removed from the political scene, it was now time for the cut. The Pacific Yew Act, it will be recalled, included a 'sunset' clause. On 14 February 1995, the Secretary of Health and Human Services notified the Secretaries of Agriculture and Interior that enough taxol was now being made from alternative sources, thereby bringing the Act's requirements to an end.[211]

Bristol-Myers Squibb's decision to withdraw from the Pacific Northwest cut networks that had been built so painstakingly with *Taxus brevifolia* as the key actor. Once cut, the networks disintegrated, leaving the tree without network support.[212] In terms of its identity, *Taxus brevifolia* had been transformed through network effects from a waste product to a valuable species. Now, in a world of cut networks, its identity was lost, left to float free. After more than thirty years, during which taxol and *Taxus brevifolia* were inseparable, the tie that bound them was severed.

Notes

1 For an interesting analysis of how network news treated the subject of old-growth forests and the spotted owl in the early 1990s see Liebler and Bendix, 'Old-growth forests' and Gilbert, 'A response'.

2 In the latter part of the 1980s and continuing to the present, a large number of books, conference proceedings and articles were published linking bio-diversity with the conservation of medicinal agents. See, for example, the following: Aylward and Barbier, 'What is biodiversity worth?'; Myers, *The Sinking Ark*; Newman, 'Earth's vanishing medicine cabinet'; Soejarto and Rivier, 'Intellectual property rights'; Plotkin and Famolare, *Sustainable Harvest*; Myers, *The Primary Source*; Grifo and Rosenthal, *Biodiversity and Human Health*; Eisner, 'Chemical prospecting'; Akerele, Heywood and Synge, *The Conservation'*; Takacs, *The Idea of Biodiversity*; and Wilson and Peter, *Biodiversity.*

3 A good collection of essays that bears directly on this point is Cronon, *Uncommon Nature.*

4 The literature on this is now vast. A seminal book was Hecht and Cockburn, *The Fate of the Forest.*

5 Caufield, *In the Rainforest*, p. 287. The book was originally published in 1984 but the Afterword, from which this quotation is taken, was added in 1991.

6 A sense of this can be gained from the following examples of publications: Caufield, 'The ancient forest'; Mitchell, 'War in the woods'; Findley, 'Will we save our own?'; Knize, 'The mismanagement'; Maser, *Forest Primeval*; Dietrich, *The Final Forest*; and Ervin, *Fragile Majesty.*

7 The chief estimates were those of: Spies and Franklin, 'Characteristics of old-growth'; Haynes, 'Inventory and value'; and Morrison, *Old Growth*. For a discussion of these, see Norse, *Ancient Forests*, pp. 243–252. See also Booth, 'Estimating'.

8 Booth, 'Estimating', p. 29.

9 Yaffee, *The Wisdom of the Spotted Owl*, p. 132.

10 Proctor and Pincetl, 'Nature', p. 693.

11 Proctor and Pincetl, 'Nature', p. 691 and Yaffee, *The Wisdom of the Spotted Owl*, pp. 140–151. Late-successional reserves are those areas of old-growth plus those areas beginning to show old-growth characteristics, as they were described in Old-Growth Definition Task Group, 'Interim definitions'. A full designation of federal lands as outlined in Option 9 can be found in Tuchmann et al., *The Northwest Forest Plan*, p. 78. Events since 1993 can be followed in Marcot and Ward, 'Of spotted owls' and Durbin, *Tree Huggers.*

12 Data from Forest Service, Region 6, 'Timber cut and sold, 1909–1997'.

13 See Dietrich, *The Final Forest* for a discussion of both kinds of attitudes.

14 *Time*, for one, made this point clearly in their coverage of the debate: see Lemonick, 'Whose woods are these?'.

15 This and the following exchange is from Subcommittee on Fisheries, etc. *Joint Hearing: Pacific Yew Act of 1991*, pp. 36–37.

16 Subcommittee on Fisheries, etc. *Joint Hearing: Pacific Yew Act of 1991*, p. 41.

17 A year before Chabner appeared as a witness in this hearing, the Division of Cancer Treatment had already recognized the problems in leaving supply considerations until the point when a particular compound showed anti-cancer activity. See Cragg et al., 'The taxol supply crisis'.

18 Chabner's response seems to have satisfied his interrogators as they neither pursued the issue any further nor asked representatives of these agencies the same question.

19 There is a good discussion of actor–network theory and identity in Michael, *Constructing*, pp. 79–104, 131–152.

20 See Callon, 'The state and technical innovation', Callon, 'Some elements' and Callon and Law, 'Agency'.

21 Callon and Law, 'Agency', pp. 502–504.

22 There is, in Callon and others' works, a veiled criticism of a whole literature dedicated to understanding symbols. For forests and trees, see, for example: Rival, *The Social Life of Trees*; Harrison, *Forests*; Schama, *Landscape and Memory*; Pakenham, *Meetings*; Smith, 'The value'; and Rolston 'Aesthetic experience'.

23 See Dietrich, *The Final Forest*, Robbins, 'The social context', and Dumont, 'The demise of community'.

24 Bolsinger and Jaramillo, '*Taxus brevifolia*'.

25 Other identities existed. Fencepost makers and firewood collectors, for example, valued *Taxus brevifolia* for its special characteristics and frequently salvaged what was left of the tree from slash piles or littering the floor of the clear-cut forest. *Taxus brevifolia* played a major part in Native American cultural history in this region and into British Columbia and Alaska. See Hartzell, *The Yew Tree*, and United States Department of Agriculture, Forest Service, *Pacific Yew: Final EIS*, Appendix, pp. L-1–L-8. A recent collection of essays on tree symbolism continues to reinforce the idea that identity is constructed at a point and not within a network of relations of people and things. See Rival, *The Social Life of Trees*, especially the essay by Bloch, 'Why trees'.

26 Not everyone's voice was heard. In particular, Native Americans, at least as they were represented by the Karuk Tribe of California, felt that their voice did not count, and that what they intended as prescriptive was taken merely as suggestive. See their comment on the Draft Environmental Impact Statement in United States Department of Agriculture, Forest Service, *Pacific Yew: Final EIS*, pp. A-298–A-303. On the issue of whose voices get to be heard in claims over the old-growth forests, see the excellent study on British Columbia by Willems-Braun, 'Buried epistemologies'.

27 Annual Report to the Food and Drug Administration, March 1991, p. 18.

28 Grever to various, 24 October 1990, NPB2/2 and Taxol Status Report, 8 January 1991, p. 11. Saul Schepartz, Deputy Associate Director of the Developmental Therapeutics Program of the Division of Cancer Treatment, in a letter of 12 February 1992, stated that Sam Broder, the Director of the National Cancer Institute referred to the supply problem as a 'national emergency' – GCB1.

29 Taxol Status Report, 27 November 1990, p. 9, NPBII.

30 Taxol Status Report, 8 January 1991, p. 11, NPBII and Annual Report to the Food and Drug Administration, Taxol, March 1991, p. 18.

31 Holmes et al., 'Phase II trial of taxol'.

32 The response rate varied from twenty-two per cent for the pretreated patients to sixty-two per cent for those untreated – Taxol Status Report, 4 August 1992, p. 5. The results were reported at the 1992 annual meeting of the American Society of Clinical Oncology and published in the following year – see Reichman et al., 'Taxol'.

33 Notes, 1988, NPBI/2.
34 Destito to Vishnuvajjala, 15 November 1989, DST.
35 Jackson to Downes, 21 November 1989, NPBIV.
36 Snader to Cragg, 8 November 1989, NPBIII.
37 Snader to Cragg, 8 November 1989, NPBIII.
38 Jackson to Downes, 21 November 1989, NPBIV.
39 Destito to Vishnuvajjala, 15 November 1989, DST.
40 Jackson to Downes, 21 November 1989, NPBIV.
41 This is all contained in Destito to Vishnuvajjala, 15 November 1989, DST.
42 Jones (Director of Timber Management, Forest Service) to Forest Supervisors, 23 August 1989, DST.
43 Jackson to Destito, 13 December 1989, NPBIV.
44 Destito to Jackson, 31 December 1989, DST.
45 Jackson to Downes, 29 January 1990, NPBIV.
46 Connolly to Downes, 28 February 1990, CON.
47 Destito to Jackson, 31 December 1989 and Destito to Jackson, 24 February 1990, both in DST.
48 Destito to Jackson, 14 March 1990, DST and Jackson to Anderson, 15 March 1990, NPBIV.
49 Jans to Destito, 3 April, 1990, DST. The actual amount of bark that Hauser received was 7,294 pounds.
50 Taxol Status, April 1990, FRD4; Cragg to Stull, 4 April 1990 and Cragg to 'To whom it may concern', 4 April 1990, both in NPBIII.
51 Cragg to 'To whom it may concern', 4 April 1990, NPBIII.
52 Cragg to 'To whom it may concern', 4 April 1990, NPBIII.
53 Cragg to Stull, 5 April 1990, NPBIII. And Taxol Status, April 1990, FRD4. This letter from Cragg is further proof that, in 1990, at least, forestry practices were still treating *Taxus brevifolia* as waste, whatever forestry officials were saying in public.
54 Jans to Destito, 6 April 1990, DST.
55 Jans to Destito, 6 April 1990, DST.
56 Destito to Jackson, 30 April 1990, DST.
57 Destito to Jackson, 30 April 1990, DST.
58 Schepartz to Broder, 9 May 1990, 'Progress Report on Taxol, FRD4 and Daughenbaugh to Snader, 9 May 1990, NPBII.
59 Jans to Connolly, 23 April 1990 and Jans to 'To whom it may concern', 24 April 1990, both in CON.
60 Agreement, Connolly and Hauser, 23 April 1990, CON.
61 See, for example, Jones (FS) to West Side Forest Supervisors, 2 May 1990, Jans to Norlin (BLM), 7 May 1990 and Jans to 'To whom it may concern', 7 May 1990, all in CON.
62 Agreement, Connolly and Hauser, 23 April 1990, CON.
63 Destito to Jackson, 30 April 1990, DST.
64 Jackson to Destito, 20 May 1990, DST.
65 Destito to Jackson, 14 June 1990, DST.
66 Taxus Survey Trip, 11–15 June 1990, Kenneth M. Snader and Gordon M. Cragg, 21 June 1990, FRD2.
67 This part of the visit revealed some extremely important specific information about how taxol varied in its concentration by part, season and species.
68 Thomas to Raub and Broder, 7 June 1990, DST.
69 Thomas to Raub and Broder, 7 June 1990, DST.

70 Thomas to Raub and Broder, 14 June 1990, DST.
71 Taxus Survey Trip, 11–15 June 1990, Kenneth M. Snader and Gordon M. Cragg, 21 June 1990, FRD2 and interview with John Destito, 26 February 1998.
72 Cragg and Snader to Brown (General Counsel, NCI), 5 July 1990, NPBIV.
73 Destito to Jans, 19 July 1990, DST.
74 Springer to Raub and Broder, 11 July 1990, DST. On the day before, Destito's lawyers finally received a letter from William Raub, the NCI's Acting Director, responding to the charges made in the two letters they had previously received. Raub maintained that the NCI did not have a bark contract with Hauser nor did it receive bark from any other supplier during the term of the contract with Advanced Molecular Technologies. He also remarked that Bristol-Myers Squibb had asked Hauser 'to explore potential sources for bark collection' as part of the overall CRADA negotiations. Raub to Thomas, 10 July 1990, DST.
75 Jans to Destito, 13 July 1990 and Jans to Destito, 28 August 1990, both in DST. By the end of November, nothing had changed in this regard. Destito told Dianne DeFuria of the Licensing Group at Bristol-Myers Squibb that working as part of the Hauser network was unlikely – DeFuria to Destito, 20 November 1990, DST.
76 Destito, 'Outline of events', in DST.
77 Jans, 'Bark collection report', 20 August 1990, CON. The NCI thought the target amount was 400,000 pounds – Cragg and Snader to Grever, 26 September 1990, GCB2.
78 Cragg and Snader to Grever, 26 September 1990, GCB2 and Canetta and Kuhn (Bristol-Myers Squibb) to file, 29 October 1990.
79 Snader, Notes, 'Taxol Project Meeting II', 18 October 1990, NPBII.
80 Connolly to Jans, 17 September 1990, NPBII.
81 Connolly to Jackson, 1 October 1990, NPBII.
82 Connolly to Jackson, 1 October 1990, NPBII and Connolly to DeFuria, 21 October 1990.
83 Jans told Destito that the company had suspended the collection of limbs and needles while they awaited further investigation of their suitability as a raw material – Jans to Destito, 13 July 1990, DST. It is not known when Hauser informed Connolly and Ehrheart but by the end of August, Ehrheart was complaining to Jans about the change in the nature of the contract – Ehrheart to Jans, 28 August 1990, CON.
84 Ehrheart to Jans, 28 August 1990, CON.
85 Jans to Ehrheart, 30 August 1990, CON.
86 Connolly to Jans, 24 September 1990, CON.
87 Connolly to Jans, 24 September 1990, CON.
88 Connolly to Jans, 24 September 1990, CON.
89 Connolly to DeFuria, 21 October 1990 and Connolly's notes, October 1990, both in CON. Connolly was in debt at this point to the tune of $40,000 and admits he had no real option but to sell up – Interview with Connolly, 17 April 1997.
90 Interview with Ehrheart, 12 April 1999. According to his own records, Ehrheart collected over 470,000 pounds of green bark in 1992 and over 600,000 pounds in 1993.
91 'Taxol Status Report', 8 January 1991, NPBII and Canetta and Kuhn to List, 29 October 1990, NPBII.

92 Sander's notes, 18 October meeting, FRD4.
93 The amount of bark that could be harvested from a single *Taxus brevifolia* tree was a very contentious issue and figures varied wildly. The estimate here uses seven pounds of bark per tree – Blume, 'Investigators'. Comprehensive data on the bark poundage distribution according to tree diameter were not assembled until late in 1992. The data showed a huge difference in the average amount of bark depending on diameter. For example, a three-inch diameter tree yielded two to five pounds of bark; a ten-inch tree yielded thirty to forty pounds while a twenty-inch tree yielded eighty to 120 pounds of bark. See United States Department of Agriculture, Forest Service, *Pacific Yew: Draft EIS*, p. III-17.
94 Information on what was discussed at this meeting is in a memo, Schepartz to Grever, 17 July 1990, FRD1 and in Interview with Michael Bean, 8 April 1997 and Interview with Bruce Manheim, 9 April 1997.
95 An 'endangered' species is 'any species which is in danger of extinction throughout all or a significant portion of its range': a 'threatened species' is 'any species which is likely to become an endangered species within the foreseeable future throughout all or a significant portion of its range' – Coggins and Harris, 'The greening of American law' p. 278. On the politics of endangered species and a critique of the bureaucratic machinery involved, see the fascinating case study of the black-footed ferret in Clark and Westrum, 'Paradigms and ferrets'.
96 Schepartz to Grever, 17 July 1990, FRD1.
97 Environmental Defense Fund, Fact Sheet.
98 Coggins and Harris, 'The greening of American law'. This article provides an excellent overview of the nature of the Endangered Species Act as it evolved and was practised with respect to plants and animals until the late 1980s.
99 Interview with Michael Bean, 8 April 1997 and Interview with Bruce Manheim, 9 April 1997.
100 Norse, *Ancient Forests*, pp. 110–111.
101 Manheim to Cragg/Snader, 6 August 1990, NPB(S).
102 Interview with Bruce Manheim, 9 April 1997.
103 Manheim et al. to Lujan, 19 September 1990, EDF.
104 The following discussion draws on the response by the Fish and Wildlife Service of the Department of the Interior to the petition. See *Federal Register*, 56, no. 159, 16 August 1991.
105 Philpot (Station Director, Forest Service PNW) to Deputy Chief for Research, 30 October 1990, including Chuck Bolsinger's notes on *Taxus brevifolia* for 28 September 1990. See also Bolsinger's notes 18 May 1988, BOL and Bolsinger and Jaramillo, '*Taxus brevifolia*'.
106 Interview with Michael Bean, 8 April 1990.
107 Kenneth M. Snader, Speaker abstract, 'Workshop on Taxol and *Taxus*: Current and future perspectives', 26 June 1990, Bethesda, MD.
108 Kenneth M. Snader, Speaker abstract, 'Workshop on Taxol and *Taxus*: Current and future perspectives', 26 June 1990, Bethesda, MD.
109 Charles L. Bolsinger, Speaker abstract, 'Workshop on Taxol and *Taxus*: Current and future perspectives', 26 June 1990, Bethesda, MD.
110 Edward M. Croom, Jr., Speaker abstract, 'Workshop on Taxol and *Taxus*: Current and future perspectives', 26 June 1990, Bethesda, MD.
111 Interview with Stanley Scher and Shimon Schwarzschild, 31 October 1998.

112 Statement, 'Yew group urges conservation of a strategic resource', 13 July 1990, CON.
113 Bruno Latour introduced this idea in his book on Pasteur. See Latour, *The Pasteurization*, pp. 43–49.
114 Meeting notes, Yew Conservation Group Meeting, 24 August 1990, DST.
115 The following is adapted from Meeting notes, Yew Conservation Group Meeting, 24 August 1990, DST.
116 Stan Scher told the meeting that before it began he had received a telephone call from someone who would only identify himself as a member of the medical community. The caller wanted to know why this conservation group wanted to stop the taxol programme by blocking the collections. The debate over taxol over the next year or so became highly polarized. A typical headline, 'Is a tree worth a life?', was used in a much-quoted *Newsweek* article from October 1991.
117 Material emanating from the Medford meeting can be found in CON.
118 Schulz and Luoma to Bean and Kerr (Oregon Natural Resource Council), 5 October 1990.
119 The quote is from an interview with Michael Bean, 8 April 1997. Bruce Manheim made a very similar point – interview, 9 April 1997.
120 These tests are discussed in Chapters 3–5.
121 Witherup et al., *'Taxus* spp. needles'.
122 This paper was pre-circulated as 'The yew – a renewable economic resource for the Pacific Northwest'.
123 J. Rust, 'The yew – a renewable economic resource for the Pacific Northwest', p. 7.
124 J. Rust, 'The yew – a renewable economic resource for the Pacific Northwest', p. 1.
125 NYCC update, 'Taxofile', vol. 1, no. 1, Spring 1992, p. 1.
126 Hauser Northwest, '1991 yew harvest report: harvest from U.S.F.S. land', 6 November 1991, GCB2.
127 NYCC update, 'Taxofile', vol. 1, no. 1, Spring 1992, p. 1.
128 NYCC update, 'Taxofile', vol. 1, no. 1, Spring 1992, p. 2.
129 Vidensek et al., 'Taxol content'.
130 The letter is Snader to Connolly, 16 January 1991, CON. It was published in 'The Taxol *Taxus* Newsletter', vol. 1, issue 4, 18 June 1991, pp. 5–6, and sent to all members of the Council.
131 Hartzell, *The Yew Tree*.
132 Rust to BonFonte, 31 December 1991, CON.
133 Profiles of both men and their activities with the Oregon Natural Resources Council can be found in Durbin, *Tree Huggers* and Dietrich, *The Final Forest*.
134 Dietrich, *The Final Forest*, p. 211.
135 Subcommittee on Regulation, Business Opportunities, and Energy, *Hearing: Exclusive Agreements*, 29 July 1991, p. 172 and Monteith to Kaufman, 15 January 1988, WOD.
136 Interview with Wendell Wood, 15 April 1997.
137 This, and the following, when not cited specifically, is based on an interview with Wendell Wood, 15 April 1997.
138 An excellent outline of how these legislative statements contained the legal framework for changing forest practices so that a management plan could emerge specifically for *Taxus brevifolia* can be found in Heiken, 'The Pacific yew and taxol'.

139 Subcommittee on Regulation, Business Opportunities, and Energy, *Hearing: Exclusive Agreements*, 29 July 1991, pp. 172–173 and Borman, 'Scientists mobilize', p. 14. See also Oregon Natural Resources Council, Press Release, 'Yew needles, not bark, hold the most promise for future taxol production', 1991, WOD.

140 Statement of Wendell Wood, 5 November 1991, WOD.

141 Press Release, 15 November 1991, WOD.

142 The media were not the only ones to construct the events of the day in confrontational terms. Academics did it too. See, for example, Day and Frisvold, 'Medical research'. For an analysis of the events that takes a different perspective, see Walsh and Goodman, 'Cancer chemotherapy'.

143 Marilyn Chase, *Wall Street Journal*, 9 April 1991.

144 Press Release, Office of Congressman Gerry E. Studds, 'Studds bill would help cancer victims, conserve trees', 20 November 1991.

145 Congress of the United States, House of Representatives, *Pacific Yew Act of 1991*, 'Statement of the Honorable Gerry E. Studds', 20 November 1991.

146 Pacific Yew Act, H.R. 3836, p. 4.

147 Subcommittee on Fisheries, etc., *Joint hearing: Pacific Yew Act of 1991*, 'Statement of Bruce S. Manheim, Jr', 4 March 1992, pp. 211–221.

148 Calculated from Subcommittee on Fisheries, etc., *Joint hearing: Pacific Yew Act of 1991*, 'Statement of Bruce S. Manheim, Jr', 4 March 1992, pp. 215–216.

149 United States General Accounting Office, 'Cancer treatment: actions taken to more fully utilize the bark of Pacific yews on Federal land', 4 March 1992, in Subcommittee on Fisheries, etc., *Joint Hearing: Pacific Yew Act of 1991*, pp. 164–166.

150 Section 8 required that the Secretary of Health and Human Services inform the Secretary of Agriculture and the Secretary of the Interior of her/his intentions. Once they all agreed, then, after notifying the appropriate committees, the Act expired.

151 There was another Bill doing the rounds at about the same time as the Pacific Yew Act. Called The Ancient Forest Protection Act, it sought to conserve all old-growth-dependent species, including *Taxus brevifolia*.

152 Wendell Wood was quoted as saying that the theft issue was a smoke screen and diverting attention from the real issue – wasted bark resources from decades of clear cutting and slash burning. See Eric Nalder, 'Yew-bark "gold rush" prompts sting', *The Seattle Times*, 20 October 1991, p. A15.

153 Kathleen Monje, '$6,000 reward offered after bark stripped from 56 Pacific yews', *The Oregonian*, 30 May 1991, p. B4.

154 'Yew bark theft reported', *The Oregonian*, 21 October 1991, p. A8.

155 Eric Nalder, 'Yew-bark "gold rush" prompts sting', *The Seattle Times*, 20 October 1991, p. A15.

156 Devlin, 'Resource protection', Bradley, 'Resource protection'.

157 Pat Kight, 'Pacific yew bark theft declines sharply, officials say', *The Oregonian*, 4 August 1992, p. B4.

158 The data come from United States Department of Agriculture, Forest Service, *Pacific Yew: Draft EIS*, p. III-107 and Hauser Northwest, 'Taxol and Yew', 21 August 1992.

159 The data come from United States Department of Agriculture, Forest Service, *Pacific Yew: Draft EIS*, p. III-107 and Hauser Northwest, 'Taxol and

Yew', 21 August 1992. These are not the only data for bark harvests. Many other figures were bandied about. *The Oregonian* of 28 April 1993, for example, reported that 1.8 million pounds of bark was collected from Federal forests in 1992. It is interesting how the numbers vary even where documents are produced by the same organization. For example, at the 1993 Congressional Hearing on the pricing of drugs, one document from Bristol-Myers Squibb referred to 825,000 pounds of bark collected in 1991 as a result of their efforts on Forest Service and Bureau of Land Management lands, and a similar amount from private lands. In the press release dated the same time, the figure of 825,000 was taken as the total harvest from all land. See pp. 121 and 134.

160 Hauser Northwest, 'Taxol and Yew', 14 August 1992.

161 At the Second National Cancer Institute Workshop on Taxol and *Taxus*, held on 23 and 24 September 1992, Dean Stull and Neil Jans of Hauser Chemical Research reported that the company's production technology was capable of yielding one kilogram of taxol from 16,000 pounds of bark. In the company's in-house document, *Taxol: From Research to Reality*, originally published in 1992 and revised in 1994, they were able to report that the yield was now 13,000 pounds of bark per kilogram of taxol (p. 7).

162 Using similar data, Ed Croom has estimated taxol production between 200 and 246 kilograms – see Croom, '*Taxus* for taxol', p. 45.

163 This figure is calculated on the basis of an estimate of 20–25 kilograms of taxol needed to treat 12,000 women annually with ovarian cancer – see Cragg and Snader, 'Taxol: the supply issue', p. 233.

164 The clinical information is from Arbuck, 'Current status'.

165 See Hauser Northwest, 'Taxol and Yew', 31 July 1992. Gerry Kordon quoted in *Logger's World*, October 1991.

166 Gerry Kordon, a log buyer for Hauser Northwest, quoted in *Logger's World*, October 1991. Another estimate for the daily income of bark harvesters is between $100 and $150 – see United States Department of Agriculture, Forest Service, *Pacific Yew: Final EIS*, p. III-112.

167 Data from Debra Warren, *Production, Prices, Employment and Trade in Northwest Forest Industries, Second Quarter 1997*, Resource Bulletin PNW-RB-228. Portland, OR: US Department of Agriculture, Forest Service, Pacific Northwest Research Station, 1998, p. 25; Freudenburg, Wilson and O'Leary, 'Forty years of spotted owls?', p. 14; and Tuchmann et al., *The Northwest Forest Plan*, p. 150. The lumber and wood products industry includes logging, lumber and plywood. The major decline in employment was in logging and milling.

168 Croom, '*Taxus* for taxol', p. 45.

169 Boly, 'Wishing on a falling star'.

170 Boly, 'Wishing on a falling star', p. 64.

171 Daniel Luoma, past Vice-President, Native Plant Society of Oregon, e-mail, 18 November 1998.

172 *The Cancer Letter*, 18 October 1991, p. 3.

173 *The Cancer Letter*, 18 October 1991, p. 3.

174 Largely because of the difficult experiences with taxol, in 1991, the National Cancer Institute hosted a workshop on the large-scale production of natural products. The workshop brought together experts from a range of fields concerned with natural product drug development, but it also sought to develop strategies to avert the supply crisis that infected the taxol

programme. The workshop recommended that the Decision Network be revised in cases when a natural compound was passing through it; specifically to build into the Decision Network Points provisions for supply appropriate to those points. See Developmental Therapeutics Program, Division of Cancer Treatment, National Cancer Institute, 'Workshop on Large-Scale Production of Natural Products', Rockville, Maryland, 4 March 1991. See also Cragg et al., 'The taxol supply crisis' and Cragg and Snader, 'Taxol: the supply issue'.

175 Eric Nalder, 'Trials of taxol promising cancer drug is stalled in the forest – how the bureaucracy stalled the process of harvesting product from yew-tree bark', *Seattle Times*, 15 December 1991, A1.

176 Subcommittee of Regulation, Business Opportunities and Energy, *Hearing: Exclusive Agreements*, p. 158.

177 Subcommittee of Regulation, Business Opportunities and Energy, *Hearing: Exclusive Agreements*, p. 113.

178 USDA, Forest Service, Pacific Northwest Region, Forest Service News, 8 December 1992.

179 Richard Cockle, 'BLM finds yew trees in variety of areas', *The Oregonian*, 9 December 1992, B13. As it turned out, and unmentioned in the press, eighty per cent of the ten million figure was made up of yew shrubs with diameters less than one inch and too small to harvest for bark. The Bureau of Land Management estimated that just over two million trees of diameter exceeding one inch – possible to harvest – grew on their land. See United States Department of Agriculture, Forest Service, *Pacific Yew: Final EIS*, Appendix F-19.

180 United States Department of Agriculture, Forest Service, *Pacific Yew: Final EIS*, Appendices, vol. 2, F-22.

181 Spies, 'Conservation biology research', p. 11. Spies and Jerry Franklin had co-authored an extremely important and highly cited paper on forest dynamics of old-growth in which they proposed the idea of 'old-growthness' – see Spies and Franklin, 'Old growth'.

182 United States Department of Agriculture, Forest Service, *Pacific Yew: Final EIS*, pp. III-47–85. The available knowledge on the yew's ecosystem was collected in USDA, Forest Service, Pacific Northwest Region, 'An interim guide to the conservation and management of Pacific yew', March 1992, pp. 17–21.

183 Spies, 'Conservation biology research', p. 11.

184 Subcommittee on Regulation, Business Opportunities and Technology, *Hearing: Pricing of Drugs*, p. 9.

185 Subcommittee on Regulation, Business Opportunities and Technology, *Hearing: Pricing of Drugs*, p. 91.

186 This is not the place to go into the intricacies of legislation and its differential effects on public and private lands. For a rich and rewarding analysis as it pertains to the spotted owl issue, see Proctor and Pincetl, 'Nature'.

187 Under the terms of the National Environmental Planning Act (NEPA), whenever a Federal agency proposes an action that may have a significant impact on the environment, that agency is required to provide an Environmental Impact Statement (EIS). In 1991, in response to the bark harvest plans for that year of 750,000 pounds, the Forest Service, the Bureau of Land Management and the Food and Drug Administration joined co-operatively to prepare the EIS. On the background to and specific nature

of the document, see Campbell and Whitney, 'Pacific yew' and Heiken, 'The Pacific yew', pp. 221–228.

188 Harry Esteve, 'Taxol maker won't require public's trees', *The Register-Guard*, 30 January 1993.

189 There are many examples in United States Department of Agriculture, Forest Service, *Pacific Yew: Final EIS*, Appendix, vol. 1.

190 Quoted in Harry Esteve, 'Taxol maker won't require public's trees', *The Register-Guard*, 30 January 1993.

191 David Pilz, 'Where to now?', *Taxofile*, 1 June 1993, vol. 1/3, p. 2.

192 Pilz to Connolly, 17 April 1993, Native Yew Conservation Council, Heart of the Valley Environmental Conference, 'Yew harvesting/taxol update (not out of the woods yet, folks!)', CON.

193 B. Shimon Schwarzschild and Stanley Scher, 'NYCC convenes First International Yew Conference', *Taxofile*, 1 June 1993, vol. 1/3, p. 3.

194 Interview with Shimon Schwarzschild and Stan Scher, 31 October 1998.

195 'Hauser Chemical's share price plunges 29%', *The New York Times*, 2 February 1993, p. D4.

196 Milt Freudenheim, 'Bristol-Myers won't renew Hauser pact', *The New York Times*, 14 August 1993, p. 1/35.

197 'Hauser reaches taxol capacity at new plant', *Scrip*, 15 January 1993, no. 1786, p. 12.

198 Lance Robertson, 'Out of the woods: the frenzy over the taxol-producing yew tree fades', *The Register-Guard*, 28 September 1993.

199 Nelson (Acting State Director for Resource Planning, Use & Protection) to District Managers (Bureau of Land Management), 28 May 1998. This point appears to have been well-understood – see Pilz to Connolly, 17 April 1993, Native Yew Conservation Council, Heart of the Valley Environmental Conference, 'Yew harvesting/taxol update (not out of the woods yet, folks!)', CON.

200 Hauser Chemical Research, *Taxol: From Research to Reality*, p. 8.

201 'Yew harvest to go on despite synthetic find', *Seattle Times*, 28 April 1993, p. B2.

202 Bureau of Land Management, 'Yew bark sales and harvests, 1989–1998'.

203 Forest Service, 'Pacific Yew Harvest, USDA Forest Service, Fiscal year 1993', Pacific yew files, USFS, Portland, Oregon.

204 Hauser Chemical Research, *Taxol: from research to reality*, pp. 8 and 16 and 'Taxol and yew', vol. 2, issue 2, 1993 quoting Phil Hassrick.

205 Hauser Chemical Research, *Taxol: from research to reality*, p. 8.

206 Bristol-Myers Squibb was quoted as saying that 'it had a stockpile of 1.6 million pounds of yew bark' in February 1993 – 'Harvesting Pacific yew bark halted for year: no more needed', *Seattle Times*, 13 February 1993, p. A20.

207 'Bristol-Myers Squibb (BMS) signs taxol deal with Indena', *Scrip*, 8 July 1992, no. 1733, p. 11. Interview with Ezio Bombardelli, 22 November 1995.

208 Phil Hassrick, for example, was quoted as saying that Bristol-Myers Squibb was going to a cheaper supplier. He explained that Federal regulations on utilization (those promulgated by the Pacific Yew Act) were forcing Hauser to increase the labour intensity of their harvesting procedures because they were required to strip the small limbs in addition to the trunk of the tree. The rising marginal costs of labour, therefore, were driving Bristol-Myers Squibb out of the domestic market – see Lance

Robertson, 'Out of the woods: the frenzy over the taxol-producing yew tree fades', 28 September 1993.

209 Bristol-Myers Squibb, 'The development of Taxol® (paclitaxel)', March 1997, p. 10. See also 'New version of taxol is approved by F.D.A.', *The New York Times*, 13 December 1994, p. C6.

210 Milt Freudenheim, 'Bristol-Myers won't renew Hauser pact', *The New York Times*, 14 August 1993, p. 1/35.

211 Bureau of Land Management, 'Questions and answers; Pacific Yew Act', 12 February 1998.

212 Marilyn Strathern discusses how ownership, or the appropriation of things, cuts networks. One can think of Bristol-Myers Squibb doing the same through its ownership of taxol, lock, stock and barrel. See Strathern, 'Cutting the network' and also the discussion in Chapter 5 on ownership and trademark.

References and Bibliography

Abbott, B.J. 'Bioassay of plant extracts for anticancer activity.' *Cancer Treatment Reports* **60** (1976), 1007–1010.

Adair, John R. 'The bioprospecting question: should the United States charge biotechnology companies for the commercial use of public wild genetic resource?' *Ecology Law Quarterly* **24** (1997), 131–171.

Adams, Jonathan D., Flora, Karl P., Goldspiel, Barry R., Wilson, James W., Arbuck, Susan G., and Finely, Rebecca. 'Taxol: a history of pharmaceutical development and current pharmaceutical concerns.' *Journal of the National Cancer Institute Monographs* **15** (1993), 141–147.

Akerle, Olayiwola, Heywood, Vernon, and Synge, Hugh. *The Conservation of Medicinal Plants.* Cambridge: Cambridge University Press, 1991.

Anon. 'Photo-finish to artificial taxol.' *Chemistry and Industry* (21 February 1994), 125.

Arbuck, Susan G. 'Current status of the clinical development of taxol.' Speaker Abstract, Second National Cancer Institute Workshop on Taxol and *Taxus*, Alexandria: VA, 23–24 September 1992.

Arbuck, Susan G. and Blaylock, Barbara A. 'Taxol: clinical results and current issues in development.' In Suffness, Matthew (ed.), *Taxol®: Science and Applications*. Boca Raton, FL: CRC Press, 1995, 379–415.

Artuso, Anthony. 'Capturing the chemical value of biodiversity: economic perspectives and policy prescriptions.' In Grifo, Francesca and Rosenthal, Joshua (eds), *Biodiversity and Human Health*. Washington, DC: Island Press, 1997, 184–204.

Asbury, Carolyn H. 'Evolution and current status of the Orphan Drug Act.' *International Journal of Technology Assessment in Health Care* **8** (1992), 573–582.

Aylward, Bruce A. and Barbier, Edward B. 'What is biodiversity worth to a developing country? Capturing the pharmaceutical value of species information.' London Environmental Economics Centre, Discussion Paper DP 92-05, November 1992.

Averette, Hervy E., Janicek, Mike F., and Menck, Herman R. 'The national cancer data base report on ovarian cancer.' *Cancer* **76** (1995), 1096–1103.

Baker, C.G. 'Cancer research program strategy and planning – the use of contracts for program implementation.' *Journal of the National Cancer Institute* **59**, Supplement 2 (1977), 651–670.

Balandrin, Manuel F., Klocke, James A., Wurtele, Eve Syrkin, and Bollinger, Wm. Hugh. 'Natural plant chemicals: sources of industrial and medicinal materials.' *Science* **228** (1985), 1154–1160.

Balandrin, Manuel F., Kinghorn, A. Douglas, and Farnsworth, Norman R. 'Plant-derived natural products in drug discovery and development: an overview.' In Kinghorn, A. Douglas and Balandrin, Manuel F. (eds), *Human Medicinal Agents from Plants*. Washington, DC: American Chemical Society, 1993, 2–12.

Balick, Michael J. 'Botany with a human face.' *Garden* **14** (1990), 2–3.

Barclay, Arthur S. and Perdue, Robert E. Jr. 'Distribution of anticancer activity in higher plants.' *Cancer Treatment Reports* **60** (1976), 1081–1113.

Barclay, Arthur S., Gentry, Howard S., and Jones, Quentin. 'The search for new industrial crops II: *Lesquerella* (Cruciferae) as a source of new oil seeds.' *Economic Botany* **16** (1962), 95–100.

Barker, Tracey. 'Merck accelerates, Glaxo falters.' *Scrip Magazine* (January 1999), 39–40.

Bechtel, W. 'Integrating sciences by creating new disciplines: the case of cell biology.' *Biology and Philosophy* **8** (1993), 277–299.

Bechtel, W. 'Deciding on the data: epistemological problems surrounding instruments and research techniques in cell biology.' *PSA 1994: 2* Philosophy of Science Association: East Lansing, 1995, 167–178.

Belkin, Morris and Fitzgerald, Dorothea B. 'Tumor-damaging capacity of plant materials. I. Plants used as cathartics.' *Journal of the National Cancer Institute* **13** (1952), 139–155.

Belkin, Morris and Fitzgerald, Dorothea B. 'Tumor-damaging capacity of plant materials. III. Plants used as pesticides.' *Journal of the National Cancer Institute* **13** (1953), 889–893.

Belkin, Morris, Fitzgerald, Dorothea B., and Felix, Marie D. 'Tumor-damaging capacity of plant materials. II. Plants used as diuretics.' *Journal of the National Cancer Institute* **13** (1952), 741–744.

Ben-Menahem, Yemima. 'Historical contingency.' *Ratio* **10** (1997), 99–107.

Bennett, J.W. and Bentley, Ronald, 'What's in a name? – microbial secondary metabolism.' *Advances in Applied Microbiology* **34** (1989), 1–28.

Bentley, Ronald. 'Microbial secondary metabolites play important roles in medicine; prospects for discovery of new drugs.' *Perspectives in Biology and Medicine* **40** (1997), 364–394.

Bentley, Ronald. 'Secondary metabolites play primary roles in human affairs.' *Perspectives in Biology and Medicine* **40** (1997), 197–221.

Berman, Evan Michael. 'Technology transfer and the federal laboratories: a midterm assessment of cooperative research.' *Policy Studies Journal* **22** (1995), 338–348.

Bissery, M.-C. and Lavelle, F. 'The taxoids.' In Teicher, B.A. (ed.), *Cancer Therapeutics: Experimental and Clinical Agents*. Totowa, NJ: Humana Press, 1997, 175–193.

Bloch, Maurice. 'Why trees, too, are good to think with: towards an anthropology of the meaning of life.' In Rival, Laura (ed.), *The Social Life of Trees*. Oxford: Berg, 1998, 39–55.

Blume, Elaine. 'Investigators seek to increase taxol supply.' *Journal of the National Cancer Institute* **81** (1989), 1122–1123.

Bolsinger, Charles L. and Jaramillo, Annabelle E. '*Taxus brevifolia* Nutt.: Pacific yew.' In Burns, Russell M. and Honkala, Barbara H. (eds), *Silvics of North America*. Agricultural Handbook 654. Washington, DC: United States Department of Agriculture, Forest Service, 1990, 573–579.

Bolsinger, Charles L. and Waddell, Karen L. *Area of Old-growth Forests in California, Oregon, and Washington*. USDA, Forest Service, Pacific Northwest Research Station, Resource Bulletin PNW-RB-197, December 1993.

Boly, William. 'Wishing on a fallen star.' *Health* (September 1993), 63–69.

Booth, Douglas E. 'Estimating prelogging old-growth in the Pacific Northwest.' *Journal of Forestry* **89** (1991), 25–29.

Boring, Daniel and Doninger, Chris. 'The need for balancing regulation of pharmaceutical trademarks between the Food and Drug Administration and the Patent and Trademark Office.' *Food and Drug Journal* **52** (1997), 109–116.

Borman, Stu. 'Anticancer drug: boost to taxol supply planned.' *Chemical and Engineering News* **70** (9 March 1992), 4.

Borman, Stu. 'Scientists mobilize to increase supply of anticancer drug taxol.' *Chemical and Engineering News* **69** (2 September 1991), 11–18.

Borman, Stu. 'Total synthesis of anticancer agent taxol achieved by two different routes.' *Chemical and Engineering News* **72** (21 February 1994), 32–34.

Boyd, Michael R. 'Status of implementation of the NCI human tumor cell line *in vitro* primary drug screen.' *Proceedings of the American Association for Cancer Research* **30** (1989), 652–654.

Bradley, William L. 'Resource protection and accountability on Federal land.' In *Pacific Yew: A Resource for Cancer Treatment*. Conference: Oregon State University, Corvallis, OR, 3–5 August 1992, 17.

Brody, Baruch. 'Public goods and fair prices: balancing technological innovation with social well-being.' *Hastings Center Report* **26** (1996), 5–11.

Brooks, Browning. 'Tree holds hope in cancer war.' *Philadelphia Inquirer* (4 October 1987), A5.

Brush, Stephen B. and Stabinsky, Doreen (eds). *Valuing Local Knowledge: Indigenous People and Intellectual Property Rights*. Washington, DC: Island Press, 1996.

Bud, R.F. 'Strategy in American cancer research after World War II: a case study.' *Social Studies of Science* **8** (1978), 425–459.

Bugos, Glenn E. and Kevles, Daniel J. 'Plants as intellectual property: American practice, law, and policy in world context.' *Osiris* **7** (1992), 75–104.

Bull, J.P. 'The historical development of clinical therapeutic trials.' *Journal of Chronic Diseases* **10** (1959), 218–248.

Burk, D. 'Foreword.' In Moulton, Forest Ray (ed.), *Approaches to Tumor Chemotherapy*. Washington, DC: American Association for the Advancement of Science, 1947.

Callon, Michel. 'The state and technical innovation: a case study of the electrical vehicle in France.' *Research Policy* **9** (1980), 358–376.

Callon, Michel. 'Some elements of a sociology of translation: domestication of the scallops and fishermen of St Brieuc Bay.' In Law, John (ed.), *Power, Action and Belief: a New Sociology of Knowledge?* London: Routledge, 1986, 196–229.

Callon, Michel. 'Society in the making: the study of technology as a tool for sociological analysis.' In Bijker, W.E., Hughes, T.P., and Pinch, T.J. (eds), *The Social Construction of Technological Systems: New Directions in the Sociology and History of Technology.* Cambridge, MA: The MIT Press, 1987, 83–103.

Callon, Michel and Law, John. 'Agency and the hybrid *collectif*.' *The South Atlantic Quarterly* **94** (1995), 481–507.

Campbell, S.J. and Whitney, S.A. 'The Pacific Yew Environmental Impact Statement.' In Georg, Gunda I., Chen, Thomas T., Ojima, Iwao, and Vyas, Dolatrai M. (eds), *Taxane Anticancer Agents: Basic Science and Current Status.* Washington, DC: American Chemical Society, 1995, 58–71.

Cantor, D. 'Cortisone and the politics of drama, 1949–55.' In Pickstone, John V. (ed.), *Medical Innovations in Historical Perspective.* Basingstoke: Macmillan, 1992, 165–184.

Cantor, D. 'Cortisone and the politics of empire: imperialism and British medicine, 1918–1955.' *Bulletin of the History of Medicine* **67** (1993), 463–493.

Caporale, Lynn Helena. 'Chemical ecology: a view from the pharmaceutical industry.' *Proceedings of the National Academy of Science USA* **92** (1995), 75–82.

Capron, Terence F. and Strong, Carson M. 'Ethics of Phase I clinical trials.' *Journal of the American Medical Association* **249** (1983), 882–883.

Carter, Stephen K. and Livingston, Robert B. 'Plant products in cancer chemotherapy.' *Cancer Treatment Reports* **60** (1976), 1141–1156.

Carter, Stephen L. 'The trouble with trademark.' *Yale Law Journal* **99** (1990), 759–800.

Cassileth, Barrie R., Lusk, Edward J., Miller, David S., and Hurwitz, Shelley. 'Attitudes toward clinical trials among patients and the public.' *Journal of the American Medical Association* **248** (1982), 968–970.

Caufield, Catharine. *In the Rainforest.* Chicago: University of Chicago Press, 1984.

Caufield, Catharine. 'The ancient forest.' *The New Yorker* (14 May 1990), 46–84.

Chandler, A.D., Jr. *Scale and Scope: The Dynamics of Industrial Capitalism.* Cambridge, MA: Harvard University Press, 1990.

Chauvière, Gérard, Guénard, Daniel, Picot, Françoise, Sénilh, Véronique, and Potier, Pierre. 'Analyse structurale et étude biochimique de produits isolés de l'If.' *Comptes rendus de l'Académie des Sciences de Paris, Série II* **293** (1981), 501–503.

Clark, Tim and Westrum, Ron. 'Paradigms and ferrets.' *Social Studies of Science* **17** (1987), 3–33.

Clary, David A. *Timber and the Forest Service.* Lawrence, KS: University of Kansas Press, 1986.

Coggins, George Cameron and Harris, Anne Fleishel. 'The greening of American law?: the recent evolution of Federal law for preserving floral diversity.' *Natural Resources Journal* **27** (1987), 247–307.

Coghill, R.D. 'Preclinical program: plan of action – its philosophy and implementation.' *Cancer Chemotherapy Reports* **7** (1960), 29–41.

Cohen, Dorothy. 'Trademark strategy revisited.' *Journal of Marketing* **55** (1991), 49–59.

Colin, M., Guénard, D., Guéritte-Voegelein, F., Mangatal, L., and Potier, P. 'Preparation of baccatin III derivatives as antitumour agents.' *European Patent Application EP 336851, 11.10.1989* and *French Patent Application 884513, 6.4.1988.*

Commerçon, A., Bezard, D., Bernard, F., and Bourzat, J.D. 'Improved protection and esterification of a precursor of the Taxotere® and taxol side-chains.' *Tetrahedron Letters* **33** (1992), 5185–5188.

Condon-Rall, Mary Ellen. 'The Army's war against malaria: collaboration in drug research during World War II.' *Armed Forces & Society* **21** (1994), 129–143.

Corner, G.W. *A History of the Rockefeller Institute 1901–1953: Origins and Growth.* New York: The Rockefeller Institute Press, 1964.

Correll, D.S., Schubert, B.G., Gentry, H.S., and Hawley, W.O. 'The search for plant precursors of cortisone.' *Economic Botany* **9** (1955), 307–375.

Cragg, Gordon. 'Paclitaxel (Taxol®): a success story with valuable lessons for natural product drug discovery and development.' *Medicinal Research Reviews* **18** (1998), 315–331.

Cragg, Gordon M. and Snader, Kenneth M. 'Taxol: the supply issue.' *Cancer Cells* **3** (1991), 233–235.

Cragg, Gordon M., Boyd, Michael R., Cardellina, John H. II, Grever, Michael R., Schepartz, Saul A., Snader, Kenneth M., and Suffness, Matthew. 'Role of plants in the National Cancer Institute drug discovery and development program.' In Kinghorn, A. Douglas and Balandrin, Manuel F. (eds), *Human Medicinal Agents from Plants.* Washington, DC: American Chemical Society, 1993, 80–95.

Cragg, Gordon M., Schepartz, Saul A., Suffness, Matthew, and Grever, Michael R. 'The taxol supply crisis. New NCI policies for handling the large-scale production of novel natural product anticancer and anti-HIV agents.' *Journal of Natural Products* **56** (1993), 1657–1668.

Cragg, Gordon M., Newman, David J., and Snader, Kenneth M. 'Natural products in drug discovery and development.' *Journal of Natural Products* **60** (1997), 52–60.

Cragg, Gordon M., Newman, David J., and Weiss, Raymond B. 'Coral reefs, forests and thermal vents: the worldwide exploration of nature for novel antitumor agents.' *Seminars in Oncology* **24** (1997), 156–163.

Creech, John L. 'Tactics of exploration and collection.' In Frankel, O.H. and Bennett, E. (eds), *Genetic Resources in Plants – Their Exploration and Conservation.* Oxford: Blackwell Scientific Publications, 1970, 221–229.

Cronon, William (ed.). *Uncommon Ground.* New York: Norton, 1995.

Croom, Edward M. Jr. 'Taxus for taxol and taxoids.' In Suffness, Matthew (ed.), *Taxol®: Science and Applications.* Boca Raton, FL: CRC Press, 1995, 37–70.

Culliton, Barbara J. 'NIH, Inc.: the CRADA boom.' *Science* **245** (1989), 1034–1036.

Culp, O.S., Magid, M.A., and Kaplan, I.W. 'Podophyllin treatment of condylomata acuminata.' *Journal of Urology* **51** (1944), 655–659.

Danishefsky, Samuel J., Masters, J.J., Young, W.B., Link, J.T., Snyder, L.B., Magee, T.V., Jung, D.K., Isaacs, R.C.A., Bornmann, W.G., Alaimo, C.A., Coburn, C.A., and Di Grandi, M.J. 'Total synthesis of baccatin III and taxol.' *Journal of the American Chemical Society* **118** (1996), 2843–2859.

Dann, Kevin and Mitman, Gregg. 'Essay review: Exploring the borders of environmental history and the history of ecology.' *Journal of the History of Biology* **30** (1997), 291–302.

Daugherty, Christopher, Ratain, Mark J., Grochowski, Eugene, Stocking, Carol, Kodish, Eric, Mick, Rosemarie, and Siegler, Mark. 'Perceptions of cancer patients and their physicians involved in Phase I trials.' *Journal of Clinical Oncology* **13** (1995), 1062–1072.

David, Paul A. 'Clio and the economics of QWERTY.' *American Economic Review* **75** (1985), 332–337.

Day, K.A. and Frisvold, G.B. 'Medical research and genetic resources management: the case of taxol.' *Contemporary Policy Issues* **11** (1993), 1–11.

DeBell, Dean S. and Curtis, Robert O. 'Silviculture and new forestry in the Pacific Northwest.' *Journal of Forestry* **91** (1993), 25–30.

Deignan, S.L. and Miller, E. 'The support of research in medical and allied fields for the period 1946 through 1951.' *Science* **115** (1952), 321–343.

Demain, Arnold L. 'Functions of secondary metabolites.' In Hershberger, Charles, L., Queener, Stephen W., and Hegeman, George (eds), *Genetics and Molecular Biology of Industrial Microorganisms*. Washington, DC: American Society for Microbiology, 1989, 1–11.

Demain, Arnold L. 'Microbial secondary metabolism for academia and industry.' In *Secondary Metabolites: Their Function and Evolution*. Ciba Foundation Symposium 171. Chichester: John Wiley, 1992, 3–23.

Denis, Jean-Noël, Greene, Andrew E., Aarão-Serra, A., and Luche, Marie-Jacqueline. 'An efficient enantioselective synthesis of the taxol side chain.' *Journal of Organic Chemistry* **51** (1986), 46–50.

Denis, Jean-Noël, Greene, Andrew E., Guénard, Daniel, Guéritte-Voegelein, Françoise, Mangatal, Lydia, and Potier, Pierre. 'A highly efficient practical approach to natural taxol.' *Journal of the American Chemical Society* **110** (1988), 5917–5919.

Dennis, M.A. 'Accounting for research: new histories of corporate laboratories and the social history of American science.' *Social Studies of Science* **17** (1987), 479–518.

Devall, Bill (ed.). *Clearcut: The Tragedy of Industrial Forestry.* Washington, DC: Sierra Club Books/Earth Island Press, 1993.

DeVita, V.T., Oliverio, V.T., Muggia, F.M., Wiernik, P.W., Ziegler, J., Goldin, A., Rubin, D., Henney, J., and Schepartz, S. 'The drug development and clinical trials programs of the Division of Cancer Treatment, National Cancer Institute.' *Cancer Clinical Trials* **2** (1979), 195–216.

Devlin, Robert. 'Resource protection and accountability on Federal land.' In *Pacific Yew: A Resource for Cancer Treatment.* Conference: Oregon State University, Corvallis, OR, 3–5 September 1992, 16.

Dietrich, William. *The Final Forest: The Battle for the Last Great Trees of the Pacific Northwest.* New York: Penguin, 1993.

DiMasi, Joseph A., Seibring, Mark A., and Lasagna, Louis. 'New drug development in the United States from 1963 to 1992.' *Clinical Pharmacology & Therapeutics* 55 (1994), 609–622.

Donehower, Ross C. 'The clinical development of paclitaxel.' *Stem Cells* 14 (1995), 25–28.

Donehower, Ross C., Rowinsky, Eric K., Grochow, Louise B., Longnecker, Stephen M., and Ettinger, David S. 'Phase I trial of taxol in patients with advanced cancer.' *Cancer Treatment Reports* 71 (1987), 1171–1177.

Douros, John and Suffness, Matthew. 'The National Cancer Institute's natural products antineoplastic development program.' In Carter, Stephen, K. and Sakurai, Yoshio (eds), *New Anticancer Drugs.* Berlin: Springer-Verlag, 1980, 21–44.

Driscoll, John S. 'The preclinical new drug research program of the National Cancer Institute.' *Cancer Treatment Reports* 68 (1984), 63–76.

Dumont, Clayton W. Jr. 'The demise of community and ecology in the Pacific Northwest: historical roots of the ancient forest conflict.' *Sociological Perspectives* 39 (1996), 277–300.

Durbin, Kathie. *Tree Huggers: Victory, Defeat and Renewal in the Northwest Ancient Forest Campaign.* Seattle, WA: The Mountaineers, 1996.

Dustin, Pierre. 'Microtubules.' *Scientific American* 243 (1980), 59–68.

Dyer, H.M. *An Index of Tumor Chemotherapy.* Washington, DC: Public Health Service, 1949.

Eagle, Harry. 'Propagation in a fluid medium of a human epidermoid carcinoma, strain KB.' *Proceedings of the Society for Experimental Biology and Medicine* 89 (1955), 362–364.

Einzig, A.I., Wiernik, P.H., Sasloff, J., and Gorowski, E. 'Phase II trial of taxol in patients with metastatic renal cell carcinoma.' *Cancer Investigation* 9 (1991), 133–136.

Eisenberg, Rebecca S. 'Public research and private development: patents and technology transfer in government-sponsored research.' *Virginia Law Review* 82 (1996), 1663–1727.

Eisner, Thomas. 'Chemical prospecting: a proposal for action.' In Bormann, F. Herbert and Kellert, Stephen R. (eds), *Ecology, Economics, Ethics: The Broken Circle.* New Haven, CT: Yale University Press, 1991, 196–202.

Eisner, Thomas. 'Chemical prospecting: a global imperative.' *Proceedings of the American Philosophical Society* 138 (1994), 385–392.

Endicott, K.M. 'The chemotherapy program.' *Journal of the National Cancer Institute* 19 (1957), 275–293.

Endicott, K.M. and Allen, E.M. 'The growth of medical research 1941–1953 and the role of public health service research grants.' *Science* 118 (1953), 337–343.

Erickson, Deborah. 'Secret garden: cell culture may provide a unique route to taxol.' *Scientific American* (October 1991), 121–122.

Eriksson, JoAnn H. and Walczak, Janet Ruth. 'Ovarian cancer.' *Seminars in Oncology Nursing* **6** (1990), 214–227.

Ervin, Keith. *Fragile Majesty: The Battle for North America's Last Great Forest.* Seattle, WA: The Mountaineers, 1989.

Erwin, D.O. 'The militarization of cancer treatment in American society.' In Baer, H.A. (ed.), *Encounters with Biomedicine: Case Studies in Medical Anthropology.* New York: Gordon and Breach, 1987, 201–227.

Estey, E., Hoth, D., Simon, R., Marsoni, S., Leyland-Jones, B., and Wittes, R. 'Therapeutic response in Phase I trials of antineoplastic agents.' *Cancer Treatment Reports* **70** (1986), 1105–1115.

Farnham, Timothy J. and Mohai, Paul. 'National forest timber management over the past decade: a change in emphasis for the Forest Service?' *Policy Studies Journal* **23** (1995), 268–280.

Farnsworth, Norman R. 'The pharmacognosy of the periwinkles: vinca and catharanthus.' *Lloydia* **24** (1961), 105–138.

Farnsworth, Norman R. 'How can the well be dry when it is filled with water?' *Economic Botany* **38** (1984), 4–13.

Farnsworth, Norman R. and Soejarto, Djaja Doel. 'Potential consequence of plant extinction in the United States on the current and future availability of prescription drugs.' *Economic Botany* **39** (1985), 231–240.

Farnsworth, N.R., Henry, L.K., Svoboda, G.H., Blomster, R.N., Yates, M.J., and Euler, K.L. 'Biological and phytochemical evaluation of plants. I. Biological test procedures and results from two hundred accessions.' *Lloydia* **29** (1966), 101–122.

Farnsworth, N.R., Akerele, O., Bingel, A.S., Soejarto, D.D., and Guo, Z.-G. 'Medicinal plants in therapy.' *Bulletin of the World Health Organization* **63** (1985), 965–981.

Fellers, Li. 'The medicine market.' *The Washington Post Magazine* (31 May 1998), 10–27.

Fett-Neto, Arthur, DiCosmo, Frank, Reynolds, W.F., and Sakata, Ko. 'Cell culture of *Taxus* as a source of the antineoplastic drug taxol and related taxanes.' *Bio/Technology* **10** (1992), 1572–1575.

Findley, Rowe. 'Will we save our own?' *National Geographic* (September 1990), 106–136.

Fitzgerald, Dorothea B., Belkin, Morris, Felix, Marie, D., and Carroll, Mary K. 'Tumor-damaging capacity of plant materials. IV. Conifers.' *Journal of the National Cancer Institute* **13** (1953), 895–903.

Fitzgerald, D.B., Hartwell, J.L., and Leiter, J. 'Distribution of tumor-damaging lignans among conifers.' *Journal of the National Cancer Institute* **18** (1957), 83–99.

Flam, Faye. 'Race to synthesize taxol ends in a tie.' *Science* **263** (1994), 91.

Flanagan, S.P. '"Nude", a new hairless gene with pleiotropic effects in the mouse.' *Genetic Research* **8** (1966), 295–309.

Flournoy, Alyson C. 'Beyond the "spotted owl problem": learning from the old-growth controversy.' *Harvard Environmental Law Review* **17** (1993), 261–332.

Franklin, Jerry F. and Spies, Thomas A. 'Characteristics of old-growth Douglas-fir forests.' In *New Forests for a Changing World*. Bethesda, MD: Society of American Foresters, 1984, 328–334.

Franklin, Jerry F., Cromack, Kermit Jr., Denison, William, McKee, Angus, Maser, Chris, Sedell, James, Swanson, Fred, and Juday, Glen. *Ecological Characteristics of Old-growth Douglas-fir Forests*. United States Department of Agriculture, Forest Service, Pacific Northwest Forest and Range Experiment Station, General Technical Report PNW-118, 1981.

Franklin, Jerry F., Hall, F., Laudenslayer, W., Maser, C., Nunan, J., Poppino, J., Ralph, C.J., and Spies, T. 'Interim definitions for old-growth Douglas-fir and mixed-conifer forests in the Pacific Northwest and California.' United States Department of Agriculture, Forest Service, Pacific Northwest Research Station, Research Note PNW-447, July 1986.

Franklin, Sarah. 'Science as culture, culture as science.' *Annual Review of Anthropology* **24** (1995), 163–184.

Freudenburg, William R., Wilson, Lisa J., and O'Leary, Daniel J. 'Forty years of spotted owls? A longitudinal analysis of logging industry job losses.' *Sociological Perspectives* **41** (1998), 1–26.

Fuchs, David A. and Johnson, Randall K. 'Cytological evidence that taxol, an antineoplastic agent from *Taxus brevifolia*, acts as a mitotic spindle poison.' *Cancer Treatment Reports* **62** (1978), 1219–1222.

Fujimura, Joan H. 'The molecular biological bandwagon in cancer research: where social worlds meet.' *Social Problems* **35** (1988), 261–283.

Gartler, Stanley M. 'Apparent HeLa cell contamination of human heteroploid cell lines.' *Nature* **217** (1968), 750–751.

Gaudillière, Jean-Paul. 'Essay review: Cancer and science: the hundred years war.' *Journal of the History of Biology* **31** (1998), 279–288.

Gentry, Howard S. with Hadley, Diana. ' "Listening to my mind": Howard Scott Gentry's recollections of the Río Mayo.' *Journal of the Southwest* **37** (1995), 178–245.

Geran, R.I., Greenberg, N.H., Macdonald, M.M., Schumacher, A.M., and Abbott, B.J. 'Protocols for screening chemical agents and natural products against animal tumors and other biological systems (third edition).' *Cancer Chemotherapy Reports* **3** (1972), 1–103.

Gibson, D.M., Ketchum, R.E.B., Vance, N.C., and Christen, A.A. 'Initiation and growth of cell lines of *Taxus brevifolia* (Pacific yew).' *Plant Cell Reports* **12** (1993), 479–482.

Gibson, Donna M., Ketchum, Raymond E.B., Hirasuna, Thomas J., and Shuler, Michael L. 'Potential of plant cell culture for taxane production.' In Suffness, Matthew (ed.), *Taxol®: Science and Applications*. Boca Raton, FL: CRC Press, 1995, 71–95.

Gilbert, Sarah Ann. 'A response to "Old-growth forests on network news: news sources and the framing of an environmental controversy".' *Journalism & Mass Communication Quarterly* **74** (1997), 883–885.

Gillis, Anna Maria. 'The new forestry: an ecosystem approach to land management.' *BioScience* **40** (1990), 558–562.

Gilman, A. and Philips, F.S. 'The biological actions and therapeutic application of the β-chloroethyl amines and sulfides.' *Science* **103** (1946) 409–415.

Giovanella, B.C., Yim, S.O., Morgan, A.C., Stehlin, J.S., and Williams, L.J. Jr. 'Metastases of human melanomas transplanted in "nude" mice.' *Journal of the National Cancer Institute* **50** (1973), 1051–1053.

Giovanella, B.C. and Stehlin, J.S. 'Heterotransplantation of human malignant tumors in "nude" thymusless mice. I. Breeding and maintenance of "nude" mice.' *Journal of the National Cancer Institute* **51** (1973), 615–619.

Goldin, Abraham and Venditti, John M. 'Progress report on the screening program at the Division of Cancer Treatment, National Cancer Institute.' *Cancer Treatment Reviews* **7** (1980), 167–176.

Goldin, Abraham, Carter, Stephen, and Mantel, Nathan. 'Evaluation of antineoplastic activity: requirements of test systems.' In Sartorelli, Alan C. and Johns, David G. (eds), *Antineoplastic and Immunosuppressive Agents*. Berlin: Springer-Verlag, 1974, 12–32.

Goldin, Abraham, Schepartz, Saul A., Venditti, John M., and DeVita, Vincent T. 'Historical development and current strategy of the National Cancer Institute drug development program.' In DeVita, Vincent T. and Busch, Harris (eds), *Methods in Cancer Research*, Vol. XVI: *Cancer Drug Development*. New York: Academic Press, 1979, 165–245.

Golley, Frank Benjamin. *A History of the Ecosystem Concept in Ecology: More Than the Sum of the Parts*. New Haven, CT: Yale University Press, 1993.

Goodman, Jordan. 'Can it ever be pure science? Pharmaceuticals, the pharmaceutical industry and biomedical research in the twentieth century.' In Gaudillière, Jean-Paul and Löwy, Ilana (eds), *The Invisible Industrialist: Manufactures and the Production of Scientific Knowledge*. Basingstoke: Macmillan, 1998, 143–166.

Goodman, Jordan. 'Plants, cells and bodies: the molecular biography of colchicine, 1930–1975.' In de Chadarevian, Soraya and Kamminga, Harmke (eds), *Molecularizing Biology and Medicine: New Practices and Alliances, 1910s–1970s*. Amsterdam: Harwood Academic Publishers, 1998, 17–46.

Goodman, Jordan. 'The pharmaceutical industry in the twentieth century.' In Pickstone, John and Cooter, Roger (eds), *Medicine in the Twentieth Century*. Harwood Academic Publishers, 2000, 143–156.

Goodman, Jordan and Walsh Vivien. 'Attaching to things: property and the making of an anti-cancer drug.' Paper presented at 'ANT and After Workshop', Keele University, July 1997.

Goodman, L.S., Wintrobe, M.M., Dameshek, W., Goodman, M.J., Gilman, A., and McLennan, M.T. 'Nitrogen mustard therapy. Use of methyl-bis (betachloroethyl) amine hydrochloride for Hodgkin's disease, lymphosarcoma, leukemia and certain allied and miscellaneous disorders.' *Journal of the American Medical Association* **132** (1946), 126–132.

Gordon, A.S. 'Introductory remarks.' *Annals of the New York Academy of Sciences* **69** (1957), 527.

Gosselin, Raymond A. 'The status of natural products in the American pharmaceutical market.' *Lloydia* **25** (1962), 241–243.

Gould, Stephen Jay. *Wonderful Life: The Burgess Shale and the Nature of History.* London: Penguin Books, 1991.

Grabowski, H. and Vernon, J. 'Longer protection for increased generic competition in the US – the Waxman-Hatch Act after one decade.' *Pharmacoeconomics* **10** (1996), 110–123.

Grifo, Francesca, and Rosenthal, Joshua (eds), *Biodiversity and Human Health.* Washington, DC: Island Press, 1997.

Grifo, Francesca, Newman, David, Fairfield, Alexandra, S., Bhattacharya, Bhaswati, and Grupenhoff, John T. 'The origins of prescription drugs.' In Grifo, Francesca and Rosenthal, Joshua (eds), *Biodiversity and Human Health.* Washington, DC: Island Press, 1997, 131–163.

Grindey, Gerald B. 'Current status of cancer drug development: failure or limited success?' *Cancer Cells* **2** (1990), 163–171.

Grindley, June. 'The natural approach to pharmaceuticals.' *Scrip Magazine* (December 1993), 30–33.

Griswold, D.P. Jr. 'Consideration of the subcutaneously implanted B16 melanoma as a screening model for potential anticancer agents.' *Cancer Chemotherapy Reports* **3/2** (1972), 315–324.

Guéritte-Voegelein, F., Sénilh, David, B., Guénard, D., and Potier, P. 'Chemical studies of 10-deacetyl baccatin III. Hemisynthesis of taxol derivatives.' *Tetrahedron* **42** (1986), 4451–4460.

Haffner, Marlene E. 'Orphan products: origins, progress, and prospects.' *Annual Review of Pharmacology and Toxicology* **31** (1991), 603–620.

Hagen, Joel B. *An Entangled Bank: The Origins of Ecosystem Ecology.* New Brunswick, NJ: Rutgers University Press, 1992.

Hakala, Marie T. and Rustum, Y.M. 'The potential value of *in vitro* screening.' In DeVita, Vincent T. and Busch, Harris (eds), *Methods in Cancer Research.* Vol XVI: *Cancer Drug Development.* New York: Academic Press, 1979, 247–287.

Hamel, Ernest. 'Antimitotic drugs and tubulin-nucleotide interactions.' In Glazer, Robert I. (ed.), *Developments in Cancer Chemotherapy.* Boca Raton, FL: CRC Press, 1984, 131–164.

Hansen, Robert C., Cochran, Kenneth D., Keener, Harold M. Jr., and Croom, Edward M. Jr. '*Taxus* populations and clippings yields at commercial nurseries.' *HortTechnology* **4** (1994), 372–377.

Haraway, Donna. 'Universal donors in a vampire culture: it's all in the family: biological kinship categories in the twentieth-century United States.' In Cronon, William (ed.), *Uncommon Ground.* New York: W.W. Norton, 1996, 321–366.

Harrison, Robert Pogue. *Forests: The Shadow of Civilization.* Chicago: University of Chicago Press, 1992.

Hartwell, Jonathan L. 'Plants used against cancer. A survey.' *Lloydia* **30** (1967), 379–436.

Hartwell, Jonathan L. 'Types of anticancer agents from plants.' *Cancer Treatment Reports* **60** (1976), 1031–1067.

Hartwell, Jonathan L. *Plants Used Against Cancer. A Survey.* Lawrence, MA: Quarterman Publications, 1982.

Hartwell, Jonathan L. and Abbott, Betty J. 'Antineoplastic principles in plants: recent developments in the field.' In Garattini, S., Goldin, A., Hawking, F., and Kopin, I.J. (eds), *Advances in Pharmacology and Chemotherapy.* New York: Academic Press, 1969, 117–209.

Hartzell, Hal. *Birth of a Cooperative: Hoedads, Inc. a Worker Owned Forest Labor Co-op.* Eugene, OR: Hulogosi, 1987.

Hartzell, Hal. *The Yew Tree: A Thousand Whispers.* Eugene, OR: Hulogosi Press, 1991.

Hartzell, Hal and Rust, Jerry. *Yew.* Eugene, OR: Private, 1983.

Haynes, Richard W. *Inventory and Value of Old-growth in the Douglas-fir Region.* United States Department of Agriculture, Forest Service, Pacific Northwest Research Station, Research Note PNW-437, January 1986.

Hays, Finley, 'Advanced Molecular Technologies, Inc.' *Loggers World* **26** (February 1990), 29–33.

Hays, Samuel P. *Beauty, Health, and Permanence: Environmental Politics in the United States, 1955–1985.* Cambridge: Cambridge University Press, 1987.

Hecht, Susanna and Cockburn, Alexander. *The Fate of the Forest: Developers, Destroyers and Defenders of the Amazon.* New York: HarperCollins, 1990.

Heidemann, Steven R. and Gallas, Peter T. 'The effect of taxol on living eggs of *Xenopus laevis*.' *Developmental Biology* **80** (1980), 489–494.

Heiken, Douglas O. 'The Pacific yew and taxol: Federal management of an emerging resource.' *Journal of Environmental Law and Litigation* **7** (1992), 175–246.

Helfand, W.H., Woodruff, H.B., Coleman, K.M.H., and Cowen, D.L. 'Wartime industrial development of penicillin in the United States.' In Parascandola, John (ed.), *The History of Antibiotics: A Symposium.* Madison, WI: American Institute of the History of Pharmacy, 1980, 31–56.

Heller, J.R. 'The National Cancer Institute: a twenty-year retrospect.' *Journal of the National Cancer Institute* **19** (1957), 147–190.

Hess, David J. *Can Bacteria Cause Cancer? Alternative Medicine Confronts Big Science.* New York: New York University Press, 1997.

Hirt, Paul W. *A Conspiracy of Optimism: Management of the National Forests Since World War II.* Lincoln, NB: University of Nebraska Press, 1994.

Hodge, W.H. and Erlanson, C.O. 'Plant introduction as a federal service to agriculture.' *Advances in Agronomy* **7** (1955), 189–211.

Holmes, F.A., Kudelka, A.P., Kavanagh, J.J., Huber, M.H., Ajani, J.A., and Valero, V. 'Current status of clinical trials with paclitaxel and docetaxel.' In Georg, Gunda I., Chen, Thomas T., Ojima, Iwao, and Vyas, Dolatrai M. (eds), *Taxane Anticancer Agents: Basic Science and Current Status.* Washington, DC: American Chemical Society, 1995, 31–57.

Holmes, F.A., Walters, R.S., Thierault, R.L., Forman, A.D., Newton, L.K., Raber, M.N., Buzdar, A.U., Frye, D.K., and Hortobagyi, G.N. 'Phase II trial of taxol, an active drug in the treatment of metastatic breast cancer.' *Journal of the National Cancer Institute* **83** (1991), 1797–1805.

Holton, R.A. 'Synthesis of the taxane ring system.' *Journal of the American Chemical Society* **106** (1984), 5731–5732.

Holton, R.A., Juo, R.R., Kim, H.-B., Williams, A.D., Harusawa, S., Lowenthal, R., and Yogai, S. 'A synthesis of taxusin.' *Journal of the American Chemical Society* **110** (1988), 6558–6560.

Holton, R.A., Somoza, C., Kim, H.B., Liang, F., Biedeger, R.J., Boatman, P.D., Shindo, M., Smith, C.C., Kim, S.C., Nadizadeh, H., Suzuki, Y., Tao, C.L., Vu, P., Tang, S.H., Zhang, P.S., Murthi, K.K., Gentile, L.N., and Liu, J.H. 'First total synthesis of taxol: 1. Functionalization of the B-ring.' *Journal of the American Chemical Society* **116** (1994), 1597–1598.

Holton, R.A., Kim, H.B., Somoza, C., Liang, F., Biedeger, R.J., Boatman, P.D., Shindo, M., Smith, C.C., Kim, S.C., Nadizadeh, H., Suzuki, Y., Tao, C.L., Vu, P., Tang, S.H., Zhang, P.S., Murthi, K.K., Gentile, L.N., and Liu, J.H. 'First total synthesis of taxol: 2. Completion of the C-ring and D-ring.' *Journal of the American Chemical Society* **116** (1994), 1599–1600.

Horwitz, Susan Band. 'How to make taxol from scratch.' *Nature* **367** (1994), 593–594.

Horwitz, Susan B. and Horwitz, M.S. 'Effects of camptothecin on the breakage and repair of DNA during the cell cycle.' *Cancer Research* **33** (1973), 2834–2836.

Horwitz, Susan B. and Loike, John D. 'A comparison of the mechanism of action of VP-16-213 and podophyllotoxin.' *Lloydia* **40** (1977), 82–89.

Horwitz, S.B., Parness, J., Schiff, P.B., and Manfredi, J.J. 'Taxol: a new probe for studying the structure and function of microtubules.' *Cold Spring Harbor Symposium on Quantitative Biology* **46** (1982), 219–226.

Hounshell, D.A. 'Interpreting the history of industrial research and development: the case of E.I. du Pont de Nemours & Co.' *Proceedings of the American Philosophical Society* **134** (1990), 387–407.

Huang, Paul L., Huang, Philip L., Huang, Peter, Huang, Henry I., and Lee-Huang, Sylvia. 'Developing drugs from traditional medicinal plants.' *Chemistry and Industry* (20 April 1992), 290–293.

Infield, G.B. *Disaster at Bari*. New York: The Macmillan Co., 1971.

Jacobson, Martin J. 'Plants, insects, and man – their interrelationships.' *Economic Botany* **36** (1982), 346–354.

Joel, Simon P. 'Taxol and taxotère: from yew tree to tumour cell.' *Chemistry and Industry* (7 March 1994), 172–175.

Johnson, I.S., Wright, H.F., and Svoboda, G.H. 'Experimental basis for clinical evaluation of antitumor principles derived from *Vinca rosea* Linn.' *Journal of Laboratory and Clinical Medicine* **54** (1959), 830.

Jones, Quentin and Wolff, Ivan A. 'The search for new industrial crops.' *Economic Botany* **14** (1960), 54–68.

Joyce, Christopher. *Earthly Goods: Medicine-hunting in the Rainforest*. Boston, MA: Little, Brown and Company, 1994.

Karnofsky, David A. 'The nitrogen mustards and their application in neoplastic diseases.' *New York State Journal of Medicine* **47** (1947), 992–993.

Karnofsky, D.A. 'The bases for cancer chemotherapy.' *Stanford Medical Bulletin* **6** (1948), 257–269.

Karnofsky, David A. and Burchenal, Joseph H. 'Present status of clinical cancer chemotherapy.' *American Journal of Medicine* **8** (1950), 767–788.

Keller, E. Fox. 'Physics and the emergence of molecular biology: a history of cognitive and political synergy.' *Journal of the History of Biology* **23** (1990), 389–409.

Kelly, Margaret G. and Hartwell, Jonathan L. 'The biological effects and the chemical composition of podophyllin. A review.' *Journal of the National Cancer Institute* **14** (1957), 967–1010.

Kelsey, Rick G. and Vance, Nan C. 'Taxol and cephalomannine concentrations in the foliage and bark of shade-grown and sun-exposed *Taxus brevifolia* trees.' *Journal of Natural Products* **55** (1992), 912–917.

Kevles, D.J. 'Foundations, universities, and trends in support for the physical and biological sciences, 1900–1992.' *Daedalus* **121** (1992), 219–223.

King, Steven R. and Carlson, Thomas J. 'Biocultural diversity, biomedicine and ethnobotany: the experience of Shaman Pharmaceuticals.' *Interciencia* **20** (1995), 134–139.

Kinghorn, A. Douglas and Balandrin, Manuel F. (eds), *Human Medicinal Agents from Plants*. Washington, DC: American Chemical Society, 1993.

Kingston, David G.I., Hawkins, Douglas R., and Ovington, Liza. 'New taxanes from *Taxus brevifolia*.' *Journal of Natural Products* **45** (1982), 466–470.

Kirk, Ruth. *The Olympic Rain Forest: An Ecological Web*. Seattle, WA: University of Washington Press, 1992.

Klose, Nelson. *America's Crop Heritage: The History of Foreign Plant Introduction by the Federal Government*. Ames, IW: Iowa State College Press, 1950.

Knize, Perri. 'The mismanagement of the National Forests.' *Atlantic Monthly* (October 1991), 98–112.

Kopytoff, I. 'The cultural biography of things: commoditization as process.' In Appadurai, A. (ed.), *The Social Life of Things: Commodities in Cultural Perspective*. Cambridge: Cambridge University Press, 1986, 64–91.

Kreig, Margaret B. *Green Medicine: The Search for Plants that Heal*. London: George G. Harrap, 1965.

Kupchan, S. Morris, Komoda, Y., Court, W.A., Thomas, G.J., Smith, R.M., Karim, A., Gilmore, C.J., Haltiwanger, R.C., and Bryan, R.F. 'Maytansine, a novel antileukemic ansa macrolide from *Maytenus ovatus*.' *Journal of the American Chemical Society* **94** (1972), 1354–1356.

Lakoff, George and Johnson, Mark. *Metaphors We Live By*. Chicago: University of Chicago Press, 1980.

Landes, William M. and Posner, Richard A. 'Trademark law: an economic perspective.' *Journal of Law & Economics* **30** (1987), 265–309.

Lange, Jonathan I. 'The logic of competing information campaigns: conflict over old growth and the spotted owl.' *Communication Monographs* **60** (1993), 239–257.

Larrabee, Charles, X. *Many Missions: Research Triangle Institute's First 31 Years 1959–1990*. Research Triangle Park, NC: Research Triangle Institute, 1991.

Lasagna, Louis. 'Congress, the FDA, and new drug development: before and after 1962.' *Perspectives in Biology and Medicine* **32** (1989), 322–343.

Latour, Bruno. *Science in Action.* Cambridge, MA: Harvard University Press, 1987.

Latour, Bruno. *The Pasteurization of France.* Cambridge, MA: Harvard University Press, 1988.

Latour, Bruno. *We Have Never Been Modern.* Cambridge, MA: Harvard University Press, 1993.

Latour, Bruno. 'Do scientific objects have a history?' *Common Knowledge* **5** (1996), 76–91.

Law, John. 'Notes on the theory of the actor-network: ordering, strategy, and heterogeneity.' *Systems Practice* **5** (1992), 379–393.

Law, John. *Organizing Modernity.* Oxford: Blackwell, 1994.

Law, John and Hassard, John (eds). *Actor Network Theory and After.* Oxford: Blackwell, 1999.

Layne, Linda. 'Introduction.' *Science, Technology, & Human Values* **23** (1998), 4–23.

Leary, David E. 'Naming and knowing: giving forms to things unknown.' *Social Research* **62** (1995), 267–298.

Lehmann, Pedro A., Bolivar, Antonio, and Quintero, Rodolfo. 'Russell E. Marker: pioneer of the Mexican steroid industry.' *Journal of Chemical Education* **50** (1973), 195–199.

Lemonick, Michael D. 'Whose woods are these?' *Time* (9 December 1991), 70–75.

Lesch, John E. 'Chemistry and biomedicine in an industrial setting: the invention of the sulfa drugs.' In Mauskopf, S.H. (ed.), *Chemical Sciences in the Modern World.* Philadelphia: University of Pennsylvania Press, 1994, 158–215.

Levi, Daniel and Kocher, Sara. 'The spotted owl controversy and the sustainability of rural communities in the Pacific Northwest.' *Environment and Behavior* **27** (1995), 631–649.

Lewis, M.R. 'Inertness of sulfanilamide in relation to tumors in mice.' *American Journal of Cancer* **34** (1938), 431–433.

Lewis, M.R. 'The failure of purified penicillin to retard the growth of grafts of sarcoma in mice.' *Science* **100** (1944), 314–315.

Li, Jia-yao, Strobel, Gary, Sidhu, Rajinder, Hess, W.M., and Ford, Eugene J. 'Endophytic taxol-producing fungi from bald cypress, *Taxodium distichum.*' *Microbiology* **142** (1996), 2223–2226.

Liao, Lon-Lon, Kupchan, S. Morris, and Horwitz, Susan B. 'Mode of action of the antitumor compound bruceantin, an inhibitor of protein synthesis.' *Molecular Pharmacology* **12** (1976), 167–176.

Liebenau, Jonathan. 'Industrial R&D in pharmaceutical firms in the early twentieth century.' *Business History* **26** (1984), 329–346.

Liebenau, Jonathan. 'Paul Ehrlich as a commercial scientist and research administrator.' *Medical History* **34** (1990), 65–78.

Liebler, Carol M. and Bendix, Jacob. 'Old-growth forests on network news: news sources and the framing of an environmental controversy.' *Journalism & Mass Communication Quarterly* **73** (1996), 53–65.

Lilienfeld, Abraham M. '*Ceteris paribus*: the evolution of the clinical trial.' *Bulletin of the History of Medicine* **56** (1982), 1–18.

Lipsett, Mortimer B. 'On the nature and ethics of Phase I clinical trials of cancer chemotherapies.' *Journal of the American Medical Association* **248** (1982), 941–942.

Little, C.C. 'James Bumgardner Murphy.' *Biographical Memoirs of the National Academy of Sciences* **34** (1960), 183–203.

Little, Elbert L. Jr. 'To know the trees: important forest trees of the United States.' *1949 Yearbook of Agriculture*. Washington, DC: United States Department of Agriculture, GPO (n.d.), 763–814.

Löwy, I. 'Biomedical research and the constraints of medical practice: James Bumgardner Murphy and the early discovery of the role of lymphocytes in immune reactions.' *Bulletin of the History of Medicine* **63** (1989), 356–391.

Löwy, Ilana. 'Innovation and legitimation strategies: the story of the New York Cancer Research Institute.' In Löwy, Ilana (ed.), *Medicine and Change: Historical and Sociological Studies of Medical Innovation*. Paris: Editions John Libbey Eurotext, 1993, 337–358.

Löwy, Ilana. ' "Nothing more to be done": palliative care versus experimental therapy I advanced cancer.' *Science in Context* **8** (1995), 209–229.

Löwy, Ilana. *Between Bench and Bedside: Science, Healing, and Interleukin-2 in a Cancer Ward*. Cambridge, MA: Harvard University Press, 1996.

Löwy, Ilana. 'Cancer: the century of the transformed cell.' In Krige, John and Pestre, Dominique (eds), *Science in the 20th Century*. Amsterdam: Harwood Academic, 1997, 461–477.

Löwy, Ilana and Gaudillière, Jean-Paul. 'Disciplining cancer: mice and the practice of genetic purity.' In Gaudillière, Jean-Paul and Löwy, Ilana (eds), *The Invisible Industrialist: Manufactures and the Production of Scientific Knowledge*. Macmillan: Basingstoke, 1998, 209–249.

Luce, J.K., Thurman, W.G., Isaacs, B.L., and Talley, W.R. 'Clinical trials with the antitumor agent 5-(3,3-dimethyl-1-triazeno)imidazole-4-carboxamide (NSC-45388).' *Cancer Chemotherapy Reports* **54** (1970), 119–124.

Lythgoe, B. 'The *Taxus* alkaloids.' In Manske, R.H.F. and Holmes, H.L. (eds), *The Alkaloids: Chemistry and Pharmacology*, Vol. 10. New York: Academic Press, 1967, 597–626.

Lythgoe, B., Nakanishi, K., and Uyeo, S. 'Taxane.' *Proceedings of the Chemical Society* (1964), 301.

McCracken, R.J. 'Introduction.' *Cancer Treatment Reports* **60** (1976), 973–974.

McEvoy, Arthur F. *The Fisherman's Problem: Ecology and Law in the California Fisheries*. Cambridge: Cambridge University Press, 1986.

Macgregor, A.B. 'The search for a chemical cure for cancer.' *Medical History* **10** (1966), 374–385.

McGuire, William P., Rowinsky, Eric K., Rosenshein, Neil B., Grumbine, Francis C., Ettinger, David S., Armstrong, Deborah K., and Donehower, Ross C. 'Taxol: a unique antineoplastic agent with significant activity in advanced ovarian epithelial neoplasms.' *Annals of Internal Medicine* **111** (1989), 273–279.

MacKenzie, D. 'Marx and the machine.' *Technology and Culture* **25** (1984), 473–502.

McLaughlin, Jerry L., Miller, Roger W., Powell, Richard G., and Smith, Cecil R. Jr. '19-hydroxybaccatin III, 10-deacetylcephalomannine, and 10-deacetyltaxol: new antitumor taxanes from *Taxus wallichiana*.' *Journal of Natural Products* **44** (1981), 312–319.

Maasen, Sabine. 'Who is afraid of metaphors?' In Maasen, Sabine, Mendelsohn, Everett, and Weingart, Peter (eds), *Biology as Society, Society as Biology: Metaphors*. Dordrecht: Kluwer Academic Publishers, 1995, 11–35.

Mandelbaum-Shavit, Frederika, Wolpert-DeFilippes, Mary K., and Johns, David G. 'Binding of maytansine to rat brain tubulin.' *Biochemical and Biophysical Research Communications* **72** (1976), 47–54.

Marcot, Bruce G. and Thomas, Jack Ward. *Of Spotted Owls, Old Growth, and New Policies: A History Since the Interagency Scientific Committee Report*. United States Department of Agriculture, Forest Service, Pacific Northwest Research Station, General Technical Report, PNW-GTR-408, September 1997.

Marcus, Alan I. 'From Ehrlich to Waksman: chemotherapy and the seamed web of the past.' In Garber, Elizabeth (ed.), *Beyond History of Science: Essays in Honor of Robert E. Schofield*. Bethlehem, PA: Lehigh University Press, 1990, 266–283.

Marcus, G.E. 'Ethnography in/of the world system: the emergence of multi-sited ethnography.' *Annual Review of Anthropology* **34** (1995), 95–117.

Marks, Harry M. 'Cortisone, 1949: a year in the political life of a drug.' *Bulletin of the History of Medicine* **66** (1992), 419–439.

Marks, Harry M. *The Progress of Experiment: Science and Therapeutic Reform in the United States, 1900–1990*. Cambridge: Cambridge University Press, 1997.

Marks, Michelle. 'NIH CRADA panel hears complaints, recommends removal of "reasonable price" clause.' *Biotechnology Law Report* **13** (1994), 485–487.

Maser, Chris. *Forest Primeval: The Natural History of an Ancient Forest*. Toronto: Stoddart, 1991.

Max, Hannah L. 'Action woman: a portrait of Susan Band Horwitz.' *Taxane Journal* **2** (1996), 14–18.

Mendelsohn, R. and Balick, M.J. 'The value of undiscovered pharmaceuticals in tropical forests.' *Economic Botany* **49** (1995), 223–228.

Michael, Mike. 'Constructing a constructive critique of social constructionism: finding a narrative space for the non-human.' *New Ideas in Psychology* **14** (1996), 209–244.

Michael, Mike. *Constructing Identities*. London: Sage, 1996.

Miller, Roger W. 'A brief survey of *Taxus* alkaloids and other taxane derivatives.' *Journal of Natural Products* **43** (1980), 425–437.

Miller, Roger W., Powell, Richard G., and Smith, C.R. Jr. 'Antileukemic alkaloids from *Taxus wallichiana*.' *Journal of Organic Chemistry* **46** (1981), 1469–1474.

Mitchell, John G. 'War in the woods.' *Audubon* (January 1990), 82–121.

Montgomery, Scott L. 'Codes and combat in biomedical discourse.' *Science as Culture* **2** (1991), 341–390.

Morelli, I. 'Costituenti di *Taxus baccata* L.' *Fitoterapia* **47** (1976), 31–38.

Morrison, Peter H. *Old Growth in the Pacific Northwest: A Status Report.* Washington, DC: The Wilderness Society, 1988.

Moss, Ralph W. *The Cancer Industry.* Brooklyn, NY: Equinox Press, 1996.

Muggia, Franco M., McGuire, William P., and Rozencweig, Marcel. 'Rationale, design, and methodology of Phase II clinical trials.' In DeVita, Vincent T. Jr. and Busch, Harris (eds), *Methods in Cancer Research.* Vol. XVII. *Cancer Drug Development.* New York: Academic Press, 1979, 199–214.

Murdoch, Jonathan. 'Inhuman/nonhuman/human: actor-network theory and the prospects for a nondualistic and symmetrical perspective on nature and society.' *Environment and Planning D: Society and Place* **15** (1997), 731–756.

Murphy, J.B. 'An analysis of the trends in cancer research.' *Journal of the American Medical Association* **120** (1942), 107–111.

Myers, Norman. *The Sinking Ark: A New Look at the Problem of Disappearing Species.* Oxford: Pergamon Press, 1979.

Myers, Norman. *The Primary Source: Tropical Forests and our Future.* New York: W.W. Norton, 1984.

Nalder, Eric. 'Trials of taxol. Promising cancer drug is stalled in the forest – how the bureaucracy stalled the process of harvesting product from yew-tree bark.' *Seattle Times* (15 December 1991), A1.

Nelkin, Dorothy. 'Science controversies: the dynamics of public disputes in the United States.' In Jasanoff, Sheila, Markle, Gerald E., Petersen, James C., and Pinch, Trevor (eds), *The Handbook of Science and Technology Studies.* Thousand Oaks, CA: Sage, 1995, 444–456.

Nelson-Rees, W.A., Daniels, D.W., and Flandermeyer, R.R. 'Cross-contamination of cells in culture.' *Science* **212** (1981), 446–452.

Neushul, P. 'Science, government, and the mass production of penicillin.' *The Journal of the History of Medicine and Allied Sciences* **48** (1993), 371–395.

Neuss, N. and Neuss, M.N. 'Therapeutic use of bisindole alkaloids from *Catharanthus.*' In Brossi, A. and Suffness, M. (eds), *The Alkaloids. Antitumor Bisindole Alkaloids from* Catharanthus roseus (*L.*). New York: Academic Press, 1990, 229–239.

Neuss, N., Johnson, I.S., Armstrong, J.G., and Jansen, C.J. 'The *vinca* alkaloids.' *Advances in Cancer Chemotherapy* **1** (1964), 133–174.

Neuss, Norbert, Gorman, Marvin, and Johnson, Irving S. 'Natural products in cancer chemotherapy.' In Busch, Harris (ed.), *Methods in Cancer Research.* New York: Academic Press, 1967, 633–702.

Newman, Daniel. 'The great taxol giveaway.' *Multinational Monitor* **13** (1992), 17–21.

Newman, David J. 'Mother nature's pharmacy: a source of novel chemical structures.' *Society for Industrial Microbiology News* **44** (1994), 277–283.

Newman, Erin B. 'Earth's vanishing medicine cabinet: rain forest destruction and its impact on the pharmaceutical industry.' *American Journal of Law and Medicine* **20** (1994), 479–501.

Nicolaou, K.C. and Guy, R.K. 'The conquest of taxol.' *Angewandte Chemie International Edition English* **34** (1995), 2079–2090.

Nicolaou, K.C., Dai, W.-M., and Guy, R.K. 'Chemistry and biology of taxol.' *Angewandte Chemie International Edition English* **33** (1994), 15–44.

Nicolaou, K.C., Yang, Z., Liu, J.J., Ueno, H., Nantermet, P.G., Guy, R.K., Claiborne, C.F., Renaud, J., Couladouros, E.A., Paulvannan, K., and Sorensen, E.J. 'Total synthesis of taxol.' *Nature* **367** (1994), 630–634.

Nicolaou, K.C., Guy, R.K., and Potier, Pierre. 'Taxoids: new weapons against cancer.' *Scientific American* **274** (1996), 84–88.

Noble, David F. 'Social choice in machine design: the case of the automatically controlled machine tools, and a challenge for labor.' *Politics and Society* **8** (1978), 313–347.

Noble, Robert L. 'The discovery of the vinca alkaloids – chemotherapeutic agents against cancer.' *Biochemistry and Cell Biology* **68** (1990), 1344–1351.

Noble, R.L., Beer, C.T., and Cutts, J.H. 'Role of chance observations in chemotherapy: *vinca rosea*.' *Annals of the New York Academy of Sciences* **76** (1958), 882–894.

Norse, Elliott A. *Ancient Forests of the Pacific Northwest*. Washington, DC: Island Press, 1990.

O'Neill, Melanie J. and Lewis, Jane A. 'The renaissance of plant research in the pharmaceutical industry.' In Kinghorn, A. Douglas and Balandrin, Manuel F. (eds), *Human Medicinal Agents from Plants*. Washington, DC: American Chemical Society, 1993, 48–55.

Olmsted, Joanna B. and Borisy, Gary G. 'Microtubules.' *Annual Review of Biochemistry* **42** (1973), 507–540.

Ozawa, Connie P. 'Science in environmental conflicts.' *Sociological Perspectives* **39** (1996), 219–230.

Pakenham, Thomas. *Meetings with Remarkable Trees*. London: Weidenfeld & Nicolson, 1996.

Pantelouris, E.M. 'Absence of thymus in a mouse mutant.' *Nature* **217** (1968), 370–371.

Parks, Jean A. 'Taxol: a case study of biomedical research and pharmaceutical development in the United States.' Unpublished M.A. thesis, Michigan State University, 1994.

Patterson, James T. *The Dread Disease: Cancer and Modern American Culture*. Cambridge, MA: Harvard University Press, 1987.

Pauly, Philip J. 'The beauty and menace of the Japanese cherry trees: conflicting visions of American ecological independence.' *Isis* **87** (1996), 51–73.

Pazdur, Richard, Kudelka, Andrzej P., Kavanagh, John J., Cohen, Philip R., and Raber, Martin N. 'The taxoids: paclitaxel (Taxol®) and docetaxel (Taxotere®).' *Cancer Treatment Reviews* **19** (1993), 351–386.

Perdue, Robert E., Jr. 'Procurement of plant materials for antitumor screening.' *Cancer Treatment Reports* **60** (1976), 987–998.

Perdue, Robert E., Jr. 'KB cell culture. I. Role in discovery of antitumor agents from higher plants.' *Journal of Natural Products* **45** (1982), 418–426.

Perdue, Robert E., Jr. and Christenson, Gudrun G. 'Plant exploration.' In Janick, Jack (ed.), *The National Germplasm System of the United States*. Portland, OR: Timber Press, 1989, 67–94.

Perdue, Robert E., Jr. and Hartwell, Jonathan L. 'The search for plant sources of anticancer drugs.' *Morris Arboretum Bulletin* **20** (1969), 35–53.

Perdue, Robert E., Jr., Abbott, Betty J., and Hartwell, Jonathan L. 'Screening plants for antitumor activity. II. A comparison of two methods of sampling herbaceous plants.' *Lloydia* **33** (1970), 1–6.

Persinos, Georgia J. 'Bryostatin 1 – a winner from out of the blue.' *Washington Insight* **3** (15 December 1990), 7.

Persinos, Georgia J. 'The Pacific yew and cancer.' *The World and I (Washington Times)* (January 1991), 335–339.

Persinos, Georgia J. 'Taxol – thirty years in the wings.' *Washington Insight* **3** (15 September 1990), 7.

Pettit, George R. 'The scientific contributions of Jonathan L. Hartwell, Ph.D.' *Journal of Natural Products* **58** (1995), 359–364.

Plotkin, Mark and Famolare, Lisa. *Sustainable Harvest and Marketing of Rain Forest Products*. Washington, DC: Island Press, 1992.

Potier, Pierre. 'Contribution of an organic chemist to the resolution of some biological problems – consequences.' *Pure and Applied Chemistry* **58** (1986), 737–744.

Potier, Pierre. 'Search and discovery of new antitumour compounds: Rhône-Poulenc Lecture.' *Chemical Society Reviews* **21** (1992), 113–119.

Powell, Richard G., Miller, Roger W., and Smith, Cecil R. Jr. 'Cephalomannine; a new antitumor alkaloid from *Cephalotaxus mannii*.' *Journal of the Chemical Society: Chemical Communications* (1979), 102–104.

Price, Jennifer. 'Looking for nature at the mall: a field guide to the Nature Company.' In Cronon, William (ed.), *Uncommon Ground*. New York: W.W. Norton, 1996, 186–203.

Princen, L. H. 'New oilseed on the horizon.' *Economic Botany* **37** (1983), 478–492.

Proctor, James D. 'The owl, the forest, and the trees: eco-ideological conflict in the Pacific Northwest.' Unpublished Ph.D. dissertation, University of California, Berkeley, 1992.

Proctor, James D. 'Whose nature? The contested moral terrain of ancient forests.' In Cronon, William (ed.), *Uncommon Ground*. New York: W.W. Norton, 1996, 269–297.

Proctor, James D. and Pincetl, Stephanie. 'Nature and the reproduction of endangered space: the spotted owl in the Pacific Northwest and southern California.' *Environment and Planning D: Society and Space* **14** (1996), 683–708.

Proctor, Robert N. *Cancer Wars: How Politics Shapes What we Know and Don't Know About Cancer*. Basic Books: New York, 1995.

Prout, Alan. 'Actor-network theory, technology and medical sociology: an illustrative analysis of the metered dose inhaler.' *Sociology of Health & Illness* **18** (1996), 198–219.

Rabinow, Paul. *Making PCR: A Story of Biotechnology.* Chicago: University of Chicago Press, 1996.

Rachel, J. 'Acting and passing, actants and passants, action and passion.' *American Behavioral Scientist* **37** (1994), 809–823.

Rader, K. 'Making mice: C.C. Little, the Jackson Laboratory and the standard-ization of *mus musculus* for research.' Unpublished Ph.D. dissertation, University of Indiana, 1995.

Raffauf, Robert F. 'Plants as sources of new drugs.' *Economic Botany* **14** (1960), 276–279.

Raffauf, Robert F. 'Mass screening of plants for alkaloids.' *Lloydia* **25** (1962), 255–256.

Rasmussen, N. 'Facts, artifacts, and mesomes: practising epistemology with the electron microscope.' *Studies in the History and Philosophy of Science* **24** (1993), 227–265.

Rasmussen, N. 'Mitochondrial structure and the practice of cell biology in the 1950s.' *Journal of the History of Biology* **28** (1995), 381–429.

Reichman, B.S., Seidman, A.D., Crown, J.P.A., Hoolan, R., Hakee, T.B., Lebwohl, E.E., Gilewski, T.A., Surbono, A., Currie, V., Hudis, C.A., Yoo, T.J., Klecker, R., Jamis-Dow, C., Quinlivan, S., Berkery, R., Toomasi, F., Canetta, R., Fisherman, J., Arbuck, S., and Norton, L. 'Paclitaxel and recombinant human granulocyte colony-stimulating factor as initial chemotherapy for metastatic breast cancer.' *Journal of Clinical Oncology* **11** (1993), 1943–1951.

Remillard, Stephen, Rebuhn, Lionel I., Howie, Gary A., and Kupchan, S. Morris. 'Antimitotic activity of the potent tumor inhibitor maytansine.' *Science* **189** (1975), 1002–1005.

Rettig, R.A. *Cancer Crusade: The Story of the National Cancer Act.* Princeton, NJ: Princeton University Press, 1977.

Rhoads, C.P. 'Nitrogen mustards in the treatment of neoplastic disease. Official statement.' *Journal of the American Medical Association*, **131** (1946), 656–658.

Rhoads, C.P. 'The sword and the ploughshare.' *Journal of the Mount Sinai Hospital* **13** (1947) 299–309.

Rhoads, C.P. 'Rational cancer chemotherapy.' *Science* **119** (1954), 77–80.

Rival, Laura (ed.). *The Social Life of Trees.* Oxford: Berg, 1998.

Robbins, William G. 'The social context of forestry: the Pacific Northwest in the twentieth century.' *Western Historical Quarterly* **16** (1985), 411–427.

Rolston, Holmes III. 'Aesthetic experience in forests.' *Journal of Aesthetics and Art Criticism* **56** (1998), 157–166.

Rorty, R. *Contingency, Irony, and Solidarity.* Cambridge: Cambridge University Press, 1989.

Ross, Judith Wilson. 'The militarization of disease: do we really want a war on AIDS?' *Soundings* **72** (1989), 39–58.

Ross, Ronald B. 'Recent advances in chemotherapy of cancer.' *Journal of Chemical Education* **36** (1959), 369–377.

Rothenberg, L. and Terselic, R.A. 'Management of the National Cancer Institute's drug research program through application of the linear array concept.' *Cancer Chemotherapy Reports* **54** (1970), 303–310.

Rouhi, A. Maureen. 'Seeking drugs in natural products.' *Chemical and Engineering News* (7 April 1997), 14–29.

Rous, Peyton. 'Concerning the cancer problem.' *American Scientist* **34** (1946), 329–358.

Rowinsky, E.K., Donehower, R.C., Rosenshein, N.B., Ettinger, D.S., and McGuire, W.P. 'Phase II study of taxol in advanced epithelial malignancies.' *Proceedings of the Association of Clinical Oncology* **7** (1988), 136.

Rusch, Harold P. 'The beginnings of cancer research centers in the United States.' *Journal of the National Cancer Institute* **74** (1985), 391–403.

Russell, C.A. 'The changing role of synthesis in organic chemistry.' *Ambix* **34** (1987), 169–180.

Rygaard, J. and Poulsen, C.O. 'Heterotransplantation of a human malignant tumor to "nude" mice.' *Acta Pathologica et Microbiologica Scandinavica* **77** (1969), 758–760.

Satterfield, Theresa. ' "Voodoo science" and common sense: ways of knowing old-growth forests.' *Journal of Anthropological Research* **53** (1997), 443–459.

Schama, Simon. *Landscape and Memory.* New York: HarperCollins, 1995.

Schepartz, Saul A. 'Screening.' *Cancer Chemotherapy Reports* **2** (1971), part 3, 3–8.

Schepartz, Saul A. 'History of the National Cancer Institute and the plant screening program.' *Cancer Treatment Reports* **60** (1976), 975–977.

Schiff, Peter B., Fant, Jane, Auster, Lori A., and Horwitz, Susan B. 'Effects of taxol on cell growth and *in vitro* microtubule assembly.' *Journal of Supramolecular Structure* **8**, Supplement 2 (1978a), 328.

Schiff, Peter B., Kende, Andrew S., and Horwitz, Susan B. 'Steganacin: an inhibitor of HeLa cell growth and microtubule assembly *in vitro*.' *Biochemical and Biophysical Communications* **85** (1978b), 737–746.

Schiff, Peter B., Fant, Janet, and Horwitz, Susan B. 'Promotion of microtubule assembly *in vitro* by taxol.' *Nature* **277** (1979), 665–667.

Schultes, Richard Evans. 'Tapping our heritage of ethnobotanical lore.' *Economic Botany* **14** (1960), 257–262.

Schultes, Richard Evans. 'The role of the ethnobotanist in the search for new medicinal plants.' *Lloydia* **25** (1962), 257–266.

Schultes, R.E. and Raffauf, R. *The Healing Forest.* Portland, OR: Dioscorides Press, 1991.

Seidl, Peter Rudolph, Gottlieb, Otto Richard, and Kaplan, Maria Auxiliadora Coelho. *Chemistry of the Amazon: Biodiversity, Natural Products, and Environmental Issues.* Washington, DC: American Chemical Society, 1995.

Sénilh, Véronique, Guéritte, Françoise, Guénard, Daniel, Colin, Michel, and Potier, Pierre. 'Hémisynthèses de nouveaux analogues du taxol. Étude de leur interaction avec la tubuline.' *Comptes rendus de l'Académie des Sciences de Paris, Série II* **299** (1984), 1039–1043.

Sessoms, Stuart M. 'Review of the Cancer Chemotherapy National Service Center program.' *Cancer Chemotherapy Reports* **7** (1960), 25–28.

Shannon, Colleen. 'Chemists fight cancer without felling trees.' *New Scientist* (2 May 1992), 19.

Shapin, S. 'History of science and its sociological reconstructions.' *History of Science* **20** (1982), 157–211.

Shear, M.J. 'Some aspects of a joint institutional research program on chemotherapy of cancer: current laboratory and clinical experiments with bacterial polysaccharide and synthetic organic compounds: I. Scope of the program.' In Moulton, Forest Ray (ed.), *Approaches to Tumor Chemotherapy.* Washington, DC: American Association for the Advancement of Science, 1947, 236–241.

Shear, M.J. 'Role of the chemotherapy research laboratory in clinical cancer research.' *Journal of the National Cancer Institute* **12** (1951), 569–581.

Shelanski, M.L., Gaskin, F., and Cantor, C.R. 'Microtubule assembly in the absence of added nucleotides.' *Proceedings of the National Academy of Sciences* **70** (1973), 765–768.

Shuler, M.L. 'Production of secondary metabolites from plant tissue culture – problems and prospects.' *Annals of the New York Academy of Sciences* **369** (1981), 65–79.

Shuler, Michael L. 'Bioreactor engineering as an enabling technology to tap biodiversity: the case of taxol.' *Annals of the New York Academy of Sciences* **745** (1994), 455–461.

Shulman, Sheila, Bienz-Tadmor, Brigitta, Seo, Pheak Son, DiMasi, Joseph A., and Lasagna, Louis. 'Implementation of the Orphan Drug Act: 1983–1991.' *Food and Drug Law Journal* **47** (1992), 363–403.

Simpson, R. David, Sedjo, Roger A., and Reid, John W. 'Valuing biodiversity for use in pharmaceutical research.' *Journal of Political Economy* **104** (1996), 163–185.

Singleton, V. and Michael, M. 'Actor-networks and ambivalence: general practitioners in the UK Cervical Screening Programme.' *Social Studies of Science* **23** (1993), 227–264.

Skipper, H.E. 'Improvement in model systems.' *Cancer Research* **29** (1969), 2329–2333.

Smith, J.K. Jr. 'The scientific tradition in American industrial research.' *Technology and Culture* **31** (1990), 121–131.

Smith, Michael B. 'The value of a tree: public debates of John Muir and Gifford Pinchot.' *The Historian* **60** (1998), 758–778.

Snader, Kenneth M. 'Detection and isolation.' In Suffness, Matthew (ed.), *Taxol®: Science and Applications.* Boca Raton, FL: CRC Press, 1995, 277–286.

Soejarto, Djaja Djendoel and Rivier, Laurent (eds). 'Intellectual property rights, naturally derived bioactive compounds and resource conservation.' *Journal of Ethnopharmacology* **51** (1996), Special issue, nos 1–3.

Sontag, Susan. *Illness as Metaphor.* London: Penguin Books, 1991.

Spencer, R. R. 'The meaning of cancer research.' *Journal of the American Medical Association* **137** (1946), 1361–1364.

Spies, Thomas A. 'Conservation biology research.' In *Pacific Yew: A Resource for*

Cancer Treatment. Conference: Oregon State University, Corvallis, OR, 3–5 September 1992, 11.

Spies, Thomas A. and Franklin, Jerry F. 'Old growth and forest dynamics in the Douglas-fir region of western Oregon and Washington.' *Natural Areas Journal* 8 (1988), 190–201.

Spjut, Richard W. 'Limitations of a random screen: search for new anticancer drugs in higher plants.' *Economic Botany* 39 (1985), 266–288.

Spjut, Richard W. and Perdue, Robert E., Jr. 'Plant folklore: a tool for predicting sources of antitumor activity?' *Cancer Treatment Reports* 60 (1976), 979–985.

Stacey, Jackie. *Teratologies: A Cultural Study of Cancer*. London: Routledge, 1997.

Statz, DuWayne and Coon, Francis B. 'Preparation of plant extracts for anti-tumor screening.' *Cancer Treatment Reports* 60 (1976), 999–1005.

Steiner, Paul E. 'Emphasis in cancer research.' *Journal of the National Cancer Institute* 14 (1954), 1205–1221.

Stierle, Andrea, Strobel, Gary, and Stierle, Donald. 'Taxol and taxane production by *Taxomyces andreanae*, an endophytic fungus of Pacific yew.' *Science* 260 (1993), 214–216.

Stierle, Andrea, Strobel, Gary, Stierle, Donald, Grothaus, Paul, and Bignami, Gary. 'The search for a taxol-producing microorganism among the endophytic fungi of the Pacific yew, *Taxus brevifolia*.' *Journal of Natural Products* 58 (1995), 1315–1324.

Stock, C.C. 'Aspects of approaches in experimental cancer chemotherapy.' *American Journal of Medicine* 8 (1950), 658–674.

Stock, C.C., Clarke, D.A., Philips, F.S., and Barclay, R.K. 'Sarcoma 180 inhibition screening data.' *Cancer Research* 15, Supplement 2 (1955), 179–331.

Stock, C.C. Clarke, D.A., Philips, F.S., Barclay, R.K. and Myron, S.A. 'Sarcoma 180 screening data.' *Cancer Research* 20, no. 5/2 (1960), 193–382.

Stone, Christopher D. 'What to do about biodiversity: property rights, public goods, and the earth's biological riches.' *Southern California Law Review* 68 (1995), 577–620.

Strathern, Marilyn. 'Cutting the network.' *Journal of the Royal Anthropological Institute* 2 (1997), 517–535.

Strathern, Marilyn. 'What is intellectual property after?' In Law, John and Hassard, John (eds), *Actor Network Theory and After*. Oxford: Blackwell Publishers, 1999, 156–180.

Strickland, S.P. *Politics, Science, and Dread Disease*. Cambridge, MA: Harvard University Press, 1972.

Strobel, G.A., Hess, W.M., Ford, E., Sidhu, R.S., and Yang, X. 'Taxol from fungal endophytes and the issue of biodiversity.' *Journal of Industrial Microbiology* 17 (1996), 417–423.

Strobel, Gary, Yang, Xianshu, Sears, Joe, Kramer, Robert, Sidhu, Rajinder S., and Hess, W.M. 'Taxol from *Pestalotiopsis microspora*, an endophytic fungus of *Taxus wallichiana*.' *Microbiology* 142 (1996), 435–440.

Strong, Donald R. (ed.). 'Special feature–spotted owl.' *Ecology* 68 (1987), 766–779.

Strycker, Lisa. 'Cancer cure may be in common yew.' *The Register-Guard* (7 April 1987), 1B.

Subcommittee on Fisheries and Wildlife Conservation and the Environment, Committee on Merchant Marine and Fisheries; Subcommittee on Forests, Family Farms, and Energy, Committee on Agriculture; and Subcommittee on National Parks and Public Lands, Committee on Interior and Insular Affairs, House of Representatives. *Joint Hearing: The Pacific Yew Act of 1991.* Washington, DC, 4 March 1992, Serial No. 102-71 and Serial No. 102-61.

Subcommittee on Regulation, Business Opportunities, and Energy, Committee on Small Business, House of Representatives. *Hearing: Exclusive Agreements Between Federal Agencies and Bristol-Myers Squibb Co. for Drug Development: Is the Public Interest Protected?* Washington, DC, 29 July 1991, Serial No. 102-35.

Subcommittee on Regulation, Business Opportunities, and Technology, Committee on Small Business, House of Representatives. *Hearing: Pricing of Drugs by Federal Laboratories and Private Companies.* Washington, DC, 25 January 1993, Serial No. 103-2.

Suffness, Matthew. 'The discovery and development of antitumor drugs from natural products.' In Vlietinck, Arnold J. and Dommisse, Roger A. (eds), *Advances in Medicinal Plant Research.* Stuttgart: Wissenschaftliche Verlagsgesellschahft, 1985, 101–133.

Suffness, Matthew. 'New approaches to the discovery of antitumor agents.' In Hostettmann, K. and Lea, P.J. (eds), *Biologically Active Natural Products.* Oxford: Oxford University Press, 1987, 85–104.

Suffness, Matthew. 'Development of antitumor natural products as the National Cancer Institute.' *Gann Monograph on Cancer Research* **36** (1989), 21–44.

Suffness, Matthew. 'Taxol: from discovery to therapeutic use.' *Annual Reports in Medicinal Chemistry* **28** (1993), 305–314.

Suffness, Matthew. 'Overview of paclitaxel research: progress on many fronts.' In Georg, Gunda I., Chen, Thomas T., Ojima, Iwao, and Vyas, Dolatrai M. (eds), *Taxane Anticancer Agents: Basic Science and Current Status.* Washington, DC: American Chemical Society, 1995, 1–17.

Suffness, Matthew and Cordell, Geoffrey A. 'Antitumor alkaloids.' In Brossi, Arnold (ed.), *The Alkaloids: Chemistry and Pharmacology,* Vol. XXV: New York: Academic Press, 1985, 1–369.

Suffness, Matthew and Douros, John. 'Drugs of plant origin.' In DeVita, Vincent T. and Busch, Harris (eds), *Methods in Cancer Research,* Vol. XVI: *Cancer Drug Development.* New York: Academic Press, 1979, 73–126.

Suffness, Matthew and Douros, John. 'Current status of the NCI plant and animal product program.' *Journal of Natural Products* **45** (1982), 1–14.

Suffness, Matthew and Wall, Monroe E. 'Discovery and development of taxol.' In Suffness, Matthew (ed.), *Taxol®: Science and Applications.* Boca Raton, FL: CRC Press, 1995, 3–25.

Svoboda, Gordon H. 'Alkaloids of vinca rosea (*Catharanthus roseus*). IX. Extraction and characterization of leurosidine and leurocristine.' *Lloydia* **24** (1961), 173–178.

Swann, John P. 'The search for synthetic penicillin during World War II.' *British Journal for the History of Science* **16** (1983), 155–190.

Swann, John P. 'Biomedical research and government support: the case of drug development.' *Pharmacy in History* **31** (1989), 103–116.

Swann, John P. 'The biomedical industries.' In Pickstone, John and Cooter, Roger (eds), *Medicine in the Twentieth Century.* Cambridge: Cambridge University Press, 2001.

Swindell, C. 'Taxane diterpene synthesis strategies – a review.' *Organic Preparations and Procedures International* **23** (1991), 465–543.

Takacs, David. *The Idea of Biodiversity: Philosophies of Paradise.* Baltimore, MD: Johns Hopkins University Press, 1996.

Taylor, Joseph E. III. 'Making salmon: the political economy of fishery science and the road not taken.' *Journal of the History of Biology* **31** (1998), 33–59.

Temin, Peter. 'Technology, regulation, and market structure in the modern pharmaceutical industry.' *Bell Journal of Economics* **10** (1979), 429–446.

Temin, Peter. *Taking Your Medicine: Drug Regulation in the United States.* Cambridge, MA: Harvard University Press, 1980.

Tuchmann, E. Thomas, Connaughton, Kent P., Freedman, Lisa E., and Moriwaki, Clarence B. *The Northwest Forest Plan: A Report to the President and Congress.* Portland, OR: USDA, Office of Forestry and Economic Assistance, 1996.

Tyler, Varro E. 'Note on the occurrence of taxine in *Taxus brevifolia.*' *Journal of the American Pharmaceutical Association* **49** (1960), 683–684.

Tyler, Varro E. 'Plight of plant-drug research in the United States today.' *Economic Botany* **33** (1980), 377–383.

Tyler, Varro E. 'Plant drugs in the twenty-first century.' *Economic Botany* **40** (1986), 279–288.

Tyler, Varro E. 'Medicinal plant research: 1953–1987.' *Planta Medica* **54** (1988), 95–100.

United States Department of Agriculture, Forest Service; United States Department of the Interior, Bureau of Land Management; and United States Department of Health and Human Services, Food and Drug Administration. *Pacific Yew: Draft Environmental Impact Statement.* January 1993.

United States Department of Agriculture, Forest Service; United States Department of the Interior, Bureau of Land Management; and United States Department of Health and Human Services, Food and Drug Administration. *Pacific Yew: Final Environmental Impact Statement.* September 1993.

Vallee, Richard, B. 'The use of taxol in cell biology.' In Suffness, Matthew (ed.), *Taxol®: Science and Applications.* Boca Raton, FL: CRC Press, 1995, 259–274.

Van der Geest, S., White, S.R., and Hardon, A. 'The anthropology of pharmaceuticals: a biographical approach.' *Annual Review of Anthropology* **25** (1996), 153–178.

Venditti, John M. 'Relevance of transplantable animal-tumor systems to the selection of new agents for clinical trials.' In *Pharmacological Basis of Cancer Chemotherapy.* Baltimore, MD: Williams and Wilkins, 1975, 245–270.

Venditti, John M. and Abbott, Betty J. 'Studies on oncolytic agents from natural sources. Correlations of activity against animal tumors and clinical effectiveness.' *Lloydia* **30** (1967), 332–348.

Venditti, John M., Wesley, Robert A., and Plowman, Jacqueline. 'Current NCI preclinical antitumor screening *in vivo*: results of tumor panel screening, 1976–1982, and future directions.' *Advances in Pharmacology and Chemotherapy* **20** (1984), 1–20.

Vidensek, N., Lim, P., Campbell, A., and Carlson, C. 'Taxol content in bark, wood, root, leaf, twig, and seedling from several *Taxus* species.' *Journal of Natural Products* **53** (1990), 1609–1610.

Vining, Leo C. 'Roles of secondary metabolites from microbes.' In *Secondary Metabolites: Their Function and Evolution*. Ciba Foundation Symposium 171. Chichester: John Wiley, 1992, 184–194.

Von Hoff, Daniel D., Rozencweig, Marcel, Soper, William T., Helman, Lee J., Penta, John S., Davis, Hugh L., and Muggia, Franco M. 'Whatever happened to NSC———?' *Cancer Treatment Reports* **61** (1977), 759–768.

Wagner, L.J. and Flores, H.E. 'Effect of taxol and related compounds on growth of plant pathogenic fungi.' *Phytopathology* **84** (1994), 1173–1178.

Wainwright, M. 'Streptomycin: discovery and resultant controversy.' *History and Philosophy of the Life Sciences* **13** (1991), 97–124.

Waksman, S.A. and Woodruff, H.B. 'Bacteriostatic and bactericidal substance produced by a soil actinomyces.' *Proceedings of the Society for Experimental Biology and Medicine* **45** (1940), 609–614.

Wall, Monroe E. and Wani, Mansukh C. 'Camptothecin and taxol: discovery to clinic.' *Cancer Research* **55** (1995), 753–760.

Wall, Monroe E. and Wani, Mansukh C. 'Paclitaxel: from discovery to clinic.' In Georg, Gunda I., Chen, Thomas T., Ojima, Iwao, and Vyas, Dolatrai M. Vyas (eds), *Taxane Anticancer Agents: Basic Science and Current Status*. Washington, DC: American Chemical Society, 1995, 18–30.

Wall, Monroe E. and Wani, Mansukh C. 'Camptothecin: discovery to clinic.' *Annals of the New York Academy of Sciences* **803** (1996), 1–12.

Wall, Monroe E., Krider, Merle M., Krewson, C.F., Eddy, C. Rowland, Willaman, J.J., Corell, D.S., and Gentry, H.S. 'Steroidal sapogenins. VII. Survey of plants for steroidal sapogenins and other constituents.' *Journal of the American Pharmaceutical Association* **43** (1954), 1–7.

Wall, Monroe E., Wani, M.C., and Taylor, Harold. 'Isolation and chemical characterization of antitumor agents from plants.' *Cancer Treatment Reports* **60** (1976), 1011–1030.

Walsh, Vivien. 'Invention and innovation in the chemical industry: demand-pull or discovery-push?' *Research Policy* **13** (1984), 211–234.

Walsh, Vivien. 'Industrial R&D and its influence on the organization and management of the production of knowledge in the public sector.' In Gaudillière, Jean-Paul and Löwy, Ilana (eds), *The Invisible Industrialist: Manufactures and the Production of Scientific Knowledge*. Basingstoke: Macmillan, 1998, 301–344.

Walsh, Vivien and Goodman, Jordan. 'Cancer chemotherapy, biodiversity, public and private property: the case of the anti-cancer drug Taxol.' *Social Science and Medicine* **49** (1999), 1215–1225.

Wani, M.C., Taylor, H.L., Wall, M.E., Coggon, P., and McPhail, A.T. 'Plant antitumor agents. VI. The isolation and structure of taxol, a novel antileukemic and antitumor agent from *Taxus brevifolia*.' *Journal of the American Chemical Society* **93** (1971), 2325–2327.

Waring, R.H. and Franklin, J.F. 'Evergreen coniferous forests of the Pacific Northwest.' *Science* **204** (1979), 1380–1386.

Waterman, Peter G. 'Roles of secondary metabolites in plants.' In *Secondary Metabolites: Their Function and Evolution*. Ciba Foundation Symposium 171. Chichester: John Wiley, 1992, 255–269.

Weatherall, Miles. *In Search of a Cure: A History of Pharmaceutical Discovery*. Oxford: Oxford University Press, 1990.

Weisenthal, Larry M. '*In vitro* assays in preclinical antineoplastic drug screening.' *Seminars in Oncology* **8** (1981), 362–376.

Wender, Paul and Mucciaro, Thomas. 'A new and practical approach to the synthesis of taxol and taxol analogues: the pinene path.' *Journal of the American Chemical Society* **114** (1992), 5878–5879.

Wender, Paul, Natchus, Michael, and Shuker, Anthony. 'Toward the total synthesis of taxol and its analogues.' In Matthew Suffness (ed.), *Taxol®: Science and Applications*. Boca Raton, FL: CRC Press, 1995.

Wender, Paul A., Badham, Neil F., Conway, Simon P., Floreancig, Paul E., Glass, Timothy E., Houze, Jonathan B., Krauss, Nancy E., Lee, Daesung, Marquess, Daniel G., McGrane, Paul L., Meng, Wei, Mucciaro, Thomas P., Mühlebach, Michel, Natchus, Michael G., Ohkuma, Takeshi, Peschke, Bernd, Rawlins, David B., Shuker, Anthony J., Sutton, Jim C., Taylor, Richard E., Tomooka, Katsuhiko, and Wessjohann, Ludger A. 'The pinene path to taxanes: genesis and evolution of a strategy for synthesis.' In Georg, Gunda I., Chen, Thomas T., Ojima, Iwao, and Vyas, Dolatrai M. (eds), *Taxane Anticancer Agents: Basic Science and Current Status*. Washington, DC: American Chemical Society, 1995, 326–339.

Wheeler, N.C., Stonecypher, R.W., Jech, K.S., Masters, S.A., O'Brien, C., and Dettmering, A. 'Genetic variation in the Pacific yew (*Taxus brevifolia*): practical application.' Abstract, Second National Cancer Institute Workshop on Taxol and *Taxus*, 23–24 September 1992.

White, Neil and Cohen, Simon. 'Trademarks must not go generic.' *Nature* **375** (1995), 432.

Wiernik, P.H., Dutcher, J.P., Lipton, R.B., Strauman, J.J., Einzig, A., and Schwartz, E.L. 'Phase I trial of taxol given as a 24-hour infusion every 21 days: responses observed in metastatic melanoma.' *Journal of Clinical Oncology* **5** (1987), 1232–1239.

Wilcove, David S. 'Turning conversation goals into tangible results: the case of the spotted owl and old-growth forests.' In Edwards, P.J., May, R.M., and Webb, N.R. (eds), *Large-scale Ecology and Conservation Biology*. Oxford: Blackwell Scientific Publications, 1994, 313–329.

Willaman, J.J. and Schubert, Bernice G. 'Alkaloid hunting.' *Economic Botany* **9** (1955), 141–150.

Willems-Braun, Bruce. 'Buried epistemologies: the politics of nature in (post)-

colonial British Columbia.' *Annals of the Association of American Geographers* **87** (1997), 3–31.

Williams, Dudley H., Stone, Martin J., Hauck, Peter R., and Rahman, Shirley K. 'Why are secondary metabolites (natural products) biosynthesized?' *Journal of Natural Products* **52** (1989), 1189–1208.

Williams, Michael. *Americans and Their Forests: A Historical Geography.* Cambridge: Cambridge University Press, 1989.

Wilson, E.O. and Peter, Frances M. *Biodiversity.* Washington, DC: National Academy Press, 1988.

Wilson, Leslie. 'Pharmacological and biochemical properties of microtubule proteins: Symposium.' *Federation Proceedings* **33** (1974), 151.

Wilson, Leslie, Bamburg, James R., Mizel, Steven B., Grisham, Linda M., and Creswell, Karen M. 'Interaction of drugs with microtubule proteins.' *Federation Proceedings* **33** (1974), 158–166.

Witherup, Keith M., Look, Sally A., Stasko, Michael W., Ghiorzi, Thomas J., and Muschik, Gary M. '*Taxus* spp. Needles contain amounts of taxol comparable to the bark of *Taxus brevifolia*: analysis and isolation.' *Journal of Natural Products* **53** (1990), 1249–1255.

Wolf, E. and Wortman, D. 'Pacific yew management on national forests: a biological and policy analysis.' *The Northwest Environment Journal* **8** (1992), 347–366.

Wolff, Ivan A. and Jones, Quentin. 'Cooperative new crops research – what the program has to involve.' *Chemurgic Digest* **17** (1958), 4–8.

Wood, H.B., Jr. 'Selection of agents for the tumor screen of potential new antineoplastic drugs.' In Saunders, Joseph F. and Carter, Stephen K. (eds), *Methods of Development of New Anticancer Drugs.* National Cancer Institute Monograph 45, 1977, 15–35.

Woolley, Paul V. and Schein, Philip S. 'Clinical pharmacology and Phase I trial design.' In DeVita, Vincent T. Jr. and Busch, Harris (eds), *Methods in Cancer Research*, Vol. XVII: *Cancer Drug Development.* New York: Academic Press, 1979, 177–198.

Yaffee, Steven L. *The Wisdom of the Spotted Owl: Policy Lessons for a New Century.* Washington, DC: Island Press, 1994.

Youngken, H.W., Jr. 'Botany and medicine.' *American Journal of Botany* **43** (1956), 862–869.

Zubrod, C.G. 'The chemical control of cancer.' *Proceedings of the National Academy of Sciences of the USA* **69** (1972), 1042–1047.

Zubrod, C.G. 'Historic milestones in curative chemotherapy.' *Seminars in Oncology* **6** (1979), 490–505.

Zubrod, C.G., Schepartz, S., Leiter, J., Endicott, K.M., Carrese, L.M., and Baker, C.G. 'The chemotherapy program of the National Cancer Institute: history, analysis, and plans.' *Cancer Chemotherapy Reports* **50**, no. 7 (1966), 349–540.

Zurer, Pamela. 'Chemists closing in on synthesis of scarce anticancer agent taxol.' *Chemical and Engineering News* **66** (10 October 1988), 22–23.

Index